R **ONE WEEK LOAN** d

Renew Books on PHONE-it: 01443 654456

Books are to be returned on or before the last date below

Glyntaff Learning Resources Centre
University of Glamorgan CF37 1DL

Review of Obesity and Bariatric Surgery

Essential Notes and Multiple Choice Questions

Subhash Kini MD, FACS, FRCS, FRCS (Ed), FRCP&S (Glas)
Assistant Professor of Surgery
Division of Metabolic, Endocrine and Minimally Invasive Surgery
Mount Sinai School of Medicine, NY, USA

Dr. Raghavendra Rao MBBS
Former Research Fellow
Division of Metabolic, Endocrine and Minimally Invasive Surgery
Mount Sinai School of Medicine, NY, USA

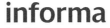

informa
healthcare

New York   London

Published in 2012 by Informa Healthcare, 119 Farringdon Road, London EC1R 3DA, UK

Simultaneously published in the USA by Informa Healthcare, 52 Vanderbilt Avenue, 7th Floor, New York NY 10017, USA.

Informa Healthcare is a trading division of Informa UK Ltd. Registered Office: 37–41 Mortimer Street, London W1T 3JH, UK. Registered in England and Wales number 1072954.

Library of Congress Cataloging-in-Publication Data

Review of obesity and bariatric surgery : essential notes and multiple choice questions / edited by Subhash Kini, Raghavendra Rao.

    p. ; cm.

    Includes bibliographical references.

    ISBN 978-1-84184-956-0 (pbk. : alk. paper)

    I. Kini, Subhash. II. Rao, Raghavendra, 1984-

    [DNLM: 1. Obesity. 2. Bariatric Surgery. WD 210]

    617.4′3--dc23

                      2011045044

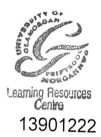

A CIP record for this book is available from the British Library.

ISBN-10: 1-84184-956-1
ISBN-13: 978-1-84184-956-0
eISBN: 978-1-84184-957-7

Orders may be sent to: Informa Healthcare, Sheepen Place, Colchester, Essex CO3 3LP, UK
Telephone: +44 (0)20 7017 6682
Email: Books@Informa.com
Informa Healthcare Website: informahealthcarebooks.com
Informa website: www.informa.com

For corporate sales please contact: CorporateBooksIHC@informa.com
For foreign rights please contact: RightsIHC@informa.com
For reprint permissions please contact: PermissionsIHC@informa.com

Typeset by MPS Limited, India.
Printed and bound in the United Kingdom.

Foreword

All of medicine, and certainly every specialty in surgery, evolves with time. First, there is a discovery phase, which identifies the importance of a problem and then develops potential new therapies to provide a cure. The next phase involves proving that the new therapy actually provides reliable and effective treatment for the disorder. From this point on, a specialty begins to define the limits of the new form of therapy as its application to the treatment of a disease becomes widespread. Education is folded into each one of these phases and reaches maturity when a new therapy becomes the standard of care. The story of bariatric surgery clearly follows this pattern of evolution. Over the past 30 years, we have learned a vast amount about morbid obesity and how surgical therapies can provide meaningful treatment for this multisystem disorder. As surgery for treating morbid obesity grows, so do the surgical programs across the nation that are charged with training increasing numbers of surgeons to combat this significant health care problem. Standardized protocols have been defined, and the training of surgeons to care for the bariatric patient has become almost as routine as the surgical management of inguinal hernia. This education allows acquisition of defined blocks of information, which will not only enhance our ability to diagnose and effectively treat patients with morbid obesity but also allow for the continued advancement of knowledge and analysis of new and expanding therapeutic options.

This *Review of Obesity and Bariatric Surgery*, which provides multiple choice questions in the specialized field of bariatric surgery, is the first book of its kind. Questions pertaining to this important area are now a standard part of the General Surgery Board evaluations and recertification, and stand as an important part of all in-service examinations at the residency training level. One can review the first few pages and realize that this compendium of multiple choice questions will not only benefit the young surgeons preparing for an examination but also any surgeon meaningfully participating in the field of bariatric surgery who wants to test his/her own skills and knowledge in the treatment of this difficult problem. For this reason, I strongly recommend this book to medical students, residents, fellows, and practicing surgeons who wish to enhance their learning and challenge their knowledge.

Michael L. Marin, MD
The Julius H. Jacobson II, M.D. Professor of Surgery
Chairman, Department of Surgery,
Mount Sinai School of Medicine, NY, USA

Preface

Obesity is currently one of the biggest health care problems in the United States and worldwide. Bariatric surgery has proven to be the most effective way for obese patient to lose weight and maintain this weight loss. This has led to a dramatic increase in the number of bariatric operations being performed each year and also to the creation of special fellowships in bariatric surgery. A great deal of research is being done in obesity and bariatric surgery. This book summarizes the recent advances in the field that would be useful for practicing physicians and bariatric surgeons. It also summarizes some of the basics that a bariatric/metabolic surgery fellow needs to be aware of.

The book has been organized into several chapters with each chapter consisting of a summary regarding the chapter, a set of multiple choice questions, followed by answers with explanations. Every attempt has been made to keep the material concise yet comprehensive, which is one of the biggest strengths of the book. The questions have been circulated among experts in the field, some of who have had extensive experience in setting questions for board examinations including the American Board of Surgery examinations. The chapter summaries serve as a quick reference guide for busy bariatric surgeons and trainees, and the multiple choice questions as a tool for self-assessment of knowledge and practice. The book and its future editions should also be useful for preparation of board exams in bariatric surgery or exams for certified obesity practitioners. There is an existing exam for the purpose of certifying obesity practitioners (The American Board of Bariatric Medicine exam), which uses a similar syllabus as this book. The Certified Obesity Medical Physician from Obesity Society and American Board of Bariatric Surgery is anticipated to be set up in the near future and the American Society for Metabolic and Bariatric Surgery may follow too.

The book was a result of the editors looking up several thousands of references in order to frame interesting and educational, yet noncontroversial, multiple choice questions. The questions and responses were modified with the feedback from surgeons and physicians in the field regarding the best practice standards and ways to make the questions more interesting and relevant. More than 50 experts in the field agreed to the relevancy as well as the accuracy of the presented material.

Given the original nature of the project, it will not be without shortcomings. We welcome healthy criticism from the readers, in order that the book can be improved in the future editions.

Lastly, we would like to thank the contributors, and our families, for their love and support, which were very crucial for the realization of this project.

Subhash Kini
Raghavendra Rao

Contents

Contributors

Neville Bamji   Department of Medicine, Division of Gastroenterology, Mount Sinai School of Medicine, New York, New York, U.S.A.

Stephen A. Brietzke   Division of Endocrinology, Department of Internal Medicine, Columbia School of Medicine, Columbia, University of Missouri, Missouri, U.S.A.

Edmond Cohen   Department of Anesthesiology, Mount Sinai Medical Center, New York, New York, U.S.A.

Gregory Dakin   Department of Surgery, Weill Cornell Medical College, New York, New York, U.S.A.

Ramsey Dallal   Bariatric/Minimally Invasive Surgery, Albert Einstein Healthcare Network, Philadelphia, Pennsylvania, U.S.A.

George D. Dangas   Professor of Medicine, Division of Cardiology, and Department of Surgery, Mount Sinai Medical Center, New York, New York, U.S.A.

Mervyn Deitel   Obesity Surgery, Toronto, Canada

John Dixon, MBBS, PhD   NHMRC Senior Research Fellow, Baker IDI Heart & Diabetes Institute, Melbourne, Australia

Martin Drooker   Department of Psychiatry, Mount Sinai School of Medicine, New York, New York, U.S.A.

Michael Edye   Department of Surgery, Mount Sinai School of Medicine, New York, New York, U.S.A.

Michel Gagner   Department of Surgery, Florida International University, Miami, Florida, U.S.A.

Paolo Gentileschi   Bariatric Surgery Unit, Department of Surgery, University of Rome Tor Vergata, Policlinico Tor Vergata, Rome, Italy

Jayleen Grams   Department of Surgery, University of Alabama at Birmingham, Birmingham, Alabama, U.S.A.

Giselle Hamad   Department of Surgery, University of Pittsburgh, Pittsburgh, U.S.A.

Mimi Harrison   Division of Metabolic, Endocrine and Metabolic Surgery, Mount Sinai Medical Center, New York, New York, U.S.A.

Daniel Herron   Department of Surgery, Mount Sinai Medical Center, New York, New York, U.S.A.

Donald Hess   Department of Surgery, Boston University School of Medicine, Boston, Massachusetts, U.S.A.

Jens Juul Holst   Departments of Medical Physiology and Biomedical Sciences, Health Sciences Faculty, University of Copenhagen, Denmark

William Inabnet   Department of Surgical Oncology, and Division of Metabolic, Endocrine and Minimally Invasive Surgery, Metabolism Institute, Mount Sinai Medical Center, New York, New York, U.S.A.

Brian P. Jacob   Department of Surgery, Mount Sinai School of Medicine, and Laparoscopic Surgical Center of New York, New York, U.S.A.

Mohammad K. Jamal   Department of Surgery, Division of Gastrointestinal, Bariatrics and Minimally Invasive Surgery, Department of Surgery, University of Iowa Hospitals and Clinics, Iowa City, Iowa, U.S.A.

Shahzeer Karmali   Department of Surgery, University of Alberta, Edmonton, Alberta, Canada

Kazunori Kasama   Weight loss and Metabolic Surgery Center, Yotsuya Medical Cube, Tokyo, Japan

Ashutosh Kaul   Minimally Invasive and Robotic Surgery, Westchester Medical Center, and New York Medical College, Valhalla, New York, U.S.A.

Kim Keith   Metabolic Medicine and Surgery Institute at Florida Hospital Celebration, Florida, U.S.A.

Subhash Kini   Division of Metabolic, Endocrine and Minimally Invasive Surgery, Mount Sinai School of Medicine, NY, U.S.A.

Robert Klafter   Mount Sinai School of Medicine, New York, New York, U.S.A.

Constantine E. Kosmas   Department of Medicine, Division of Cardiology, Mount Sinai School of Medicine, and Mount Sinai Advanced Cardiovascular Group, New York, New York, U.S.A.

Blandine Laferrère   Department of Medicine, St Luke's Roosevelt Hospital Center, Columbia University College of Physician and Surgeons, New York Obesity Nutrition Research Center, New York, New York, U.S.A.

James N. Lau   Section of Minimally Invasive/Bariatric Surgery, and Department of Surgery, Stanford School of Medicine, California, U.S.A.

Carel Le Roux   Imperial Weight Centre, Imperial College London, U.K.

Andrew B. Leibowitz   Department of Anesthesiology, The Mount Sinai Hospital, and Mount Sinai School of Medicine, New York, New York, U.S.A.

Sameer Mattar   Clarian North Medical Center, Indiana, U.S.A.

James McGinty   Department of Surgery, Columbia University, New York, New York, U.S.A.

Amir Mehran   Bariatric Surgery, UCLA Department of Surgery, California, U.S.A.

Kenneth Miller   Department of Medicine, Division of Gastroenterology, Mount Sinai School of Medicine, New York, New York, U.S.A.

Michel Murr   Department of Surgery, Bariatric Surgery, USF Health-Tampa General Hospital, Florida, U.S.A.

Murali Naidu   Minimally Invasive Surgery and Bariatric Surgery at the Hospital of Saint Raphael, New Haven, Connecticut, U.S.A.

Erik Naslund   Department of Surgery, Karolinska Institute, Stockholm, Sweden

Michael Albrecht Nauck   Diabeteszentrum Bad Lauterberg, Bad Lauterberg, Germany

John Oropello   Departments of Surgery and Medicine, Mount Sinai School of Medicine, New York, New York, U.S.A.

Hany Osman   Department of Medicine, Cairo University, Cairo, Egypt

Alfons Pomp   Section of Laparoscopic and Bariatric Surgery, Weill Medical College of Cornell University, New York Presbyterian Hospital, New York, New York, U.S.A.

Vasudevan Raghavan   Department of Internal Medicine, Texas A&M Health Science Center College of Medicine, College Station, Texas, U.S.A.

P. S. Venkatesh Rao   Department of Endocrine Surgery, Kadri Clinic, Bangalore, India

Raghavendra Rao   Formerly Division of Metabolic, Endocrine and Minimally Invasive Surgery, Mount Sinai School of Medicine, NY, U.S.A.

Vemuru Sunil Kumar Reddy   Bronx-Lebanon Hospital Center, New York, New York, U.S.A.

Ram Roth   Department of Anesthesiology, Mount Sinai School of Medicine, New York, New York, U.S.A.

Barry Segal   Department of Anesthesiology, Mount Sinai Medical Center, New York, New York, U.S.A.

Don Selzer   Department of Surgery, Indiana University Health North Hospital, Indiana, U.S.A.

Ranjan Sudan   Department of Surgery, Duke Universty Medical Center, Durham, North Carolina, U.S.A.

Ronald Tamler   Division of Endocrinology, Diabetes and Bone Diseases, Mount Sinai School of Medicine, New York, New York, U.S.A.

Peter Taub   Department of Plastic Surgery, Mount Sinai School of Medicine, New York, New York, U.S.A.

Alfred Trang   Albert Einstein Health Network, Philadelphia, Pennsylvania, U.S.A.

Shawn Tsuda   Division of Minimally Invasive and Bariatric Surgery, University of Nevada School of Medicine, Nevada, U.S.A.

T. Vilsboll   Department of Internal Medicine, Gentofte Hospital, University of Copenhagen, Denmark

Robert Yanagisawa   Department of Medicine, Division of Endocrinology, Diabetes and Bone Disease, Mount Sinai School of Medicine, New York, New York, U.S.A.

Jeffrey L. Zitsman   Center for Adolescent Bariatric Surgery, Morgan Stanley Children's Hospital of NY Presbyterian, and Department of Surgery, Columbia University Medical Center, New York, New York, U.S.A.

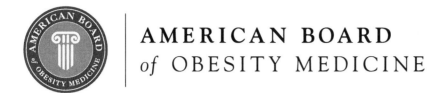

AMERICAN BOARD
of OBESITY MEDICINE

American Board of Obesity Medicine

Obesity Medicine Physician

An obesity medicine physician is a physician with expertise in the sub-specialty of obesity medicine.

This sub-specialty requires competency in and a thorough understanding of the treatment of obesity and the genetic, biologic, environmental, social, and behavioral factors that contribute to obesity.

The obesity medicine physician employs therapeutic interventions including diet, physical activity, behavioral change, and pharmacotherapy.

The obesity medicine physician utilizes a comprehensive approach, and may include additional resources such as nutritionists, exercise physiologists, psychologists and bariatric surgeons as indicated to achieve optimal results.

Additionally, the obesity medicine physician maintains competency in providing pre- peri- and post-surgical care of bariatric surgery patients, promotes the prevention of obesity, and advocates for those who suffer from obesity.

For post-fellowship qualifications for certification, and qualifications for certification without fellowship, please find full policies, procedures and applications at www.abom.org.

American Board of Obesity Medicine
3515 South Tamarac Drive, Suite 200
Denver, CO 80237
USA

Tel +1 303-770-9100; Fax +1 303-770-9104

1 | Epidemiology

CHAPTER SUMMARY
- Obesity is defined as body mass index (BMI) > 30 kg/m^2, and being overweight is defined as BMI between 25 and 30 kg/m^2.
- About 1.6 billion people in the world are overweight and 400 million are obese.
- The prevalence of obesity in the United States is about 34% (2007–2008).
- The prevalence of people being overweight or obese in the United States is about 68% (2007–2008).
- There has been no statistically significant change in the prevalence of obesity since 2003–2004.
- The Healthy People 2010 program aimed for a obesity prevalence of 15%, and this has not been attained by any state in the United States.
- The prevalence of coronary heart disease has shown a decrease, whereas the prevalence of diabetes and hypertension has shown an increase.
- During 1990–2000, there was a growth in the number of bariatric surgeries performed, with a relatively higher growth in the number of RYGB (Roux-en-Y gastric bypass) operations performed.
- Most bariatric surgeries in the world are performed laparoscopically.
- Laparoscopic adjustable gastric banding (LAGB) is the most commonly performed bariatric surgery in the world.
- The rate of growth of bariatric surgery has slowed down in the latter half of past decade when compared to initial half of the past decade.
- The etiology of obesity is genetic as well as environmental. Short nuclear polymorphisms and the fat mass and obesity associated (FTO) gene contribute to risk of obesity. Monogenic forms of obesity are however rare.
- Obesity is a major burden on the U.S. economy. It contributes to 9% of the health care spending.
- The age-adjusted prevalence of diabetes is 8.3% in the United States.
- Overall, the risk for death among people with diabetes is about twice that of people **of similar age** but without diabetes.
- The incidence of newly diagnosed diabetes is highest in the 45 to 65 years age group, while the prevalence is highest in the 65 to 75 years age group in the United States.
- The incidence of diabetes is equal in men and women with a slightly higher prevalence in men. The prevalence of obesity is very similar in men and women with a slightly higher prevalence in women.

QUESTIONS

1. **Obesity is a major epidemic in the United States. Which of the following is <u>FALSE</u> about the current obesity statistics in the United States?**
   A. Non-Hispanic blacks have a higher prevalence than the national average.
   B. About one in three persons in the United States are obese.
   C. Most states in the United States have a less than 15% prevalence of obesity.
   D. More than 60% of the people in the United States are overweight or obese.

2. **The prevalence of obesity has been progressively increasing in the United States and efforts to curb this have not been very successful. Identify the <u>FALSE</u> statements about the trends of obesity in the United States.**

   A. The prevalence of obesity has been shown to be stable among U.S. women after 2000.
   B. Obesity prevalence seems to have stabilized in men according to very recent data.
   C. Obesity trends predict the trends of the associated comorbidities.
   D. United States had stable prevalence of obesity between 1960 and 1980.

3. **The trends of prevalence of obesity-associated comorbidities do not follow that of obesity. Which of the following statements about obesity-associated comorbidities is <u>FALSE</u>?**
   A. The prevalence of coronary heart disease has been gradually decreasing.
   B. The prevalence of diabetes has been increasing.
   C. The prevalence of hypertension has been decreasing.
   D. About 25% of diabetes is undiagnosed.

4. **Over the past two decades, bariatric surgery has grown as a modality for weight loss. Identify the <u>FALSE</u> statement about the trends of this operation.**
   A. The number of bariatric procedures increased from 1990 to 2000.
   B. The number of RYGBs performed increased during the 1990s.
   C. The number of RYGBs performed relative to other bariatric procedures increased during the 1990s.
   D. Hospital stay for patients remained stable.

5. **The popularity of bariatric operations differs in different regions of the world. Identify the <u>FALSE</u> statement about the prevalence of various bariatric surgeries in the world.**
   A. The relative number of RYGBs performed has decreased all over the world.
   B. Most surgeries are performed laparoscopically all over the world.
   C. LAGB is the most commonly performed operation all over the world.
   D. The relative number of RYGBs performed has decreased in Europe, while it has increased in the United States.

6. **The cause of obesity is partly environmental and partly genetic. Identify the <u>FALSE</u> statement about the etiology of the growing pandemic.**
   A. Social networks play a role in causing obesity.
   B. Single nucleotide polymorphisms (SNPs) contribute a great extent to the burden of obesity in the entire population.
   C. The FTO gene is associated with an increased risk of type 2 diabetes mellitus (DM).
   D. No study has found a direct correlation between television viewing and obesity.

7. **Identify the <u>FALSE</u> statement about obesity trends in different parts of the world.**
   A. More than 1 billion people in the world are overweight.
   B. The prevalence of obesity varies in different parts of the world.
   C. Very few countries do have a falling trend in obesity.
   D. The global prevalence of obesity is calculated only from systematic nationally representative samples.

8. **Obesity has placed a huge economic burden on the U.S. economy. Identify the <u>FALSE</u> statement about the impact of the epidemic of obesity on the U.S. economy.**
   A. The total amount of money spent on obesity/overweight people is more than $100 billion.
   B. About 3% of health expenditure is attributable to obesity.
   C. Each person who is obese spends more than $1000 extra on his health care when compared to his lean counterpart.
   D. Obesity increases the risk of colorectal cancer.

9. A public health investigator is researching obesity in his country and finds that morbidly obese people have a two times greater mortality. The overall mortality rate in his country is 1%. Bariatric surgery has been shown to reduce mortality by 25%. He would like to know the number of obese patients he needs to treat in order to prevent one death. What is the number he needs to treat (NNT) by bariatric surgery in order to prevent one death?
   A. About 200
   B. About 500
   C. About 100
   D. Data insufficient to calculate NNT

10. Diabetes is an important comorbidity of obesity and it has also shown an increase in prevalence over time. Identify the TRUE statement about the epidemiology of diabetes in the United States.
   A. The prevalence of diabetes in the United States is about 2%.
   B. The prevalence of diabetes is slightly higher in women.
   C. The highest prevalence of diabetes is in the 45 to 64 age group when compared to age groups above 65 or younger than 45.
   D. Diabetes increases mortality of a person by two times.

ANSWER KEY

1. C	4. D	7. D	10. D
2. C	5. D	8. B	
3. C	6. D	9. A	

ANSWER KEY WITH EXPLANATION

1. **Answer: C.**

   The current prevalence of obesity in the United States is 33%. The lowest and the highest prevalence are in the states of Colorado (<20%) and Mississippi (>35%). A total of 33 states have prevalence of >30%. No state has a prevalence <15%. Obesity is more prevalent in non-Hispanic blacks and in Hispanics. The combined prevalence of obesity and overweight is about 66%.

   References:
   - Vital Signs: State-Specific Obesity Prevalence Among Adults—United States, 2009 MMWR, August 3, 2010/59 (Early Release); 1–5.
   - Flegal KM, Carroll MD, Ogden CL, et al. Prevalence and trends in obesity among US adults, 1999–2008. JAMA 2010; 303(3):235–241.

2. **Answer: C.**

   Obesity trends do not predict the trends of the obesity-associated comorbidities. This is because of improvements in health care and decrease in the risk factors associated with the comorbidities. (Please refer next question also.) The prevalence of obesity was stable between 1960 and 1980 and showed striking increases during 1980s and 1990s. The prevalence of obesity has been shown to be stable among U.S. women after 2000. Obesity prevalence seems to have stabilized in men according to recent data though there was an increase in the initial part of past decade.

   Reference:
   - Flegal KM, Carroll MD, Ogden CL, et al. Prevalence and trends in obesity among US adults, 1999–2008. JAMA 2010; 303(3):235–241.

3. **Answer: C.**

   The prevalence of hypertension has been increasing. More than 25% of diabetes is undiagnosed. It has also been shown to be increasing in prevalence (see figure). Coronary artery disease (CAD) has shown a decreasing trend for the past few decades due to improvement in the management of CAD and the public health system.

References:
- Flegal KM, Carroll MD, Ogden CL, et al. Prevalence and trends in obesity among US adults, 1999–2008. JAMA 2010; 303(3):235–241.
- http://www.cdc.gov/diabetes/statistics/prev/national/figadults.htm
- http://www.cdc.gov/diabetes/pubs/factsheet11.htm

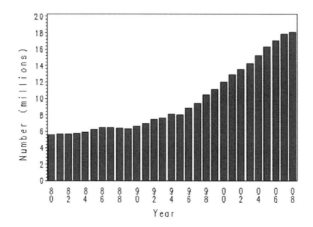

Source: http://www.cdc.gov/diabetes/statistics/prev/national/figadults.htm.

4. **Answer: D.**

   From 1990 to 2000, the national annual rate of bariatric surgery increased nearly sixfold, from 2.4 to 14.1 per 100,000 adults. Hospital stay has significantly declined from 1990 to 2000. The number of RYGBs increased from 7 procedures per 100,000 adults in 1998 to 38.6 procedures per 100,000 adults in 2002. Between 1990 and 2000, there was a ninefold increase in the use of gastric bypass procedures compared to a sixfold increase in all bariatric procedures.

   References:
   - Trus TL, Pope GD, Finlayson SR. National trends in utilization and outcomes of bariatric surgery. Surg Endosc 2005; 19(5):616–620.
   - Smoot TM, Xu P, Hilsenrath P, et al. Gastric bypass surgery in the United States, 1998–2002. Am J Public Health 2006; 96(7):1187–1189.

5. **Answer: D.**

   In 2008, 344,221 bariatric surgery operations were performed by 4680 bariatric surgeons; 220,000 of these operations were performed in United States/Canada by 1625 surgeons. The most commonly performed procedures were LAGB (42.3%), laparoscopic standard RYGB (39.7%), and total sleeve gastrectomies 4.5%. Over 90% of procedures were performed laparoscopically. Comparing the 5-year trend from 2003 to 2008, all categories of procedures, with the exception of biliopancreatic diversion/duodenal switch, increased in absolute numbers performed. However, the relative percent of all RYGBs decreased from 65.1% to 49.0%, whereas AGB increased from 24.4% to 42.3%. Markedly, different trends were found for Europe and United States/Canada: in Europe, AGB decreased from 63.7% to 43.2% and RYGB increased from 11.1% to 39.0%, whereas in United States/Canada, AGB increased from 9.0% to 44.0% and RYGB decreased from 85.0% to 51.0%. The absolute growth rate of bariatric surgery decreased over the past 5 years (135% increase), in comparison to the preceding 5 years (266% increase). Bariatric surgery continues to grow worldwide, but less so than in the past. With regard to the type of procedures, the trends in Europe versus United States/Canada are diametrically opposite.

References:

- Buchwald H, Williams S.E. Bariatric surgery worldwide 2003. Obes Surg 2004; 14 (9):1157–1164.
- Buchwald H, Oien DM. Metabolic/bariatric surgery worldwide 2008. Obes Surg 2009; 19(12):1605–1611.

6. **Answer: D**

The siblings and friends of those who are obese have a 57% increased chance of becoming obese. The monogenic forms of obesity are rare. The SNPs have modest effects on an individual's susceptibility to common forms of obesity, but because of their high frequency, they can have a large contribution to obesity on the population level. FTO has been identified in a GWA (genome-wide association) study to be associated with an increased risk of type 2 diabetes mediated through an effect on the BMI. Every hour of television watching/day has been shown to increase BMI by 2 points.

References:

- Larder R, Cheung MK, Tung YC, et al. Where to go with FTO? Trends Endocrinol Metab 2011; 22(2):53–59.
- Nguyen DM, El-Serag HB. The epidemiology of obesity. Gastroenterol Clin North Am 2010; 39(1):1–7.
- Dietz WH Jr., Gortmaker SL. Do we fatten our children at the television set? Obesity and television viewing in children and adolescents. Pediatrics 1985; 75 (5):807–812.

7. **Answer: D.**

The prevalence of obesity around the world is monitored by the WHO through the Global Database on BMI. The survey data included in the database are identified from the literature or from a wide network of collaborators. However, high-quality data from systematic nationally representative samples are sparse. As of November 2004, the database has compiled data covering approximately 86% of the adult population worldwide. The WHO estimates showed that in 2005, approximately 1.6 billion people worldwide were overweight and that at least 400 million adults were obese. There are wide variations in the prevalence of obesity throughout the world, ranging from India, where 1% or less of the population is obese, to the Pacific Islands, where the prevalence of obesity can reach up to 80% in some regions. Overall, most countries were found to have rising trends of obesity. Only 2 (Denmark and Saudi Arabia) of the 28 countries showed a falling trend in the prevalence of obesity in men, and 5 (Denmark, Ireland, Saudi Arabia, Finland, and Spain) of the 28 countries showed a falling trend in the prevalence of obesity in women.

Reference:

- Nguyen DM, El-Serag HB. The epidemiology of obesity. Gastroenterol Clin North Am 2010; 39(1):1–7.

8. **Answer: B**

Recent estimates of the annual medical costs of obesity are as high as $147 billion. On average, persons who are obese have medical costs that are $1429 more than persons of normal weight. Obesity contributes about 9% to the health care expenditure. Obesity is also associated with increased risk for numerous chronic diseases, including diabetes, hypertension, heart disease, and stroke. Furthermore, obesity is linked to several digestive diseases, including gastroesophageal reflux disease and its complications (e.g., erosive esophagitis, Barrett esophagus, and esophageal adeno-carcinoma), colorectal polyps and cancer, and liver disease (e.g., nonalcoholic fatty liver disease, cirrhosis, and hepatocellular carcinoma).

References:

- Sung MK, Bae YJ. Linking obesity to colorectal cancer: application of nutrigenomics. Biotechnol J 2010; 5(9):930–941.
- Vital Signs: State-Specific Obesity Prevalence Among Adults – United States, 2009 MMWR, August 3, 2010/59 (Early Release); 1–5.

- Nguyen DM, El-Serag HB. The epidemiology of obesity. Gastroenterol Clin North Am 2010; 39(1):1–7.

9. **Answer: A.**

The mortality rate of obese patients is 2.0 x 1% = 2%. The mortality rate after bariatric surgery is 75% of 2%, which is 1.5%. The absolute risk reduction is 2% − 1.5% = 0.5%.
The NNT is calculated by the formula: 1/absolute risk reduction = 1/0.005 = 200.

References:
- Nguyen DM, El-Serag HB. The epidemiology of obesity. Gastroenterol Clin North Am 2010; 39(1):1–7.
- Tschudy MM, Rowe PC. Research and statistics: number needed to treat and intention to treat analysis. Pediatr Rev 2010; 31(9):380–382.
- Sjöström L. Bariatric surgery and reduction in morbidity and mortality: experiences from the SOS study. Int J Obes (Lond) 2008; 32(suppl 7):S93–S97.

10. **Answer: D.**

The age-adjusted prevalence of diabetes in the United States is about 8.3%. Both men and women have a similar prevalence of diabetes with a slightly greater prevalence in men according to the 2009 data. The prevalence of diabetes is growing faster in the 65 to 74 years age group compared to younger groups. The highest prevalence of diabetes is also in the 65 to 74 years age group followed by >75 years group. However, the *incidence* of newly diagnosed diabetes is highest in the 45 to 65 years age group. This is illustrated by the following graph. Overall, the risk for death among people with diabetes is about twice that of people **of similar age** but without diabetes.

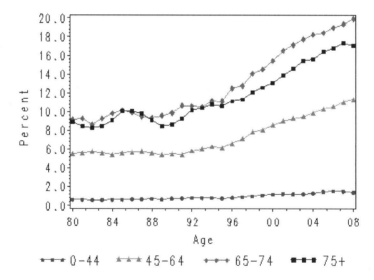

Source: http://www.cdc.gov/diabetes/statistics/prev/national/figbyage.htm.

References:
- http://www.cdc.gov/diabetes/statistics/prev/national/figbyage.htm
- http://www.cdc.gov/diabetes/statistics/meduse/fig2.htm

2 | History

CHAPTER SUMMARY
- The jejunoileal bypass (JIB) was the first ever bariatric operation performed by Kremen, Linner, and Nelson at the University of Minnesota in 1954.
- Edward Mason is the father of bariatric surgery.
- The JIB was abandoned in the 1990s due to its high incidence of metabolic complications including liver cirrhosis, nephrolithiasis and renal failure, and diarrhea.
- The first gastric bypass was performed by Mason and Ito in 1967, and it included a loop gastrojejunostomy.
- The first vertical banded gastroplasty (VBG) was performed in 1982 by Edward Mason.
- Wilkinson and Peloso were the first to place a nonadjustable band of Marlex mesh around the upper stomach in 1978.
- The first published report of placement of an adjustable gastric band was by Kuzmak in 1986.
- The first laparoscopic gastric bypass (LRYGB) was performed by Dr Alan Wittgrove in 1994.
- Lap-Band® was Food and Drug Administration (FDA) approved in June 5, 2001.
- Marceau et al. first performed the sleeve gastrectomy as a part of the biliopancreatic diversion (BPD) operation.
- The first laparoscopic biliopancreatic diversion–duodenal switch (BPD-DS) was performed by Michel Gagner.
- Leptin was isolated by Dr Jeffrey Freidman of Rockefeller University in New York in 1994. This was done by cloning the "ob" gene in mice.
- Ghrelin was discovered by Masayasu Kojima in 1999. It was discovered when the properties of growth hormone secretagogue receptors were being characterized.
- Adiponectin was discovered by Yuji Matsuzawa in 1995 while studying cells differentiating into adipocytes.

QUESTIONS

1. **A patient who had a JIB presents to a bariatric surgeon for revision to a modern bariatric procedure. Identify the <u>FALSE</u> statement about JIB.**
   A. There is increased incidence of uric acid stones.
   B. Diarrhea is a significant short-term complication.
   C. Liver disease is a significant long-term complication.
   D. The current recommendation is that all patients with a JIB need to be converted to other well-accepted bariatric procedures if able to withstand the procedure.
   E. It produces good weight loss.

2. **Dr Edward Mason is considered to be the father of bariatric surgery. Identify the <u>FALSE</u> statement about the development of Roux-en-Y gastric bypass (RYGB) as a bariatric surgical procedure.**
   A. Griffen et al. performed the first RYGB.
   B. The laparoscopic version of RYGB was developed by Dr Alan Wittgrove et al.
   C. Gastric bypass was developed after the VBG.
   D. The first gastric bypass performed by Mason and Ito consisted of a loop gastrojejunostomy.

3. **Ghrelin though discovered nearly a decade ago has not been definitively shown to be important for causing the metabolic changes involved in bariatric surgery. Identify the <u>TRUE</u> statement about the discovery of ghrelin.**
   A. Ghrelin inhibits growth hormone secretion.
   B. Ghrelin was discovered as scientists were in search of an orexigenic hormone.
   C. The concept of "orphan receptor" was used to discover ghrelin.
   D. Ghrelin in Proto-Indo-European language means hunger.

4. **Leptin was discovered nearly 15 years ago. Though identified as an anorexigenic hormone, it has never been shown to be a useful pharmacotherapy when used alone. Identify the <u>FALSE</u> statement about discovery of leptin.**
   A. The idea of a hormone secreted from the adipose tissue which regulates food intake was first proposed more than 50 years ago.
   B. The study of *ob/ob* mouse was important for the discovery of leptin.
   C. Leptin was isolated for the first time by Freidman.
   D. Leptin was first discovered by injecting adipose tissue extracts and identifying the biological effect.

5. **Gastric bands have evolved from nonadjustable to adjustable bands over the past 30 years and now they are even being placed by single incision laparoscopic surgery. All of the following are <u>TRUE</u> except:**
   A. Gastric banding was first performed in the United States in the 1970s by placing a nonadjustable Marlex band around the patient's upper stomach.
   B. The first published report of adjustable gastric band in United States was by Kuzmak in 1986.
   C. The REALIZE® band is the Swedish adjustable gastric band.
   D. Lap-Band® was approved by FDA in 1996.

6. **Leptin and adiponectin are the two most important adipokines, though a few more were recently discovered. Identify the <u>FALSE</u> statement about discovery of adiponectin.**
   A. It was discovered in 1995.
   B. It was called adipo"nectin" as the purified molecule smelled like nectar.
   C. It was discovered by studying cells differentiating into adipocytes.
   D. Before discovery of adiponectin, about 40% of proteins expressed from the adipose tissue were unknown.

7. **Glucagon-like peptide-1 (GLP-1) is an important incretin and now an indispensable armamentarium in the battle against obesity and diabetes. Identify the <u>TRUE</u> statement about discovery of GLP-1 peptide.**
   A. The insulinotropic action of GLP-1 was predicted even before its sequence was known.
   B. The existence of GLP-1 was suspected by studying its precursor molecule.
   C. Exendin-4, a GLP-1 analogue, was designed by recombinant DNA technology.
   D. The GLP-1 peptide has different sequences in mouse, rat, and human.

8. **Bariatric surgical techniques were developed mainly in the last 50 years, and they continue to be developed even today. Identify the <u>FALSE</u> statement about the development of surgical techniques in bariatric surgery.**
   A. The first LRYGB was described by Clarke and Wittgrove.
   B. Magentrasse and Mill developed a technique similar to a sleeve gastrectomy where a part of the stomach was removed.
   C. Kuzmak pioneered the adjustable band technology in the United States.
   D. The first laparoscopic BPD-DS was performed by Gagner.

9. **VBG is not a commonly performed procedure today. Identify the <u>FALSE</u> statement about VBG.**
   A. It was first performed by Edward Mason in the early 1980s.
   B. It was endorsed by the National Institutes of Health (NIH) consensus in 1991.
   C. It is covered by Medicare.
   D. Reversal of VBG is very difficult.

10. **The JIB is a procedure only of historical importance and provided valuable data about the physiology of bariatric surgery. Identify the <u>FALSE</u> statement about the history of the procedure.**
    A. The procedure was first performed by Kremen, Linner, and Nelson.
    B. The standard lengths of the jejunum and ileum in alimentary continuity are 14 and 4 in., respectively, in the most commonly performed technique.
    C. Historically a jejunocolic bypass has never been documented in humans.
    D. End-to-side JIB was discontinued by some workers due to concerns over reflux of nutrients into the bypassed ileum.

ANSWER KEY

1. A	4. D	7. B	10. C
2. C	5. D	8. B	
3. C	6. B	9. C	

ANSWER KEY WITH EXPLANATION

1. **Answer: A.**

   The JIB was first performed by Kremen et al. in 1954. It was widely performed in the 1960s and 1970s and consisted of bypassing a large segment of the jejunum and the ileum. Its most important short-term complication was diarrhea due to unabsorbed fatty acids entering the colon. In one series, the incidence of diarrhea was about 58% at 5 years. Its most significant long-term complication is liver disease and cirrhosis. In the same series, the incidence of progressive liver abnormalities was 29% and cirrhosis developed in 7%. However, it produced good weight loss (mean net weight loss was 33% at 5 years). The cause of cirrhosis after JIB is protein malnutrition (causing deficiency of amino acids). All patients with a JIB, in the presence of a metabolic complication, need to undergo conversion to another bariatric procedure.

   Bariatric surgeries (including JIB) do not increase the incidence of uric acid stones. They increase incidence of oxalate stones due to fatty acid malabsorption and formation of calcium soap, leading to decreased formation of insoluble calcium oxalate and increased absorption of oxalate with hyperoxaluria. Hyperoxaluria is nearly universal after JIB.

   References:
   - Requarth JA, Burchard KW, Colacchio TA, et al. Long-term morbidity following jejunoileal bypass. The continuing potential need for surgical reversal. Arch Surg 1995; 130(3):318–325.
   - Singh D, Laya AS, Clarkston WK, et al. Jejunoileal bypass: a surgery of the past and a review of its complications. World J Gastroenterol 2009; 15(18):2277–2279.
   - McFarland RJ, Gazet JC, Pilkington TR. A 13-year review of jejunoileal bypass. Br J Surg 1985; 72(2):81–87.
   - Hocking MP, Duerson MC, O'Leary JP, et al. Jejunoileal bypass for morbid obesity. Late follow-up in 100 cases. N Engl J Med 1983; 308(17):995–999.
   - Gonzalez R, Gallgher SF, Sarrr MG, et al. Chapter 21.8: Gastric bypass as a revisional procedure. In: Schauer PR, Schirmer BD, Brethauer SA, eds. Minimally Invasive Bariatric Surgery. New York: Springer, 2007.

2. **Answer: C.**

   Gastric bypass was first performed by laparotomy in the year 1967 by Mason and Ito, and VBG was first performed by Mason in 1982. Wittgrove et al. reported the first series of LRYGB in 1994. The gastric bypass performed by Mason in 1967 consisted of a loop gastrojejunostomy not Roux-en-Y gastrojejunostomy. The first RYGB was performed by Griffen et al. in 1977.

   References:
   - Griffen WO, Young VL, Stevenson CC. A prospective comparison of gastric and jejunoileal bypass procedures for morbid obesity. Ann Surg 1977; 186:500–507.
   - Wittgrove AC, Clark GW, Tremblay LJ. Laparoscopic gastric bypass, Roux-en-Y: preliminary report of five cases. Obes Surg 1994; 4(4):353–357.
   - Mason EE, Ito C. Gastric bypass in obesity. Surg Clin North Am 1967; 47:1345–1351.
   - Mason EE. Vertical banded gastroplasty for obesity. Arch Surg 1982; 117(5):701–706.
   - Fobi MA. Vertical banded gastroplasty vs. gastric bypass: 10 years follow-up. Obes Surg 1993; 3(2):161–164.

3. **Answer: C.**

   Ghrelin in Proto-Indo-European language means "to grow." It was identified by using the orphan receptor principle where cells expressing growth hormone secretagogue receptor were exposed to various tissue extracts to identify the ligand that binds to it. Ghrelin was discovered when scientists were in search of growth hormone secretagogues. It was discovered by Kojima et al. in 1999. Ghrelin was found to stimulate growth hormone secretion.

   References:
   - Kojima M. The discovery of ghrelin—a personal memory. Regul Pept 2008; 145 (1–3):2–6 [Epub September 21, 2007].
   - Kojima M, Hosoda H, Matsuo H, et al. Ghrelin: discovery of the natural endogenous ligand for the growth hormone secretagogue receptor. Trends Endocrinol Metab 2001; 12(3):118–122.

4. **Answer: D.**

   The leptin molecule was first produced by positional cloning of the *ob* gene in 1994. This involves the use of linkage analysis and chromosome walking. The idea of this adipokine came from studies of *ob/ob* and *db/db* mice. Though it was isolated by Freidman (Rockefeller University), the idea of existence of such a hormone secreted from adipose tissue was proposed by Kennedy in 1953. Though injections of the "*ob* protein" were necessary to determine its properties, leptin was not discovered in this manner.

   References:
   - Friedman JM. Leptin at 14 y of age: an ongoing story. Am J Clin Nutr 2009; 89 (3):973S–979S.
   - Kennedy, GC. The role of depot fat in the hypothalamic control of food intake in the rat. Proc R Soc Lond B Biol Sci 1953; 140:578–596.

5. **Answer: D.**

   Wilkinson and Peloso were the first to place a nonadjustable band of Marlex mesh around the upper part of the stomach via open surgery in 1978. These nonadjustable bands failed for a variety of reasons, notably pouch and esophageal dilation and slippage, leading to the key innovation of adjustability by several groups in the 1980s. Kuzmak performed the first adjustable gastric band and published his work in 1986. The Kuzmak band is now available as the Lap-Band® (Allergan Inc., Ontario, Canada) and the Swedish adjustable gastric band is now available as the REALIZE® Band (Ethicon Endo-Surgery, Inc., Ohio, U.S.). The Lap-Band was FDA approved on June 5, 2001.

Reference:
- http://www.fda.gov/MedicalDevices/ProductsandMedicalProcedures/ DeviceApprovalsandClearances/Recently-ApprovedDevices/ucm088965.htm

6. **Answer: B.**

The term adiponectin has been coined by Matsuzawa et al. It was called adiponectin because it is a matrix-like protein that resembles some forms of collagen. It was initially discovered in 1995 while studying cells differentiating into adipocytes. Before discovery of adiponectin, about 40% of proteins expressed by the adipose tissue were unknown.

References:
- Matsuzawa Y, Funahashi T, Kihara S, et al. Adiponectin and metabolic syndrome. Arterioscler Thromb Vasc Biol 2004; 24(1):29–33.
- Scherer PE, Williams S, Fogliano M, et al. A novel serum protein similar to C1q, produced exclusively in adipocytes. J Biol Chem 1995; 270(45):26746–26749.

7. **Answer: B.**

The existence of GLP-1 was proposed after Bell et al. at University of Chicago in 1983 discovered the sequence of preproglucagon. This 180–amino acid precursor contained the sequence of glucagon and two glucagon-like polypeptides arranged in tandem. The insulinotropic action of this peptide was first shown by Habener's group at Harvard in 1987. Exendin-4 was isolated from the saliva of Gila monster. GLP-1 has same sequence in mouse, rat, and human.

References:
- Drucker DJ, Philippe J, Mojsov S, et al. Glucagon-like peptide I stimulates insulin gene expression and increases cyclic AMP levels in a rat islet cell line. Proc Natl Acad Sci U S A 1987; 84(10):3434–3438.
- Bell GI, Santerre RF, Mullenbach GT. Hamster preproglucagon contains the sequence of glucagon and two related peptides. Nature 1983; 302(5910):716–718.
- Abu-Hamdah R, Rabiee A, Meneilly GS, et al. Clinical review: the extrapancreatic effects of glucagon-like peptide-1 and related peptides. J Clin Endocrinol Metab 2009; 94(6):1843–1852.

8. **Answer: B.**

Johnston described the Magentrasse and Mill procedure where a circular stapler was fired at the antrum and linear staplers were inserted through this defect to complete the sleeve gastrectomy. No part of the stomach was removed. Marceau et al. described the sleeve gastrectomy as an improvement over the distal gastrectomy procedure done in BPD of Scopinaro.

Michel Gagner reported the first series of laparoscopic BPD-DS patients. Gagner et al. also described a two-stage procedure for BPD-DS which reduced morbidity and mortality of this procedure.

The first LRYGB was done by Clarke and Wittgrove.

The concept for the gastric band was first developed in 1985 by Professor Dag Hallberg. Soon thereafter, Dr Lubomyr I. Kuzmak pioneered the technology in the United States. Clinical trials in the U.S. centers began in June 1995. The Lap-Band system was approved by the FDA in June 2001.

References:
- Steffen R. The history and role of gastric banding. Surg Obes Relat Dis 2008; 4(3 suppl):S7–S13.
- Ren CJ, Patterson E, Gagner M. Early results of laparoscopic biliopancreatic diversion with duodenal switch: a case series of 40 consecutive patients. Obes Surg 2000; 10(6):514–523; discussion 524.

9. **Answer: C.**

VBG, commonly referred to as "stomach stapling," was first performed in 1982 by Edward E. Mason, who is regarded as the father of obesity surgery. NIH consensus in 1991 endorsed both VBG and RYGB. It has poor long-term weight loss and several complications associated with the band. It is not covered by Medicare. Reversal of VBG is a challenging and complex procedure and hence associated with a high complication rate.

References:

- Gallhager SF, Sarr GS, Mur MM. Chapter 19: Indications for revisional bariatric surgery. In: Inabnet WB, DeMaria EJ, Ikramuddin S, eds. Laparoscopic Bariatric Surgery. Vol 1. Philadelphia: Lippincott Williams & Wilkins, 2004.
- National Institutes of Health. Gastrointestinal surgery for severe obesity. NIH consensus statement online 1991 Mar 25–27; 9(1):1–20. Available at: http://consensus.nih.gov/1991/1991GISurgeryObesity084html.htm. Accessed May 26, 2011.
- Balsinger BM, Poggio JL, Mai J, et al. Ten and more years after vertical banded gastroplasty as primary operation for morbid obesity. J Gastrointest Surg 2000; 4:598–605.
- Scozzari G, Toppino M, Famiglietti F, et al. 10-year follow-up of laparoscopic vertical banded gastroplasty: good results in selected patients. Ann Surg 2010; 252(5):831–839.
- Decision memo for bariatric surgery for the treatment of morbid obesity. Available at: http://www.cms.hhs.gov/mcd/viewdecisionmemo.asp?id=160. Accessed April 27, 2011.
- Mason EE. Vertical banded gastroplasty for obesity. Arch Surg 1982; 117(5):701–706.

10. **Answer: C.**

In 1954, Kremen, Linner, and Nelson performed the first JIB on dogs. The standard "14+4" technique was established by Payne and Dewind (14 in. of jejunum anastomosed 4 in. from the ileocecal valve). During the early 1960s, jejunum was anastomosed to the transverse colon, which resulted in a high rate of metabolic complications. Failure of weight loss was attributed to reflux of nutrients into the bypassed ileum and hence end workers started performing the end-to-end jejunoileostomy with drainage of the bypassed segment into the colon, instead of an end-to-side jejunoileostomy.

Reference:

- Buchwald H, Buchwald JN. Chapter 1. Evolution of surgery for morbid obesity. In: Pitombo C, Jones K, Higa K, et al., eds. Obesity Surgery: Principles and Practice. McGraw-Hill: New York, 2007. Available at: http://www.accesssurgery.com/content.aspx?aID=140000.

3 | Medical weight loss

CHAPTER SUMMARY
- Medical weight loss methods include dietary weight loss, exercise, and pharmacotherapy. They are also commonly used in combination.
- Low-calorie diets (LCDs) provide about 1200 kcal/day.
- Very low-calorie diet (VLCD) is a commonly used method of dietary weight loss. It is designed to provide 50% of a person's resting energy requirements. Such diets may provide up to 80 g carbohydrate/day and 15 g fat/day, and they include 100% of the recommended daily allowance for essential vitamins and minerals. The diets are designed to produce rapid weight loss while preserving lean body mass. This is accomplished by providing large amounts of dietary protein, typically 70 to 100 g/day or 0.8 to 1.5 g protein/kg ideal body weight.
- A patient is encouraged to lose weight before a bariatric procedure. Such weight loss (specifically with VLCD) has been shown to make the procedure technically simpler, resolve comorbidities, and decrease the size of the liver. In addition, it has also been shown to decrease hospital stay and produce better postoperative weight loss.
- VLCDs produce about 25% of loss of initial weight in the short term.
- Gallstones are a side effect of VLCD. About 10% of the patients present with gallstones during or within 6 months of stopping a VLCD. Ursodeoxycholic acid is given to prevent this.
- VLCD has an attrition rate of 25% to 50%.
- Atkins diet is a type of low-carbohydrate diet that is implemented in four phases. It is meant for long-term weight maintenance and is a ketogenic diet also used for epilepsy patients. There are several other low-carbohydrate diets available.
- Glycemic index (a measure of digestibility of food) is given by the following formula:
  - Glycemic index = [area under the curve (AUC) of blood glucose after ingestion of the index food]/(AUC of blood glucose after ingestion of 50 g of white bread) $\times$ 100
- The efficacy of exercise to produce weight loss is measured by "metabolic equivalent of task" (MET); 1 MET is equal to the basal metabolic rate (BMR).
- The various drugs that have been used for weight loss include sibutramine, orlistat, phentermine, rimonabant, and fenfluramine. Only orlistat and phentermine are currently approved by the Food and Drug Administration (FDA).
- Indications for obesity pharmacotherapy in adults:
  - Body mass index (BMI) > 30 kg/m^2 or BMI > 27 kg/m^2 in association with significant medical complications
  - Failure of behavioral approaches, including diet and exercise regimens
  - No strong contraindications to the medication used
  - For continued treatment, weight loss of 4 lb/mo for each of the first 3 months
- Fenfluramine has been linked with drug-induced valvulopathy and is not prescribed anymore. This side effect is related to the cumulative dose.
- Phentermine is free of the above side effect. It is thought to act by sympathetic stimulation as it is an adrenergic agonist. FDA recommends that it should be prescribed for only 12 weeks.
- Phentermine causes tachycardia and may worsen hypertension.

- Sibutramine (a serotonin norepinephrine reuptake inhibitor) has been withdrawn from the market voluntarily by the manufacturer. This is an account of the results of the sibutramine cardiovascular outcomes trial (SCOUT), which showed increased cardiovascular events with sibutramine.
- Orlistat is licensed by the FDA for patients >12 years old and can also be used for adolescent weight loss. It acts by inhibiting gastrointestinal (GI) lipases and producing fat malabsorption which causes diarrhea. This diarrhea can be minimized by decreasing the fat intake and using psyllium mucilloid.
- Rimonabant (a cannabinoid antagonist) has been linked to suicidal tendency and was never approved by the FDA.
- Experimental drugs include oxyntomodulin analogues – Peptide YY (PYY) nasal spray.
- Metformin and glucagon-like peptide-1 (GLP-1) analogues (e.g., exenatide and liraglutide) in addition to their antidiabetic effect also promote weight loss. In contrast, insulin and thiazolidinediones (TZDs) promote weight gain.
- Certain drugs are not well tolerated by post–Roux-En-Y gastric bypass (RYGB) patients – these include nonsteroidal anti-inflammatory drugs (NSAIDs) and bisphosphonates – which can result in ulceration of the pouch.
- Absorption time of drugs is reduced in post-RYGB patients.

QUESTIONS

1. Studies indicate that the achievement and maintenance of a _____ weight loss via diet and exercise alone is a reasonable goal.
   A. 4% to 6%
   B. 5% to 10%
   C. 15% to 20%
   D. 20% to 25%

2. A patient from a foreign country has tried weight loss through pharmacological means for the past 2 years with fenfluramine. He has now come to the bariatric surgeon. The patient is asymptomatic. Chest examination reveals a 3/6 systolic murmur at the cardiac apex. Echocardiography shows mitral regurgitation. Identify the FALSE statement about this drug-induced valvulopathy.
   A. Echocardiographically the valvular abnormality resembles carcinoid syndrome.
   B. Pulmonary regurgitation is the most commonly reported abnormality.
   C. It is related to the cumulative dose.
   D. It is partially reversible on discontinuation of drug.

3. A 40-year-old woman, who has a BMI of 28 has failed diet and exercise regimens for the past 2 years and wants pharmacotherapy for achieving some weight loss. Which of the following patients would NOT be considered for obesity pharmacotherapy?
   A. A patient with BMI of 32 without comorbidities who is seeking to start medications for weight loss after failure of behavioral approaches.
   B. A patient whose BMI is 25 with no comorbidities who is seeking to start medications for weight loss after failure of behavioral approaches.
   C. A patient who has lost 5% body weight in 6 months with medications and wants to continue the same.
   D. A patient with uncontrolled diabetes who has failed diet and exercise regimens and has a BMI of 29.

4. A 28-year-old obese, but healthy woman asks you to prescribe her a weight loss medication phentermine. She heard that it is safe, most effective, and FDA approved for this indication. Identify the FALSE statement about phentermine.
   A. It does not affect the cardiac valves.
   B. It causes tachycardia and hypertension.

C. It is approved by FDA for use up to a period of 2 years.

D. Its mode of action is activation of sympathetic nervous system.

5. **A 55-year-old obese woman with a family history of premature** coronary artery disease **(CAD) and history of major depression presents to your office after reading a** *New York Times* **article about sibutramine taken off the market. Identify the** **TRUE** **statement about the efficacy of sibutramine.**
   A. It has no drug interactions.
   B. Sibutramine increases mortality.
   C. Sibutramine does not improve cardiovascular outcomes.
   D. It can cause hypertension in <1% of patients.

6. **A medical student in your office asks you about pharmacotherapy options in the pipeline for the future. Identify the** **TRUE** **statement about drugs used for pharmacotherapy for obesity.**
   A. Rimonabant has been approved by the FDA.
   B. Intranasal PYY is not effective in causing weight loss.
   C. Oxyntomodulin analogues have been shown not to be effective in causing weight loss.
   D. Exenatide though effective in causing resolution of type 2 diabetes mellitus (T2DM) does not cause weight loss.

7. **Your patient heard that there is a medication that can help him/her lose weight by blocking fat absorption. Identify the** **TRUE** **statement about orlistat.**
   A. Orlistat is not available over the counter.
   B. It affects absorption of oral antidiabetic drugs.
   C. The weight loss achieved is <5%.
   D. Patients need micronutrient supplementation while on orlistat.

8. **Much of the morbidity and mortality seen with diabetes is due to the micro- and macrovascular-associated tissue damage. The usefulness of antidiabetic drugs in preventing these complications has been questioned. Which of the following regarding the extent of antidiabetic benefit is** **TRUE?**
   A. Intensive glycemic control may be associated with increased mortality.
   B. Intensive glucose control does not reduce microvascular complications.
   C. Metformin does not improve cardiovascular outcomes in diabetic patients.
   D. There are no persistent benefits of intensive glycemic control after it is stopped.

9. **RYGB being a malabsorptive procedure has produced concerns regarding absorption of drugs. Which of the following statements is** **TRUE** **about drugs used in a post-RYGB patient?**
   A. Only extended-release formulations are recommended.
   B. Liquid solutions are not recommended.
   C. NSAIDs are safe in RYGB patients as most of their stomach is bypassed.
   D. The time of absorption of a drug is decreased in a post-RYGB patient.

10. **It is common to find that morbidly obese patients are on antidiabetic medications. Which of the following is** **TRUE** **regarding the common antidiabetic medications used?**
    A. Liraglutide causes nausea.
    B. Sitagliptin causes hypoglycemia.
    C. Pramlinitide causes weight gain.
    D. Metformin need not be stopped before surgery.

11. **A 50-year-old patient who has a BMI of 28 kg/m² presents to her endocrinologist with newly discovered T2DM. The doctor starts her on metformin. After about 3 months the patient has an Hb1AC of 8.1 and has lost 2 lb. She has been compliant with the lifestyle modifications advised by her nutritionist and her doctor but she complains of excess appetite. Which of the following medications is best started at this time?**
    A. Sitagliptin
    B. Liraglutide
    C. Glyburide
    D. Pramlinitide

12. **A 35-year-old overweight (BMI 29 kg/m²), executive who is taking orlistat 120 mg thrice daily for the past 3 weeks, comes to the office with complaints of oily stools, bloating, and excess flatus. His only other medical problem is his blood pressure which has been difficult to control despite being on three drugs. He seeks advice regarding discontinuing orlistat and switching over to sibutramine. What is the appropriate advice for this patient?**
    A. Orlistat irreversibly inhibits lipase and discontinuing the drug will not relieve his diarrhea in the near future.
    B. Tell him that these side effects will diminish with reduction of dietary fat and add psyllium mucilloid to alleviate the side effects.
    C. Discontinue orlistat and prescribe sibutramine as sibutramine is much better at weight reduction at 1 year.
    D. Recommend bariatric surgery.

13. **Preoperatively bariatric surgery patients are encouraged to undergo some weight loss. Which one of the following statements regarding obesity and medical weight loss is <u>TRUE</u>?**
    A. The loss of fat with dieting is caused predominantly by a decrease in the number of fat cells.
    B. Dieting may lead to a loss of fat-free mass.
    C. Subcutaneous fat is lost more than visceral fat in patients with central obesity.
    D. Nonsurgical weight loss does not reduce liver fat.

14. **Which one of the following statements regarding dietary interventions is <u>FALSE</u>?**
    A. A reduction in calories from saturated fatty acids as a percentage of total energy reduces the serum low-density lipoprotein (LDL) cholesterol levels and decreases the incidence of coronary heart disease (CHD).
    B. Increasing soluble fiber in the diet lowers serum LDL cholesterol.
    C. Replacing saturated fat with polyunsaturated fat in diet may significantly increase serum high-density lipoprotein (HDL) cholesterol.
    D. Substitution of carbohydrates for saturated fatty acids frequently causes a fall in serum HDL cholesterol and a rise in triglycerides.

15. **LCDs are an effective way to lose weight. Which of the following statements about dietary management of obesity is <u>TRUE</u>?**
    A. The National Heart, Lung, and Blood Institute (NHLBI) recommends starting at a diet with deficit of 1500 kcal/day to aim for a weight reduction of 0.5 lb/wk.
    B. Clinical trial evidence suggests that a low-carbohydrate, high-protein, high-fat diet is superior to a low-calorie, high-carbohydrate, low-fat (conventional) diet, 1 year after initiation.
    C. Diets with low energy density are effective in reducing hunger and decreasing weight.
    D. Portion control is best managed by the patients as the use of preprepared foods causes decreased compliance.

16. The Atkins diet has become very popular as a method of weight loss. It is also the preferred diet in epileptic patients. Which of the following statements about the Atkins diet is <u>TRUE</u>?
    A. Two phases are typically described in the institution of the Atkins diet.
    B. It is absolutely contraindicated in patients with reduced renal function.
    C. Diet initiation results in higher serum concentration of β-hydroxybutyrate and other ketone bodies.
    D. Atkins diet is not meant for long-term weight loss.

17. Various types of diet with varying outcomes have been used to achieve weight loss and maintain the weight lost. Identify the <u>FALSE</u> statement.
    A. VLCD provides 50% of the resting energy requirements of a person.
    B. Meal replacements are portion controlled and nutritionally balanced.
    C. Higher protein diet enhances weight maintenance.
    D. Low–glycemic index food items have not been found to be useful in weight maintenance when compared to high–glycemic index foods.

18. Glycemic index is an important property of food. Which of the following statements <u>CORRECTLY</u> defines the glycemic index?
    A. Percentage of carbohydrate over total number of calories.
    B. It is directly proportional to the AUC of 2-hour blood glucose response curve following the ingestion of the index food.
    C. Percentage of rise in blood glucose compared to rise after taking 100 g of sucrose.
    D. It is an estimate of the total amount of glucose in the plasma.

19. A 45-year-old stock broker has a BMI of 36 and suffers from obstructive sleep apnea and uncontrolled hypertension. He has failed previous dietary and exercise measures but shows a keen interest in trying VLCD and discusses this with his primary medical doctor (PMD). Which course of action would the PMD <u>NOT</u> advise?
    A. Recommend bariatric surgery as an alternative.
    B. Commence treatment with ursodeoxycholic acid to prevent gallstones with VLCD.
    C. Warn him that VLCD does not produce sustained weight loss.
    D. Advise him against VLCD because these proprietary formulas though good at achieving weight loss fall short of the recommended daily intake of vitamins and minerals.

20. A 50-year-old diabetic patient presents to the primary care physician after being diagnosed with hypercholesterolemia at a health fair. The dietary advice given by the physician would <u>NOT</u> include which one of the following?
    A. Limit cholesterol to 200 mg/day.
    B. Less than 7% of calories are to be from saturated fat.
    C. Limit intake of trans fat.
    D. Routine supplementation with antioxidants is required.

21. The role of preoperative weight loss on the outcomes of bariatric surgery is a topic of great interest. Identify the <u>FALSE</u> statement about preoperative weight loss in bariatric surgery.
    A. Patients who have >10% excess weight loss preoperatively have a better weight loss postoperatively.
    B. The use of VLCD before surgery makes surgery technically easier.
    C. Patients successful in losing more than 5% excess weight preoperatively have shorter hospital stays.
    D. A reduction in liver volume is not observed with VLCD.

22. **Gallstones form when there is rapid weight loss, as during VLCD therapy. Identify the <u>FALSE</u> statement about VLCD therapy–associated gallstone formation.**
    A. Limiting weight loss to about 1.5 kg/wk reduces incidence of gallstones.
    B. Administration of ursodeoxycholic acid may reduce the incidence of gallstones.
    C. Gallstones can occur as early as 4 weeks after starting VLCD.
    D. Around 1% of individuals undergoing VLCD may develop gallstones.

23. **In view of the several metabolic side effects of VLCDs, the risk-benefit ratio of VLCD has been called into question. Identify the <u>FALSE</u> statement about efficacy of VLCD.**
    A. VLCDs produce 15% to 25% of loss of *initial* weight in 6 months.
    B. VLCDs have a greater than 25% attrition rate.
    C. LCDs produce a better weight loss when compared to VLCDs due to better acceptability in the long term.
    D. Short-term weight loss of VLCD is better than LCD.

24. **Calorie counting is an important part of dietary therapy of obesity. Identify the wrong calorie content of one portion of the corresponding food item.**
    A. One egg – 90
    B. One apple – 60
    C. One banana – 100
    D. Peanuts (100 g) – 200

25. **The MET is a unit for expressing energy spent during physical activities as a multiple of the resting metabolic rate (RMR). Therefore, the basal RMR is equivalent to 1 MET. Based on this definition, a man weighing 80 kg jumping a rope (10 METs) consumes**
    A. 400 kcal/hr
    B. 2400 kcal/hr
    C. 100 kcal/hr
    D. 800 kcal/hr

ANSWER KEY

1. B	8. A	15. C	22. D
2. B	9. D	16. C	23. C
3. B	10. A	17. D	24. D
4. C	11. B	18. B	25. D
5. C	12. B	19. D	
6. B	13. B	20. D	
7. D	14. C	21. D	

ANSWER KEY WITH EXPLANATION

1. **Answer: B.**

   A weight loss of just 10% is enough to bring down high blood pressure, HbA1c levels, and improve lipid parameters.

   References:
   • Feldstein AC, Nichols GA, Smith DH, et al. Weight change in diabetes and glycemic and blood pressure control. Diabetes Care 2008; 31(10):1960–1965 [Epub June 20, 2008].
   • Wadden TA, Anderson DA, Foster GD. Two-year changes in lipids and lipoproteins associated with the maintenance of a 5% to 10% reduction in initial weight: some findings and some questions. Obes Res 1999; 7:170–178.

2. **Answer: B.**

The valvulopathy caused by fenfluramine is reversible and dose related. It occurs in about one out of eight patients who have taken the drug for more than 90 days. The valvular abnormality due to fenfluramine resembles that due to carcinoid syndrome. Aortic and mitral regurgitation are the most commonly reported abnormalities. The abnormalities are reversible with some echocardiographic improvement being reported 1 year after stopping the drug. Valvular surgery may be needed in <1% of the patients.

References:
- Hensrud DD, Connolly HM, Grogan M, et al. Echocardiographic improvement over time after cessation of use of fenfluramine and phentermine. Mayo Clin Proc 1999; 74:1191–1197.
- Droogmans S, Kerkhove D, Cosyns B, et al. Role of echocardiography in toxic heart valvulopathy. Eur J Echocardiogr 2009; 10:467–476.

3. **Answer: B.**

The indications of pharmacotherapy of obesity are as follows:
- BMI > 30 kg/m^2 or BMI > 27 kg/m^2 in association with significant medical complications
- Failure of behavioral approaches, including diet and exercise regimens
- No strong contraindications to the medication used
- For continued treatment, weight loss of 4 lb/mo for each of the first 3 months

References:
- National Institutes of Health. The Practical guide. Identification, evaluation, and treatment of overweight and obesity in adults. NIH Publication Number 02-4084. Washington DC: NIH, 2000.
- Snow V, Barry P, Fitterman N, et al., for the Clinical Efficacy Assessment Subcommittee of the American College of Physicians. Pharmacologic and surgical management of obesity in primary care: a clinical practice guideline from the American College of Physicians. Ann Intern Med 2005; 142(7):525–531.
- Hensrud DD. Pharmacotherapy for obesity. Med Clin North Am 2000; 84(2):463–476 (review).

4. **Answer: C.**

Phentermine is an adrenergic reuptake inhibitor that augments adrenergic signaling in the brain and peripheral tissues. It is therefore thought to promote weight loss by activation of the sympathetic nervous system with resulting decrease in food intake and increased resting energy expenditure. Unlike fenfluramine, phentermine has no known effects on cardiac valves. As an adrenergic agonist, however, it can be associated with tachycardia and, less commonly, hypertension. Thus, phentermine should be used with caution in people at significant risk for hemodynamic or cardiovascular complications of tachycardia and those with uncontrolled hypertension. An acceptable therapeutic response is considered as 4 lb per 4 weeks for at least the first 8 to 12 weeks of therapy, when given with or without associated dietary and exercise counseling. Although approved by the FDA for only 3 months' use, many experts advocate longer term use in patients who demonstrate a good therapeutic response during the first 3 months.

References:
- Bray GA, Greenway FL. Pharmacological treatment of the overweight patient. Pharmacol Rev 2007; 59:151–184.
- Hendricks EJ, Rothman RB, Greenway FL. How physician obesity specialists use drugs to treat obesity. Obesity (Silver Spring) 2009; 17:1730–1735.
- Kaplan LM. Pharmacologic therapies for obesity. Gastroenterol Clin North Am 2010; 39(1):69–79 (review).

5. **Answer: C.**

The SCOUT evaluated the cardiovascular outcomes after treatment with sibutramine in patients who had preexisting cardiovascular disease or T2DM or both. The study found that there were increased nonfatal myocardial infarctions (MIs) and strokes in those treated with sibutramine. Sibutramine did not cause an increase in mortality. Behavior therapy when added to sibutramine produces greater weight loss. It causes hypertension in 10% to 15% of the patients, though this rarely results in the patient stopping the drug. Sibutramine should not be used with serotonin-specific reuptake inhibitor (SSRI) or monoamine oxidase (MAO) inhibitors as it may precipitate serotonin syndrome. In view of the findings of the SCOUT, the FDA asked the manufacturers of sibutramine to voluntarily withdraw it from the market.

References:
- James WP, Caterson ID, Coutinho W, et al., for the SCOUT Investigators. Effect of sibutramine on cardiovascular outcomes in overweight and obese subjects. N Engl J Med 2010; 363(10):905–917.
- Bray GA. Medical therapy for obesity. Mt Sinai J Med 2010; 77(5):407–417.
- Kaplan LM. Pharmacologic therapies for obesity. Gastroenterol Clin North Am 2010; 39(1):69–79 (review).

6. **Answer: B.**

Rimonabant is a cannabinoid CB1 receptor antagonist. CB1 receptors are located in the central nervous system (CNS), whereas CB2 receptors are located in the periphery. Endocannabinoids act through the reward system of the brain. Rimonabant was never approved by the FDA in the United States. This is due to concerns about suicidality.

Intranasal PYY has been found to be effective in causing weight loss after 6 weeks of therapy.

Oxyntomodulin has been shown to be effective in causing weight loss in small human studies and in animal models. Larger trials are required.

Exenatide, a GLP-1 agonist has been found to be effective in causing weight loss. However, this is only FDA approved for use in patients with diabetes.

References:
- Wynne K, Park AJ, Small CJ, et al. Subcutaneous oxyntomodulin reduces body weight in overweight and obese subjects: a double-blind, randomized, controlled trial. Diabetes 2005; 54:2390–2395.
- Gantz I, Erondu N, Mallick M, et al. Efficacy and safety of intranasal peptide YY3-36 for weight reduction in obese adults. J Clin Endocrinol Metab 2007; 92:1754–1757.
- Glass LC, Qu Y, Lenox S, et al. Effects of exenatide versus insulin analogues on weight change in subjects with type 2 diabetes: a pooled post-hoc analysis. Curr Med Res Opin 2008; 24:639–644.

7. **Answer: D.**

Orlistat is a potent and selective pancreatic lipase inhibitor that reduces intestinal digestion of fat. Patients should be on a low-fat diet prior to starting this medication because they will get diarrhea if they overconsume fat with orlistat. Orlistat does not affect absorption of any drug other than acyclovir and fat-soluble vitamins absorption. It is recommended that patient take daily multivitamin supplement while on this drug. It is a prescription drug (Xenical), but half the dose (Alli) is available as an over-the-counter preparation.

In a 4-year, double-blind, randomized, placebo-controlled trial with orlistat in over 3000 overweight patients, the orlistat-treated group achieved a weight loss of 11% below baseline during the first year compared to the placebo-treated group with 6% below baseline. Among 21% of who had impaired glucose tolerance, there was a 37% reduction in the conversion of patients from impaired glucose tolerance to diabetes.

References:
- Torgerson JS, Hauptman J, Boldrin MN, et al. XENical in the prevention of diabetes in obese subjects (XENDOS) study: a randomized study of orlistat as an

adjunct to lifestyle changes for the prevention of type 2 diabetes in obese patients. Diabetes Care 2004; 27:155–161.

- Wadden TA, Berkowitz RI, Womble LG, et al. Effects of sibutramine plus orlistat in obese women following 1 year of treatment by sibutramine alone: a placebo-controlled trial. Obes Res 2000; 8:431–437.
- Kaplan LM. Pharmacologic therapies for obesity. Gastroenterol Clin North Am 2010; 39(1):69–79 (review).

8. **Answer: A.**

The United Kingdom Prospective Diabetes Study (UKPDS) was a 10-year trial of newly diagnosed T2DM patients randomized to intensive therapy with a sulfonylurea or insulin versus conventional therapy with diet modification. The intensive group achieved a lower median A_1C of 7.0% versus 7.9% in the conventional group, and a 25% reduction in microvascular complications.

Observational follow-up of the diabetic participants in UKPDS for 10 to 11 years after trial completion demonstrated that despite convergence of A_1C between the intensive and conventional groups (at year 1), individuals initially assigned to intensive control maintained persistence of microvascular benefit. Furthermore, there was an emergence of cardiovascular and mortality benefit in the intensive groups. This suggests that glycemic control early on in the course of T2DM may establish a foundation of vascular health or "metabolic programming" that protects against microvascular disease and possibly cardiovascular disease and mortality later on in life. Several observational studies have shown a decreased cardiovascular risk with the use of metformin.

References:
- Umesh M. Chapter 27: Diabetes mellitus & hypoglycemia. In: McPhee SJ, Papadakis MA, eds. Current Medical Diagnosis and Treatment. 51st ed. New York: McGraw-Hill, 2011. Available at: http://eresources.library.mssm. edu:2059/content.aspx?aID=15524.
- UK Prospective Diabetes Study (UKPDS) Group. Intensive blood glucose control with sulphonylureas or insulin compared with conventional treatment and risk of complications in patients with type 2 diabetes (UKPDS 33) [published correction appears in Lancet 1999; 354:602]. Lancet 1998; 352:837–853.
- The Diabetes Control and Complications Trial Research Group. The effect of intensive treatment of diabetes on the development of and progression of long-term complications in insulin-dependent diabetes mellitus. N Engl J Med 1993; 329:977–986.
- Holman RR, Paul SK, Bethel MA, et al. 10-year follow up of intensive glucose control in type 2 diabetes. N Engl J Med 2008; 359:1577–1589.
- The Diabetes Control and Complications Trial/Epidemiology of Diabetes Interventions and Complications (DCCT/EDIC) Study Research Group. Intensive diabetes treatment and cardiovascular disease in patients with type 1 diabetes. N Engl J Med 2005; 353:2643–2653.
- Powers AC, David DA. Chapter 43: Endocrine pancreas and pharmacotherapy of diabetes mellitus and hypoglycemia. In: Brunton LL, Chabner BA, Knollmann BC, eds. Goodman & Gilman's the Pharmacological Basis of Therapeutics, 12th ed. New York: McGraw-Hill, 2011. Available at http://www.accessmedicine. com/content.aspx?aID=16674366.

9. **Answer: D.**

The time for absorption of a drug is reduced after surgery as the surface area of the intestine is reduced. Drugs with long absorptive phases that remain in the intestine for extended periods are likely to exhibit decreased bioavailability in these patients. The reduced size of the stomach after surgery can place patients at risk for adverse events associated with some medications. Medications implicated in such adverse events include NSAIDs, salicylates, and oral bisphosphonates. A change to a liquid medication formulation could increase absorption by eliminating the need for drug dissolution.

Reference:
- Miller AD, Smith KM. Medication and nutrient administration considerations after bariatric surgery. Am J Health Syst Pharm 2006; 63(19):1852–1857.

10. **Answer: A.**

Liraglutide, long-acting GLP-1 analogue, slows gastric emptying and has nausea as a dose-limiting side effect. Sitagliptin, which is a dipeptidyl peptidase 4 (DPP-4) inhibitor, does not cause hypoglycemia. Hence they are used for patients who are nearing their goal HbA1c and those who are at risk for hypoglycemia (e.g., frail individuals, elderly, and those with renal dysfunction). Pramlinitide causes maintenance of weight or weight loss. Metformin should be stopped at least 24 hours before surgery to avoid lactic acidosis. Other oral antidiabetic drugs are also stopped before surgery.

References:
- Siram AT, Yanagisawa R, Skamagas M. Weight management in type 2 diabetes mellitus. Mt Sinai J Med 2010; 77(5):533–548.
- Bray GA. Medical therapy of obesity. Mt Sinai J Med 2010; 77:407–417.

11. **Answer: B.**

In overweight patients who are unable to achieve glycemic goals on maximum metformin therapy and lifestyle modification, and who may benefit from appetite reduction, injectable GLP-1 agonists such as exenatide and liraglutide may be added to facilitate weight loss, normalize satiety, and improve postprandial glucose excursions.

DPP-IV inhibitors such as sitagliptin are weight neutral. Sulfonylureas such as glyburide stimulate insulin secretion from pancreatic β cells and are associated with modest weight gain. TZDs induce dose-dependent HbA1c lowering, but this is also paralleled by greater weight gain. Pramlinitide reduces rate of gastric emptying and decreases appetite but it is used as an adjunct to insulin injections.

References:
- Siram AT, Yanagisawa R, Skamagas M. Weight management in type 2 diabetes mellitus. Mt Sinai J Med 2010; 77(5):533–548.
- Nathan DM, Buse JB, Davidson MB, et al. Medical management of hyperglycemia in type 2 diabetes mellitus: a consensus algorithm for the initiation and adjustment of therapy: a consensus statement from the American Diabetes Association and the European Association for the Study of Diabetes. Diabetes Care 2009; 32:193–203.
- Kahn SE, Haffner SM, Heise MA, et al. for the ADOPT Study Group. Glycemic durability of rosiglitazone, metformin, or glyburide monotherapy. N Engl J Med 2006; 355:2427–2444.
- Bray GA. Medical therapy of obesity. Mt Sinai J Med 2010; 77:407–417.

12. **Answer: B.**

Orlistat (Xenical) acts in the lumen of the stomach and small intestine by forming a covalent bond with the active site of GI lipases, thus inhibiting them. Tolerability to the drug is related to the malabsorption of dietary fat and subsequent passage of fat in the feces. GI tract adverse effects are reported in at least 10% of orlistat-treated patients. These include flatus with discharge, fecal urgency, fatty/oily stool, and increased defecation. These side effects are generally experienced early, diminish as patients control their dietary fat intake, and infrequently cause patients to withdraw from clinical trials. Psyllium mucilloid is helpful in controlling the orlistat-induced GI side effects when taken concomitantly with the medication.

The patient does not meet the criteria for bariatric surgery, and switching over to sibutramine is likely to worsen his BP control. Orlistat and sibutramine produce comparable weight loss though sibutramine has been found to be superior in some studies. Sibutramine cannot be prescribed as it is off the market.

References:
- Gursoy A, Erdogan MF, Cin MO, et al. Comparison of orlistat and sibutramine in an obesity management program: efficacy, compliance, and weight regain after noncompliance. Eat Weight Disord 2006; 11(4):e127– e132.
- Kushner RF. Chapter 75: Evaluation and management of obesity. In: Fauci AS, Braunwald E, Kasper DL, et al., eds. Harrison's Principles of Internal Medicine, 17th ed. New York: McGraw-Hill, 2008. Available at http://eresources.library.mssm.edu:2059/content.aspx?aID=2883857.
- Kaplan LM. Pharmacologic therapies for obesity. Gastroenterol Clin North Am 2010; 39(1):69–79 (review).

13. **Answer: B.**

Most, if not all, of the loss of fat is caused by a decrease in the size (lipid content) of existing fat cells although there is some evidence in humans that large, long-term fat loss can also decrease the number of fat cells. Approximately 75% to 85% of weight that is lost by dieting is composed of fat and 15% to 25% is fat-free mass. In addition, there is regional heterogeneity in the distribution of fat loss with greater relative losses of intra-abdominal than total body fat mass, particularly in men and women with increased initial intra-abdominal fat mass. Nonsurgical weight loss reduces liver fat.

References:
- Klein S, Wadden T, Sugerman HJ. AGA technical review on obesity. Gastroenterology 2002; 123:882–932.
- Magkos F. Exercise and fat accumulation in the human liver. Curr Opin Lipidol 2010; 21(6):507–517.

14. **Answer: C.**

Reduction of saturated fats in the diet has been shown to reduce LDL cholesterol levels and incidence of CHD. Conversely, every 1% increase in calories from saturated fat increases LDL cholesterol by 2%. There is evidence that soluble (viscous) forms of dietary fiber can reduce LDL cholesterol levels. In contrast, insoluble fiber does not significantly affect LDL cholesterol. Polyunsaturated fatty acids when substituted for saturated fatty acids may cause a slight decrease in HDL cholesterol and triglycerides although this response is variable. Polyunsaturated fatty acids do cause a decrease in LDL cholesterol and decrease the CHD risk. When carbohydrates are substituted for saturated fatty acids, the fall in LDL cholesterol levels equals that with monounsaturated fatty acids. However, compared with monounsaturated fatty acids, substitution of carbohydrate for saturated fatty acids frequently causes a fall in HDL cholesterol and a rise in triglyceride.

Reference:
- National Cholesterol Education Program (NCEP) Expert Panel on Detection, Evaluation, and Treatment of High Blood Cholesterol in Adults (Adult Treatment Panel III). Third Report of the National Cholesterol Education Program (NCEP) Expert Panel on Detection, Evaluation, and Treatment of High Blood Cholesterol in Adults (Adult Treatment Panel III) final report. Circulation 2002; 106(25):3143–3421.

15. **Answer: C.**

The primary focus of diet therapy is to reduce overall calorie consumption. The NHLBI guidelines recommend initiating treatment with a 500 to 1000 kcal daily caloric deficit, as compared to usual diet. This roughly translates to a 1 to 2 lb loss per week.

Convincing data for the superiority of a low-carbohydrate, high-protein, high-fat diet over low-calorie, high-carbohydrate, low-fat (conventional) diet is at present lacking. At 1 year there is no difference in weight loss when the two diets are compared. Further studies are needed to understand the safety and efficacy of low-carbohydrate, high-protein, high-fat diets.

Since portion control is one of the most difficult strategies for patients to manage, the use of preprepared products, such as meal replacements, is a simple and convenient suggestion. Examples include frozen entrees, canned beverages, and bars.

Diets containing low-energy-dense foods have been shown to control hunger and result in decreased caloric intake and weight loss.

References:

- Foster GD, Wyatt HR, Hill JO, et al. A randomized trial of a low-carbohydrate diet for obesity. N Engl J Med 2003; 348(21):2082–2090.
- Kushner RF. Chapter 75: Evaluation and management of obesity. Fauci AS, Braunwald E, Kasper DL, et al., eds. Harrison's Principles of Internal Medicine, 17th ed. New York: McGraw-Hill, 2008. Available at http://eresources.library.mssm.edu:2059/content.aspx?aID=2883857.

16. **Answer: C.**

The Atkins diet is a ketogenic diet and better tolerated by individuals with epilepsy. Atkins diet is not contraindicated in renal failure or diabetes but such persons need to be more closely monitored. Diet initiation results in higher serum concentration of β-hydroxybutyrate and other ketone bodies.

Four phases are typically described in adopting the Atkins diet:

- Phase 1: Induction: Carbohydrates are restricted to 20 g each day.
- Phase 2: Ongoing weight loss: Carbohydrates are added incrementally in the form of nutrient-dense and fiber-rich foods.
- Phase 3: Premaintenance: To make the transition from weight loss to weight maintenance, daily carbohydrate intake is increased in 10-g increments each week.
- Phase 4: Lifetime maintenance: People are instructed to select from a wide variety of foods while controlling carbohydrate intake.

References:

- Baron M. The Atkins diet. Health Care Food Nutr Focus 2004; 21(10):7, 11.
- Astrup A, Meinert LT, Harper A. Atkins and other low-carbohydrate diets: hoax or an effective tool for weight loss? Lancet 2004; 364(9437):897–899.

17. **Answer: D.**

VLCDs contain about 800 kcal/day (or about 50% of the resting energy requirements of a person). But a 400-kcal diet has not been shown to cause more weight loss. Balanced deficit diets contain a balanced profile of nutrients that are relatively low in fat, high in carbohydrate, moderate in protein, and high in fiber. One disadvantage of such diets is the relatively low rate of weight loss. Meal replacements are portion controlled and nutritionally balanced. High protein content in food after a VLCD has been shown to cause a reduction in weight regain. Low–glycemic index food has also been shown to produce better weight maintenance after a VLCD.

References:

- Chapter 64: Obesity management. In: Shils ME, Shike M, Ross AC, eds. Modern Nutrition in Health and Disease, 10th ed. Philadelphia: Lippincott Williams & Wilkins, 2006.
- Larsen TM, Dalskov SM, van Baak M, et al.; Diet, Obesity, and Genes (Diogenes) Project. Diets with high or low protein content and glycemic index for weight-loss maintenance. N Engl J Med 2010; 363(22):2102–2113.
- Dubnov-Raz G, Berry EM. Dietary approaches to obesity. Mt Sinai J Med 2010; 77 (5):488–498.
- Lopes da Silva MV, de Càssia Gonçalves Alfenas R. Effect of the glycemic index on lipid oxidation and body composition. Nutr Hosp 2011; 26(1):48–55.
- Kushner RF. Chapter 75: Evaluation and management of obesity. Fauci AS, Braunwald E, Kasper DL, et al., eds. Harrison's Principles of Internal Medicine,

17th ed. New York: McGraw-Hill, 2008. Available at: http://eresources.library. mssm.edu:2059/content.aspx?aID=2883857.

18. **Answer: B.**

The glycemic index of a starchy food is a measure of its digestibility, based on the extent to which it raises the blood concentration of glucose compared with an equivalent amount of glucose or a reference food such as white bread or boiled rice.

It is given by the formula:

Glycemic index = (AUC of the blood glucose after ingestion of the index food)/ (AUC of blood glucose after ingestion of 50 g of white bread) × 100

Reference:

- Bender DA, Mayes PA. Chapter 14: Carbohydrates of physiologic significance. Murray RK, Bender DA, Botham KM, et al., eds. Harper's Illustrated Biochemistry, 28th ed. New York: McGraw-Hill, 2009. Available at: http://eresources. library.mssm.edu:2059/content.aspx?aID=5226612.

19. **Answer: D.**

The primary purpose of a VLCD is to promote a rapid and significant (13–23 kg) short-term weight loss over a 3- to 6-month period. VLCD does not produce sustained weight loss.

The conditions that improve due to rapid weight loss associated with a VLCD include poorly controlled T2DM, hypertriglyceridemia, obstructive sleep apnea, and symptomatic peripheral edema.

The risk for gallstone formation increases exponentially at rates of weight loss >1.5 kg/wk (3.3 lb/wk). Prophylaxis against gallstone formation with ursodeoxycholic acid, 600 mg/day, is effective in reducing this risk.

Because of the need for close metabolic monitoring, these diets are usually prescribed by physicians specializing in obesity care. VLCDs include the recommended daily intake of vitamins and minerals.

The patient has a BMI > 35 with several comorbidities with failure of conservative weight loss methods and hence would be an ideal candidate for bariatric surgery.

Reference:

- Kushner RF. Chapter 75: Evaluation and management of obesity. Fauci AS, Braunwald E, Kasper DL, et al., eds. Harrison's Principles of Internal Medicine, 17th ed. New York: McGraw-Hill, 2009. Available at: http://eresources.library. mssm.edu:2059/content.aspx?aID=2883857.

20. **Answer: D.**

A well-balanced, nutritious diet remains a fundamental element of therapy in diabetic patients. The recommendations by the American Diabetes Association (ADA) include the following:

- Limit saturated fat to <7% of total calories.
- Intake of trans fat should be minimized.
- In individuals with diabetes, limit dietary cholesterol to <200 mg/day.
- Two or more servings of fish per week (with the exception of commercially fried fish filets) provide n-3 polyunsaturated fatty acids and are recommended.
- Routine supplementation with antioxidants, such as vitamins E and C and carotene, lack evidence of efficacy and there are some concerns related to long-term safety.

References:

- American Diabetes Association, Bantle JP, Wylie-Rosett J, Albright AL, et al. Nutrition recommendations and interventions for diabetes: a position statement of the American Diabetes Association. Diabetes Care 2008; 31 (suppl 1):S61–S78.
- Umesh M. Chapter 27: Diabetes mellitus & hypoglycemia. In: McPhee SJ, Papadakis MA, eds. Current Medical Diagnosis and Treatment. 51st ed. New York: McGraw-Hill, 2011. Available at: http://eresources.library.mssm. edu:2059/content.aspx?aID=15524.

21. **Answer: D.**

    Bariatric surgical outcomes in super-obese patients are optimized through preoperative VLCD. The significant reductions in liver volume, abdominal wall depth, and visceral adipose tissue and subcutaneous adipose tissue (technical factors) improve the surgical procedure. Improvements in diabetes, hypertension, and degenerative joint disease (physiologic factors) enhance the health of the patient. The reduction of liver volume correlates directly with weight lost.

    In the study by Colles et al., of the 884 subjects, 425 (48%) lost more than 10% of their excess body weight prior to the operation when on VLCD. After surgery (mean follow-up, 12 months), this group was more likely to achieve 70% loss of excess body weight. Those who lost more than 5% of excess body weight prior to surgery were statistically less likely to have a length of stay of greater than 4 days.

    References:
    - Colles SL, Dixon JB, Marks P, et al. Preoperative weight loss with a very-low-energy diet: quantitation of changes in liver and abdominal fat by serial imaging. Am J Clin Nutr 2006; 84(2):304–311.
    - Still CD, Benotti P, Wood GC, et al. Outcomes of preoperative weight loss in high risk patients undergoing gastric bypass surgery. Arch Surg 2007; 142:994–998.
    - Eid GM, Jarman BT. American College of Surgeons 94th Annual Clinical Congress. Session GS58: General Surgery I. Presented October 14, 2008.

22. **Answer: D.**

    The incidence of gallstones either during or within 6 months of a stopping a VLCD is about 10%. The risk of cholelithiasis can be decreased by administration of ursodeoxycholic acid, including a moderate amount of fat in the diet, and limiting the rate of weight loss to 1 to 1.5 kg/wk. Gallstones have been documented to occur as early as 4 weeks after initiating VLCD.

    References:
    - Festi D, Colecchia A, Orsini M, et al. Gallbladder motility and gallstone formation in obese patients following very low calorie diets: use it (fat) to lose it (well). Int J Obes 1998; 22:592–600.
    - Kamrath RO, Plummer LJ, Sadur CN, et al. Cholelithiasis in patients treated with a very-low-calorie diet. Am J Clin Nutr 1992; 56(1 suppl):255S–257S.

23. **Answer: C.**

    This is a controversial issue with many studies showing that VLCDs produce greater weight loss in the short as well as long term when compared to LCDs. But the meta-analysis by Tsai and Wadden has not shown any difference in long-term weight loss between the two groups. The weight lost by VLCDs cannot be maintained over the long term, necessitating other modalities of weight loss like medications or bariatric surgery (the latter the best choice). On the short term they produce approximately 25% of loss of *initial* weight which is better than LCD diet. VLCDs have 25% to 50% rate of attrition. Both LCDs and VLCDs have a similar rate of attrition.

    Reference:
    - Tsai AG, Wadden TA. The evolution of very-low-calorie diets: an update and meta-analysis. Obesity (Silver Spring). 2006; 14(8):1283–1293 (review).

24. **Answer: D.**

    Peanuts are high-calorie foods. Hundred grams of peanuts is about 600 cal. Other high-calorie foods are listed in the following link:

    Reference:
    - http://www.weightlossforall.com/calories-high-calorie-foods.htm

25. **Answer: D.**

    The BMR may be measured using indirect calorimetry that involves estimating the amount of energy spent through the amount of oxygen consumed, or direct calorimetry that involves measuring body heat directly. The BMR in an 80-kg adult male would be approximately 80 kcal/hr; therefore, an exercise that consumes

10 times this value (10 METs) would consume approximately 800 kcal/hr. The use of METs made it easier to describe the efficiency of a certain exercise to "burn" calories in relation to doing nothing at all.

Reference:
- Norton K, Norton L, Sadgrove D. Position statement on physical activity and exercise intensity terminology. J Sci Med Sport 2010; 13(5):496–502 [Epub December 10, 2009] (review).

4 | Benefits of bariatric surgery

CHAPTER SUMMARY

- Bariatric surgery is better than conventional methods of weight loss (diet and exercise) as it produces better weight loss in short as well as long term. Conventional weight loss methods also have an unacceptable rate of recidivism.
- Weight loss after bariatric surgery is measured most commonly by *excess weight lost*.
  - *Reinhold's classification* is most commonly used to classify degree of excess weight lost.
- Biliopancreatic diversion (BPD) produces the highest excess weight loss (EWL).
- Roux-en-Y gastric bypass (RYGB) produces maximum weight loss earlier when compared to laparoscopic adjustable gastric banding (LAGB).
- Bariatric surgery has several other benefits in addition to reducing weight.
- Bariatric surgery reduces mortality (by about 27–40% in different studies with long-term follow-up).
- Diabetes:
  - All bariatric procedures improve diabetes (overall about 70–80% resolution rate).
  - All bariatric procedures improve β-cell function and insulin resistance.
  - The long-term efficacy of BPD and biliopancreatic diversion with duodenal switch (BPD-DS) in resolving diabetes has been established. The long-term efficacy of RYGB in resolving diabetes is not certain. LAGB has reappearance of diabetes in the long term.
  - Sleeve gastrectomy is very effective for diabetes (about 60% resolution rate). No long-term data are however available. Reduction in ghrelin is hypothesized as a cause of this.
- Hypertension:
  - Bariatric surgery produces an early improvement in blood pressure.
  - Bariatric surgery resolves hypertension in over 60%.
- Heart:
  - Bariatric surgery is very beneficial in improving symptoms of heart failure.
  - Bariatric surgery improves cardiovascular risk factors including lipid profile.
  - It decreases mortality due to coronary heart disease.
- Obstructive sleep apnea (OSA):
  - Has a high prevalence among bariatric surgery candidates.
  - There is an improvement of OSA, some patients tend to have residual OSA after bariatric surgery.
- Gastroesophageal reflux disease (GERD):
  - RYGB is an effective anti-reflux operation.
  - RYGB also eliminates reflux of duodenal contents.
  - LAGB also decreases GERD but pouch formation after LAGB predisposes to GERD.
  - Sleeve gastrectomy is not as effective in resolving/improving GERD.
  - VBG (vertical banded gastroplasty) is useless for GERD.
- Nonalcoholic fatty liver disease (NAFLD):
  - Bariatric surgery is not recommended at this time for improving nonalcoholic steatohepatitis (NASH) in a bariatric surgery candidate.

- Most studies reported an improvement in inflammation and steatosis in patients with NASH.
- All bariatric procedures improve asthma, although it is not known whether this is attributed to the effect of the bariatric procedure on GERD.
- Urinary incontinence:
  - It is present in about two-third of the patients presenting for bariatric surgery.
  - Bariatric surgery improves urinary incontinence in *both* men and women.
- Economic benefits:
  - Bariatric surgery decreases health care costs.
  - It decreases hospitalization for various disorders although the same for some disorders seems to be increased. Overall, hospitalization rates are decreased.
  - Bariatric surgery is cost effective. The cost-effectiveness ratio is <$50,000 per quality-adjusted life year (QALY) in all studies.
- Bariatric surgery improves fertility and other metabolic parameters for obese women with polycystic ovarian syndrome.
- Bariatric surgery improves the inflammatory state of obesity as measured by levels of C-reactive protein (CRP) and other proinflammatory cytokines.
- Open bariatric surgery has a greater number of late complications when compared with the laparoscopic approach.
- Bariatric surgery improves osteoarthritis.
- Bariatric surgery improves serum testosterone levels and sexual quality of life in men.
- Bariatric surgery has a beneficial effect on benign intracranial hypertension and resolves most symptoms like headache, tinnitus, and cranial nerve dysfunction.

QUESTIONS

1. **Bariatric surgery has many advantages over medical therapy of weight loss. Identify the <u>FALSE</u> statement about the benefits of laparoscopic Roux-en-Y gastric bypass (LRYGB) over medical therapy.**
   A. Medical therapy of obesity is not as effective as bariatric surgery in the short term (1 year).
   B. Medical therapy has higher rates of recidivism.
   C. Calorie restriction has not been definitively shown to be inferior to gastric bypass in decreasing insulin resistance within 7 days.
   D. Surgery is not superior to medical therapy in the long term (>5 years).

2. **Investigators have looked into the mortality benefit offered by bariatric surgery. Identify the <u>FALSE</u> statement about the mortality benefit offered by bariatric surgery.**
   A. The reduction in mortality after bariatric surgery is less than 10% in the long term (≥5 years).
   B. The reduction of cause-specific mortality is higher for diabetes when compared with coronary heart disease.
   C. An increase in suicide rates was reported after bariatric surgery in a large study.
   D. There is no mortality reduction just 1 year after bariatric surgery.

3. **Identify the <u>FALSE</u> statement regarding the effect of the different bariatric surgical procedures on GERD.**
   A. RYGB decreases GERD.
   B. Pouch formation after LAGB predisposes to GERD.
   C. VBG improves GERD.
   D. The evidence of the effect of sleeve gastrectomy Laparoscopic Sleeve Gastrectomy (LSG) on GERD does not consolidate to a consensus.

4. **A 30-year-old asthmatic patient with a BMI of 40 has come for a consultation about weight loss surgery. Besides her weight, she is also concerned about her asthma**

steroid medication side effects and wants to know if bariatric surgery will also help improve her asthma. Identify the <u>TRUE</u> statement about the impact of bariatric surgery on asthma.
A. RYGB and LAGB are equally effective in decreasing asthma symptoms.
B. RYGB has been shown to decrease the need for steroid use in asthmatics.
C. Sleeve gastrectomy is better than LAGB in improving asthma.
D. BPD has not been shown to be useful in resolving asthma symptoms.

5. **Coronary artery disease is the most important cause of mortality in obese and nonobese patients. Identify the <u>TRUE</u> statement about relationship between bariatric surgery and heart failure.**
A. Bariatric surgery improves left heart systolic function in heart failure.
B. Bariatric surgery decreases left ventricular hypertrophy.
C. Bariatric surgery improves diastolic dysfunction in heart failure.
D. All of the above.

6. **A 45-year-old hypertensive male with a BMI of 50 patient has come to your office to discuss weight loss surgery and has specific questions regarding resolution of hypertension. Which of the following is <u>TRUE</u> about the resolution of hypertension after bariatric surgery?**
A. Aldosterone is decreased in obese patients.
B. Overall, hypertension has been shown to be resolved in less than 30% of the patients after bariatric surgery.
C. Hypertension (HTN) is not resolved until 1 year after RYGB in most patients.
D. Bariatric surgery has been shown to decrease elevated plasma aldosterone levels in obese patients.

7. **NAFLD is increasingly recognized as a condition associated with being overweight or obese and that it may progress to end-stage liver disease. Identify the <u>FALSE</u> statement about the effect of bariatric surgery on NAFLD.**
A. NAFLD resolution is better in patients with higher insulin resistance.
B. Improvement in liver function tests (LFTs) does not correlate well with histological improvement of NASH after bariatric surgery.
C. The degree of inflammation does not increase after RYGB.
D. Steatosis improvement has been noted in almost all studies.

8. **Nursing care can be challenging with the morbidly obese secondary to associated urinary and fecal incontinence. Identify the <u>FALSE</u> statement about urinary/fecal incontinence and bariatric surgery.**
A. Urinary incontinence is present in more than 50% of the obese female patients presenting for bariatric surgery.
B. Only 10% of the female patients have a resolution of urinary incontinence after RYGB.
C. RYGB has a greater impact on stress urinary incontinence when compared to urge/mixed incontinence.
D. Fecal incontinence is more common in the obese.

9. **Certain medical conditions do not benefit and may in fact be worsened by bariatric surgery. Identify the <u>FALSE</u> statement below.**
A. Hospitalization for hematologic disorders may increase after bariatric surgery.
B. Overall hospitalization rates are increased in bariatric surgery patients.
C. Hospitalization for digestive disorders is increased after bariatric surgery.
D. Health care costs in obese patients who do not undergo surgery are around 40% higher.

10. **The cost-effectiveness of bariatric surgery is an important consideration in setting health priorities in today's cost-conscious economy. Identify the <u>FALSE</u> statement about cost-effectiveness of bariatric surgery.**
    A. Open gastric bypass is cost effective in general when compared to conventional methods of weight loss.
    B. The incremental cost-effectiveness ratio (ICER) of bariatric surgery is >US$50,000 for every QALY.
    C. LAGB is more cost effective than open VBG.
    D. Open gastric bypass may be less cost effective for older male patients with lesser BMI.

11. **A 25-year-old obese women presents to the bariatric surgeon with gain in weight over the past 3 years. Her BMI is 50 kg/m². She has tried diet modification and exercise for the past 1 year but it has not been successful. She has been unable to conceive after her marriage 2 years ago and complains of irregular menses. She has diabetes, which was discovered at a health fair about 6 months ago, and her primary care physician (PCP) has started her on metformin for the same. Examination shows facial hair. Vital signs and skin, abdomen, and chest examinations are normal. An overnight dexamethasone suppression test is within normal limits. Additional testing shows normal thyroid-stimulating hormone (TSH) level, increased luteinizing hormone/follicle-stimulating hormone (LH/FSH) ratio and elevated free testosterone and 17-hydroxyprogesterone levels. What is the next best step in management of this patient?**
    A. Discuss bariatric surgical options.
    B. Reassure her as she is already on metformin.
    C. Send her to gynecologist for ovulation induction.
    D. Prescribe gonadotropin-releasing hormone (GnRH) agonist.

12. **Gastric banding is currently the most widely performed procedure in the world. Identify the <u>FALSE</u> statement about resolution of comorbidities after gastric banding.**
    A. There is increase in incidence of diabetes in gastric banding patients in the long term (7–10 years).
    B. Gastric banding improves pancreatic β-cell function.
    C. It has been shown to resolve/improve diabetes in more than 50% of patients in most studies.
    D. Gastric banding resolves/improves hypertension in less than 30% of the patients.

13. **Weight loss is often expressed as a percentage of excess weight lost after bariatric surgery. Percentage excess weight lost is the amount of weight lost relative to _____ body weight expressed as a percentage.**
    A. preoperative
    B. ideal
    C. preoperative lean body weight
    D. difference between the preoperative weight and the ideal

14. **EWL has been used to compare the efficacy of different bariatric surgeries. About the excess weight lost after bariatric procedures, the <u>FALSE</u> statement is:**
    A. For bariatric surgery, in general, the excess weight lost is about 60%.
    B. Overall gastric banding produces less EWL when compared to gastric bypass.
    C. Open gastric bypass produces inferior EWL when compared to laparoscopic gastric bypass.
    D. Super super-obese (BMI > 60) have less percentage EWL compared to those with BMI > 60 after LRYGB.

15. **It is interesting to know how LAGB and RYGB compare with each other. Identify the <u>TRUE</u> statement about difference in outcomes after the two procedures.**
    A. LAGB and RYGB have an equal early mortality rate.
    B. RYGB and LAGB are equally effective in causing resolution of diabetes at 1 year.
    C. LAGB is less effective than RYGB in improving the cardiovascular risk factors at 1 year.
    D. RYGB and LAGB produce similar weight loss in the short term (3 years).

16. **Sleeve gastrectomy has resolved diabetes more often compared to LAGB. Identify the <u>TRUE</u> statement about outcomes after sleeve gastrectomy.**
    A. The use of 46-Fr bougie produces inferior weight loss when compared to a 36 Fr one.
    B. A 4-cm antral pouch is desired over a 7-cm antral pouch as it produces better weight loss.
    C. Mortality of the procedure is greater than LRYGB.
    D. Morbidity of the procedure is the same as that of RYGB.

17. **Various theories have been proposed as to why sleeve gastrectomy resolves diabetes and one of them is the hormonal changes associated with sleeve gastrectomy. Identify the <u>FALSE</u> statement with regard to the same.**
    A. Ghrelin is decreased after sleeve gastrectomy.
    B. No studies have shown that sleeve gastrectomy improves insulin sensitivity within a few days.
    C. Glucagon-like peptide-1 (GLP-1) secretion is increased after both RYGB and sleeve gastrectomy at 3 months.
    D. Insulin secretion is greater than that accounted for by weight loss.

18. **Identify the <u>FALSE</u> statement about the long-term outcomes of BPD-DS (10 years).**
    A. About 50% of the patients have excellent (>80% EWL) weight loss.
    B. Another 40% of the patients have fair to good (>50% EWL) weight loss.
    C. Failure of weight loss occurs in about 10% of the patients over the long term (defined as <20% EWL).
    D. Diabetes remission occurs in almost all patients (98%).

19. **Bariatric surgery has been shown to improve cardiovascular outcomes. Identify the <u>FALSE</u> statement about improvement of cardiovascular health after bariatric surgery.**
    A. Bariatric surgery causes a decrease in the rate of progression of atherosclerosis.
    B. The "cardiotoxic" epicardial fat has been shown to be decreased in thickness after bariatric surgery.
    C. Bariatric surgery increases the risk of pulmonary edema in heart failure patients.
    D. RYGB causes a decrease in coronary artery disease mortality.

20. **Obesity is an inflammatory state. Bariatric surgery, by causing weight loss, may cause a decrease in the inflammatory state. Identify the <u>FALSE</u> statement about changes in inflammatory markers after bariatric surgery.**
    A. Gastric banding causes a decrease in CRP level.
    B. The decrease in CRP found after gastric bypass does not correlate with weight loss.
    C. Proinflammatory cytokines decrease after bariatric surgery.
    D. Tumor necrosis factor–alpha (TNF-α) levels do not significantly decrease after bariatric surgery.

21. **Though bariatric surgery is the best modality of weight loss, the efficacy of bariatric surgery in resolving GERD has been debated. Identify the <u>TRUE</u> statement about treatment of GERD in morbidly obese patients.**
    A. RYGB is not an effective anti-reflux procedure.
    B. Erosive esophagitis is more resistant to healing by proton pump inhibitors (PPIs) in overweight patients when compared to normal individuals.
    C. Patients who have previously undergone Nissen fundoplication can be converted to gastric bypass.
    D. BPD-DS and RYGB are equally effective anti-reflux procedures.

22. **Recently, few investigators have expressed a concern about the efficacy of sleeve gastrectomy in resolving GERD. Identify the <u>TRUE</u> statement about GERD and sleeve gastrectomy (LSG).**
    A. LSG removes most of the parietal cell mass.
    B. Decrease in incidence of GERD is seen in the short term after LSG (3 years).
    C. The incidence of GERD after LSG can be decreased by adding a duodenal switch procedure.
    D. GERD is almost never seen as a new complaint in patients after a sleeve gastrectomy in long-term follow-up (>5 years).

23. **OSA is a well-recognized comorbidity associated with obesity. Identify the <u>TRUE</u> statement about the relationship between OSA and bariatric surgery.**
    A. Less than 10% of the patients who undergo bariatric surgery have OSA as a comorbid condition.
    B. Less than 1% of patients have residual OSA after weight loss.
    C. BMI is correlated with severity of sleep apnea.
    D. History of OSA definitively increases the risk of desaturation during induction of anesthesia.

24. **Diabetes does not resolve after bariatric surgery in some patients and the predictors of poor outcome is a topic of research. Identify the <u>FALSE</u> statement about bariatric surgery in patients with advanced type 2 diabetes mellitus (DM).**
    A. Patients with more severe forms of diabetes have lesser EWL.
    B. Patients with more severe forms of diabetes are less likely to have diabetes well controlled post surgery.
    C. Patients with late-stage diabetes have improvement in glycemic control despite gradual loss of β-cell function.
    D. Patients with more severe diabetes have a greater length of hospital stay.

25. **Bariatric surgery has been found to benefit only heart failure patients with higher BMI, while it may actually be harmful for heart failure patients with lower BMI. Identify the <u>TRUE</u> statement about the benefit of bariatric surgery on heart failure patients.**
    A. Bariatric surgery decreases the risk of pulmonary edema in heart failure patients.
    B. Bariatric surgery improves New York Heart Association (NYHA) class in severe systolic failure.
    C. Bariatric surgery improves ejection fraction in severe systolic failure.
    D. Bariatric surgery decreases hospital readmission rate in patients with severe systolic failure.
    E. All of the above.

26. **In the United States, LRYGB is considered as the gold standard for modern bariatric surgery. Which of the following has been demonstrated as a benefit of the laparoscopic approach?**
    A. Laparoscopic approach produces a greater weight loss when compared to open surgery.
    B. Patients who have laparoscopic surgery have a lower incidence of late postoperative complications.
    C. Open surgery has a higher incidence of early postoperative complications.
    D. Laparoscopic surgery has higher total costs when compared to open surgery.

27. **LAGB has a perceived advantage that the restriction can be adjusted. Identify the FALSE statement about outcomes of LAGB when compared to outcomes of RYGB.**
    A. There is no consensus on the superiority of RYGB over LAGB in causing long-term weight loss.
    B. Maximum weight loss after both RYGB and LAGB occurs at 12 to 18 months after the operation.
    C. Sweet-eating habit is not a predictor of weight loss after either RYGB or LAGB.
    D. LAGB patients exhibit increased prevalence of diabetes over the long term (>10 years) although it is decreased in the short term.

28. **Male sex hormones favorably change after bariatric surgery. Which of the following is FALSE about sex hormones and sexual quality of life in bariatric surgery patients?**
    A. Sex hormone–binding globulin decreases after bariatric surgery.
    B. Total testosterone has been shown to be increased after bariatric surgery.
    C. Bariatric surgery has been shown to improve sexual quality of life in men.
    D. Testosterone inversely correlates with the risk of having metabolic syndrome.

29. **Benign intracranial hypertension [also known as pseudotumor cerebri (PTC)] is a misnomer as it has been known to cause visual loss. Hence, it is better termed as idiopathic intracranial hypertension (IIH). The effect of bariatric surgery on PTC has not been systematically investigated. Which of the following is TRUE?**
    A. Bariatric surgery resolves cranial nerve dysfunction.
    B. Bariatric surgery does not resolve tinnitus.
    C. Symptoms of PTC take at least 3 to 4 years to resolve.
    D. Headache has not been found to resolve in most patients undergoing bariatric surgery.

30. **Hyperlipidemia is one of the important comorbidities of obesity and is present in more than 40% of patients with obesity and in more than 50% of patients with diabetes. Identify the TRUE statement about the effect of LRYGB on hyperlipidemia.**
    A. Discontinuation of lipid-lowering medications is not possible after RYGB in dyslipidemic patients.
    B. There is no decrease in very low-density lipoprotein (VLDL) as it is produced by liver, not the adipose tissue.
    C. The percentage decrease in total cholesterol is less than percentage decrease in triglycerides.
    D. No increase in high-density lipoprotein (HDL) has been demonstrated after surgery.

ANSWER KEY

1. D	9. B	17. B	25. E
2. A	10. B	18. C	26. B
3. C	11. A	19. C	27. B
4. B	12. D	20. B	28. A
5. D	13. D	21. C	29. A
6. D	14. C	22. B	30. C
7. A	15. C	23. C	
8. B	16. C	24. D	

ANSWER KEY WITH EXPLANATION

1. **Answer: D.**

   Medical therapy has a very high rate of recidivism as patients maintain only two-third of the weight loss after 1 year. It has also been shown to be less effective than bariatric surgery in the short term (1 year) although the quality of evidence for this is modest. One study (SOS) has shown bariatric surgery to produce better weight loss at 8 and 10 years when compared to medical therapy. It is not known for certain whether decrease in insulin resistance immediately after gastric bypass can be attributed to a factor other than calorie restriction, with one study showing no difference in the decrease in insulin resistance between patients undergoing a few days of calorie restriction and patients a few days after gastric bypass.

   References:
   - Maggard MA, Shugarman LR, Suttorp M, et al. Meta-analysis: surgical treatment of obesity. Ann Intern Med 2005; 142(7):547–559.
   - Isbell JM, Tamboli RA, Hansen EN, et al. The importance of caloric restriction in the early improvements in insulin sensitivity after Roux-en-Y gastric bypass surgery. Diabetes Care 2010; 33(7):1438–1442.
   - Kennel KA. Review: sparse high-quality evidence supports surgery for obesity. ACP J Club 2005; 143(2):51.
   - Wadden TA. Treatment of obesity by moderate and severe caloric restriction. Results of clinical research trials. Ann Intern Med 1993; 119:688–693.

2. **Answer: A.**

   In their observational cohort study, Christou et al. found that the 5-year death rate in the bariatric surgical group was 0.68% compared with 6.2% in the medically managed patients – an 89% relative risk reduction. Adams et al. found a 40% decrease in mortality at 7 years after gastric bypass. The mortality rate was similar between surgical patients and control patients at 1 year after surgery in the same study. Flum and Dellinger evaluated survival after gastric bypass in a retrospective cohort study and found a 27% lower 15-year death rate in morbidly obese patients who underwent gastric bypass compared with those who did not. Sjostorm et al. also reported a decrease in adjusted mortality rate of 30% in Swedish patients undergoing bariatric surgery after a follow-up of 10 years.

   Adams reported an increase in suicide rates after bariatric surgery.

   Cause-specific mortality reduction was the highest for diabetes followed by coronary heart disease and cancer in the study by Adams et al.

   References:
   - Brethauer SA, Chand B, Schauer PR. Risks and benefits of bariatric surgery: current evidence. Cleve Clin J Med 2006; 73(11):993–1007.
   - Adams TD, Gress RE, Smith SC, et al. Long-term mortality after gastric bypass surgery. N Engl J Med 2007; 357(8):753–761.
   - Christou NV, Sampalis JS, Liberman M, et al. Surgery decreases long-term mortality, morbidity, and health care use in morbidly obese patients. Ann Surg 2004; 240(3):416–423; discussion 423–424.

- Sjöström L. Bariatric surgery and reduction in morbidity and mortality: experiences from the SOS study. Int J Obes (Lond) 2008; 32(suppl 7):S93–S97.

3. **Answer: C.**

RYGB is very effective for GERD. It has also been found to decrease GERD in nonmorbidly obese patients.

VBG is not effective in decreasing GERD. Overall, LAGB has a beneficial effect on GERD. Pouch formation after LAGB has been correlated with GERD. Himpens et al. found new appearance of GERD (21%) after 6 years of follow-up in their sleeve gastrectomy patients. There is no consensus on the effect of sleeve gastrectomy on GERD in other studies.

References:

- Himpens J, Dobbeleir J, Peeters G. Long-term results of laparoscopic sleeve gastrectomy for obesity. Ann Surg 2010; 252(2):319–324.
- Chiu S, Birch DW, Shi X, et al. Effect of sleeve gastrectomy on gastroesophageal reflux disease: a systematic review. Surg Obes Relat Dis 2011; 7(4):510–515.
- de Jong JR, Besselink MG, van Ramshorst B, et al. Effects of adjustable gastric banding on gastroesophageal reflux and esophageal motility: a systematic review. Obes Rev 2010; 11(4):297–305.
- Dixon JB, O'Brien PE. Gastroesophageal reflux in obesity: the effect of lap-band placement. Obes Surg 1999; 9(6):527–531.
- Gamagaris Z, Patterson C, Schaye V, et al. Lap-band impact on the function of the esophagus. Obes Surg 2008; 18(10):1268–1272.

4. **Answer: B.**

RYGB is more effective than LAGB in decreasing the symptoms of asthma. RYGB has been shown to decrease steroid medications but not leukotriene medications. Relief from asthma after RYGB depends neither on weight loss nor on the presence of sleep disorders as was seen after multivariate analysis.

This outcome may be due to the resolution of GERD and acid-induced bronchospasm.

Asthma medication was found to be decreased by 88% in patients after BPD-DS by Marceau et al.

Sleeve gastrectomy and LAGB have been found to be similar in improving asthma.

References:

- Reddy RC, Baptist AP, Fan Z, et al. The effects of bariatric surgery on asthma severity. Obes Surg 2011; 21(2):200–206.
- Sikka N, Wegienka G, Havstad S, et al. Respiratory medication prescriptions before and after bariatric surgery. Ann Allergy Asthma Immunol 2010; 104 (4):326–330.
- Marceau P, Biron S, Hould FS, et al. Duodenal switch: long-term results. Obes Surg 2007; 17(11):1421–1430.
- Omana JJ, Nguyen SQ, Herron D, et al. Comparison of comorbidity resolution and improvement between laparoscopic sleeve gastrectomy and laparoscopic adjustable gastric banding. Surg Endosc 2010; 24(10):2513–2517.
- Mechanick JI, Kushner RF, Sugerman HJ, et al.; American Association of Clinical Endocrinologists; Obesity Society; American Society for Metabolic & Bariatric Surgery. Executive summary of the recommendations of the American Association of Clinical Endocrinologists, the Obesity Society, and American Society for Metabolic & Bariatric Surgery medical guidelines for clinical practice for the perioperative nutritional, metabolic, and nonsurgical support of the bariatric surgery patient. Endocr Pract 2008; 14(3):318–336.

5. **Answer: D.**

Bariatric surgery improves systolic as well as diastolic function in heart failure patients. It has also been shown to decrease thickness of left ventricle. The effect of bariatric surgery on right ventricular function in obese patients is not clear.

Reference:

- Ashrafian H, le Roux CW, Darzi A, et al. Effects of bariatric surgery on cardiovascular function. Circulation 2008; 118(20):2091–2102.

6. **Answer: D.**

Hypertension has been shown to be resolved as early as 1 week after RYGB. This led to suspicion of a gut factor acting on the "enterorenal axis." Aldosterone is elevated in obese hypertensive patients. This has been attributed to adipocyte-secreted aldosterone-releasing factors (ARF). Bariatric surgery has been shown to decrease aldosterone levels.

In the meta-analysis by Buchwald et al., hypertension was found to be resolved in over 60% of the patients.

References:

- Bueter M, Ahmed A, Ashrafian H, et al. Bariatric surgery and hypertension. Surg Obes Relat Dis 2009; 5(5):615–620 [Epub April 7, 2009].
- Dall'Asta C, Vedani P, Manunta P, et al. Effect of weight loss through laparoscopic gastric banding on blood pressure, plasma renin activity and aldosterone levels in morbid obesity. Nutr Metab Cardiovasc Dis 2009; 19(2):110–114 [Epub August 20, 2008].
- Buchwald H, Avidor Y, Braunwald E, et al. Bariatric surgery: a systematic review and meta-analysis JAMA 2004; 292(14):1724–1737.

7. **Answer: A.**

The gold standard for the diagnosis of NASH is a liver biopsy and LFTs do not accurately reflect the histological damage to the liver.

Inflammation remained unchanged 5 years after surgery in one study whereas other studies have found resolution of inflammation. Almost all studies have reported improvement in steatosis. NAFLD has been correlated with insulin resistance. In one study, on multivariate analysis, the refractory insulin resistance profile independently predicted the persistence of steatosis and ballooning 5 years after surgery. There are also reports of worsening of liver fibrosis after bariatric surgery and patients with greater insulin resistance and BMI seem to be more susceptible to it.

References:

- Chavez-Tapia NC, Tellez-Avila FI, Barrientos-Gutierrez T, et al. Bariatric surgery for non-alcoholic steatohepatitis in obese patients. Cochrane Database Syst Rev 2010; (1):CD007340.
- Mathurin P, Hollebecque A, Arnalsteen L, et al. Prospective study of long-term effects of bariatric surgery on liver injury in patients without advanced disease. Gastroenterology 2009; 137:532–540.

8. **Answer: B.**

Urinary incontinence occurred in about 66% of the patients presenting for bariatric surgery and included 21% urge, 33% stress, and 46% mixed urinary incontinence. About 64% of patients have complete resolution and 92% have an improvement in the urinary incontinence at 1 year. Similar numbers have been reported by other authors and by one author who also included men in his study. RYGB has a greater impact on stress urinary incontinence compared to other types. Both urinary and fecal incontinence are common in obesity and both are resolved/improved by bariatric surgery.

References:

- Richter HE, Burgio KL, Clements RH, et al. Urinary and anal incontinence in morbidly obese women considering weight loss surgery. Obstet Gynecol 2005; 106(6):1272–1277.
- Chen CC, Gatmaitan P, Koepp S, et al. Obesity is associated with increased prevalence and severity of pelvic floor disorders in women considering bariatric surgery. Surg ObesRelat Dis 2009; 5(4):411–415.
- Laungani RG, Seleno N, Carlin AM. Effect of laparoscopic gastric bypass surgery on urinary incontinence in morbidly obese women. Surg Obes Relat Dis 2009; 5 (3):334–338.
- Greer WJ, Richter HE, Bartolucci AA, et al. Obesity and pelvic floor disorders: a systematic review. Obstet Gynecol 2008; 112(2 pt 1):341–349.

9. **Answer: B.**

Hospitalizations for hematologic disorders and digestive disorders are increased in bariatric surgery patients. Overall hospitalization rates are about 50% less in post–bariatric surgery patients. Obese patients who have not undergone bariatric surgery have health care costs that are about 45% higher when compared to operated patients.

References:

- Adams TD, Gress RE, Smith SC, et al. Long-term mortality after gastric bypass surgery. N Engl J Med 2007; 357(8):753–761.
- Christou NV, Sampalis JS, Liberman M, et al. Surgery decreases long-term mortality, morbidity, and health care use in morbidly obese patients. Ann Surg 2004; 240(3):416–423; discussion 423–424.
- Sjöström L. Bariatric surgery and reduction in morbidity and mortality: experiences from the SOS study. Int J Obes (Lond) 2008; 32(suppl 7):S93–S97.

10. **Answer: B.**

The ICER is defined as the ratio of the change in costs of a therapeutic intervention (compared to the alternative, such as doing nothing or using the best available alternative treatment) to the change in effects of the intervention. ICER is often expressed in terms of QALY. ICER is much less than US$50,000 per QALY for bariatric surgery as has been shown in many studies. ICER varies from $5400 to $35,600 per QALY depending on the patient's sex, age, preoperative BMI, and type of surgery. The lower the ICER, the greater is the cost-effectiveness. The surgery is generally considered cost effective if the ICER <$50,000 per QALY.

Open gastric bypass may be less cost effective for older male patients with lower BMI and the ICER in these patients may exceed $50,000 when the base case assumptions about some clinical effectiveness parameters are varied. LAGB has been shown to be more cost effective than open VBG in a study comparing them head to head. Open gastric bypass has been shown to be more cost effective than conventional treatment.

Reference:

- Picot J, Jones J, Colquitt JL, et al. The clinical effectiveness and cost-effectiveness of bariatric (weight loss) surgery for obesity: a systematic review and economic evaluation. Health Technol Assess 2009; 13(41):1–190, 215–357, iii–iv.

11. **Answer: A.**

The resolution of polycystic ovary syndrome (PCOS) after the marked and sustained weight loss attained after bariatric surgery makes this therapeutic option a first-line strategy in women presenting with severe obesity. In patients with lesser grades of obesity who desire fertility, a short trial of metformin, followed by classic ovulation induction and/or assisted reproductive techniques in case pregnancy is not achieved in a few months, is a reasonable approach. If fertility is not an immediate concern, third-generation oral contraceptive pills containing a neutral or anti-androgenic progestin remains the drug of choice, considering their efficacy, their excellent tolerability, and their overall metabolic safety.

Reference:

- Escobar-Morreale HF. Polycystic ovary syndrome: treatment strategies and management. Expert Opin Pharmacother 2008; 9(17):2995–3008.

12. **Answer: D.**

LAGB has been shown to improve homeostasis model assessment (HOMA)-B score, which is an indicator of β-cell function. The β-cell function has also been shown to improve when adjusted for insulin sensitivity in post-LAGB patients. Disposition index has also been shown to increase after LAGB. The rate of resolution/improvement of diabetes after LAGB is ≥60%. It also has been shown to resolve/improve HTN in ≥30% of patients. There was increase in the incidence of diabetes at 7 years and 10 years follow-up in studies by Schouten et al. and Himpens et al., respectively.

References:

- Cunneen SA. Review of meta-analytic comparisons of bariatric surgery with a focus on laparoscopic adjustable gastric banding. Surg Obes Relat Dis 2008; 4 (3 suppl):S47–S55.
- Schouten R, Wiryasaputra DC, van Dielen FM, et al. Long-term results of bariatric restrictive procedures: a prospective study Obes Surg 2010; 20:1617–1626.
- Himpens J, Cadiere GB, Bazi M, et al. Long-term outcomes of laparoscopic adjustable gastric banding. Arch Surg 2011; 146(7):802–807.
- Caiazzo R, Arnalsteen L, Pigeyre M, et al. Long-term metabolic outcome and quality of life after laparoscopic adjustable gastric banding in obese patients with type 2 diabetes mellitus or impaired fasting glucose. Br J Surg 2010; 97:884–891.
- Dixon JB, O'Brien PE. Health outcomes of severely obese type 2 diabetic subjects 1 year after laparoscopic adjustable gastric banding. Diabetes Care 2002; 25(2): 358–363.

13. **Answer: D.**

A, B, and C choices do not accurately reflect the definition of percentage excess body weight loss.

Reference:

- Brethauer SA, Chand B, Schauer PR. Risks and benefits of bariatric surgery: current evidence. Cleve Clin J Med 2006; 73(11):993–1007.

14. **Answer: C.**

In the meta-analysis of Buchwald et al., EWL for all bariatric procedures combined was 61%. Analyzed by procedure, EWL was 70% for BPD, 68% for gastroplasty, 62% for gastric bypass, and 48% for gastric banding. EWL 6 months after LRYGB is similar to that with the open procedure. Super-super-obese patients (BMI > 60) have less EWL than patients with a lower BMI after standard RYGB, even though the total number of pounds lost by super-super-obese patients is greater.

References:

- Sjöström L, Narbro K, Sjöström CD, et al.; Swedish Obese Subjects Study. Effects of bariatric surgery on mortality in Swedish obese subjects. N Engl J Med 2007; 357(8):741–752.
- Gould JC, Garren MJ, Boll V, et al. Laparoscopic gastric bypass: risks vs. benefits up to two years following surgery in super-super obese patients. Surgery 2006; 140(4):524–529; discussion 529–531.
- Buchwald H, Avidor Y, Braunwald E, et al. Bariatric surgery: a systematic review and meta-analysis. JAMA 2004; 292(14):1724–1737.

15. **Answer: C.**

LAGB has a lower mortality rate when compared to RYGB. RYGB is better than LAGB for improving cardiovascular risk factors including homocysteine and total cholesterol levels. RYGB is more effective in resolving diabetes in the short term and probably in the long term (>5 years) though there are no studies comparing them head to head in the long term. RYGB produces greater weight loss when compared to LAGB at 3 years, though there is controversy regarding how they compare with each other in the long term.

References:

- Cottam DR, Atkinson J, Anderson A, et al. A case-controlled matched-pair cohort study of laparoscopic Roux-en-Y gastric bypass and Lap-Band patients in a single US center with three-year follow-up. Obes Surg 2006; 16(5):534–540.
- Woodard GA, Peraza J, Bravo S, et al. One year improvements in cardiovascular risk factors: a comparative trial of laparoscopic Roux-en-Y gastric bypass vs. adjustable gastric banding. Obes Surg 2010; 20(5):578–582 [Epub February 26, 2010].
- Parikh MS, Laker S, Weiner M, et al. Objective comparison of complications resulting from laparoscopic bariatric procedures. J Am Coll Surg 2006; 202(2):252–261 [Epub December 19, 2005].

16. **Answer: C.**

The bougie size or the size of antral pouch does not decide weight loss. Mortality is comparable to RYGB – around 0.5%. RYGB, however, has a higher morbidity (more than three times when compared to sleeve gastrectomy). There is no consensus on the relative efficacy of RYGB and sleeve gastrectomy in causing resolution of comorbidities. Sleeve gastrectomy has a lower mortality than RYGB.

References:

- Jacobs M, Bisland W, Gomez E, et al. Laparoscopic sleeve gastrectomy: a retrospective review of 1- and 2-year results. Surg Endosc 2010; 24(4):781–785.
- Chouillard EK, Karaa A, Elkhoury M, et al.; Intercontinental Society of Natural Orifice, Endoscopic, and Laparoscopic Surgery (i-NOELS). Laparoscopic Roux-en-Y gastric bypass versus laparoscopic sleeve gastrectomy for morbid obesity: case-control study. Surg Obes Relat Dis 2011; 7(4):500–505.

17. **Answer: B.**

Peterli et al. performed a randomized study of RYGB and LAGB patients. After surgery, patients had markedly increased postprandial plasma insulin and GLP-1 levels, respectively, after both of these surgical procedures, which favor improved glucose homeostasis. Compared with LSG, LRYGB patients had early and augmented insulin responses as early as 1-week postoperative, potentially mediating improved early glycemic control. After 3 months, no significant difference was observed with respect to insulin and GLP-1 secretion between the two procedures.

A definite decrease in ghrelin is seen only after LSG, whereas there is considerable variation in the levels of ghrelin reported after RYGB. In one study, in some patients, insulin resistance has been shown to decrease as early as 3 days after LSG.

References:

- Peterli R, Wölnerhanssen B, Peters T, et al. Improvement in glucose metabolism after bariatric surgery: comparison of laparoscopic Roux-en-Y gastric bypass and laparoscopic sleeve gastrectomy: a prospective randomized trial. Ann Surg 2009; 250(2):234–241.
- Rizzello M, Abbatini F, Casella G, et al. Early postoperative insulin-resistance changes after sleeve gastrectomy. Obes Surg 2010; 20(1):50–55.
- Basso N, Capoccia D, Rizzello M, et al. First-phase insulin secretion, insulin sensitivity, ghrelin, GLP-1, and PYY changes 72 h after sleeve gastrectomy in obese diabetic patients: the gastric hypothesis. Surg Endosc 2011; 25(11):3540–3550.
- Abbatini F, Rizzello M, Casella G, et al. Long-term effects of laparoscopic sleeve gastrectomy, gastric bypass, and adjustable gastric banding on type 2 diabetes. Surg Endosc 2010; 24(5):1005–1010 [Epub October 29, 2009].

18. **Answer: C.**

The more widely used Reinhold's classification of EWL is as follows:
> \>75% – excellent

50–75% – good
25–50% – fair
<25% – poor

Diabetes resolves in about 98% of the patients after BPD-DS after a follow-up of >10 years. Only approximately 2% of patients have a failure of weight loss after BPD-DS at 10 years or more. A and B are true as per the BPD-DS series of Hess and Hess.

Reference:
- Hess DS, Hess DW, Oakley RS. The biliopancreatic diversion with the duodenal switch: results beyond 10 years. Obes Surg 2005; 15(3):408–416.

19. **Answer: C.**

Progression rate of carotid bulb intima-media thickness increases significantly in morbidly obese patients when compared with post–bariatric surgical patients.

Surgery can decrease the obesity "cardiotoxic load," and demonstrates significant decreases in epicardial fat thickness on postoperative echocardiograms. The epicardial fat is related to the visceral fat and the risk of metabolic syndrome. It can also contribute to obesity cardiomyopathy.

In addition to the positive changes on cardiac function noted on imaging after bariatric surgery, both functional and clinical symptoms have also been shown to improve, such that at 5 years after surgery, the risk of pulmonary edema remains significantly decreased.

Bariatric surgery has been shown to cause a decrease in coronary artery disease mortality.

References:
- Ashrafian H, le Roux CW, Darzi A, et al. Effects of bariatric surgery on cardiovascular function. Circulation 2008; 118(20):2091–2102.
- Adams TD, Gress RE, Smith SC, et al. Long-term mortality after gastric bypass surgery. N Engl J Med 2007; 357(8):753–761.

20. **Answer: B.**

Both RYGB and gastric banding show a decrease in hsCRP (highly sensitive CRP) post surgery. However, only RYGB shows a consistent correlation between degree of weight loss and CRP levels. In a recent meta-analysis, a linear relation was observed between weight loss following lifestyle changes or bariatric surgery and the fall in hsCRP levels, which declined by 0.13 mg/L for each 1 kg of weight loss. This marker is decreased in almost all studies and hence is the most sensitive marker of inflammation in this situation.

TNF-α has not been shown to decrease after bariatric surgery. Markers of oxidative stress decrease after bariatric surgery. Proinflammatory cytokines like IL-18 and IL-8 have been shown to decrease after bariatric surgery.

References:
- Tziomalos K, Dimitroula HV, Katsiki N, et al. Effects of lifestyle measures, antiobesity agents, and bariatric surgery on serological markers of inflammation in obese patients. Mediators Inflamm 2010; 2010:364957 [Epub March 7, 2010].
- Murri M, García-Fuentes E, García-Almeida JM, et al. Changes in oxidative stress and insulin resistance in morbidly obese patients after bariatric surgery. Obes Surg 2010; 20(3):363–368.
- Botella-Carretero JI, Alvarez-Blasco F, Martinez-García MA, et al. The decrease in serum IL-18 levels after bariatric surgery in morbidly obese women is a time-dependent event. Obes Surg 2007; 17(9):1199–1208.

21. **Answer: C.**

RYGB has a very favorable impact on GERD. Its efficacy in treating GERD is thought to be related to the relatively low acid production of the small-volume (15–30 mL) gastric pouch, reduction of esophageal biliopancreatic refluxate by use of a Roux limb measuring at least 100 cm in length, and weight loss. Patients who have undergone Nissen fundoplication can be converted to gastric bypass and, in fact,

RYGB is an option after failure of Nissen fundoplication in morbidly obese patients. One series, however, found that even though such conversion was feasible it was technically difficult and resulted in a relatively higher morbidity.

A retrospective review of a large database found similar healing rates for erosive esophagitis in overweight compared with normal patients, suggesting body weight did not affect healing of esophagitis with proton pump inhibitors.

BPD-DS is not an effective anti-reflux procedure and in fact normal patients may have appearance of new GERD symptoms in the long term after BPD-DS or sleeve gastrectomy.

References:
- Zainabadi K, Courcoulas AP, Awais O, et al. Laparoscopic revision of Nissen fundoplication to Roux-en-Y gastric bypass in morbidly obese patients. Surg Endosc 2008; 22(12):2737–2740.
- Himpens J, Dobbeleir J, Peeters G. Long-term results of laparoscopic sleeve gastrectomy for obesity. Ann Surg 2010; 252(2):319–324.
- Prachand VN, Alverdy JC. Gastroesophageal reflux disease and severe obesity: fundoplication or bariatric surgery? World J Gastroenterol 2010; 16(30):3757–3761.
- Anand G, Katz PO. Gastroesophageal reflux disease and obesity. Gastroenterol Clin North Am 2010; 39(1):39–46.

22. **Answer: B.**

Himpens et al. have reported the long-term follow-up after sleeve gastrectomy. They believe that over time the formation of a "neofundus" occurs in the sleeve. This is attributed to defective technique that leaves behind too much fundus in the first place. This causes the sleeve to assume a conical instead of cylindrical shape and hence the fundus dilates over time according to Laplace law. The conical shape results in relative stenosis of the mid-stomach. Hence, the stagnation of food in the upper sleeve along with an increase in acid-producing mucosa due to dilation of the fundus causes increase in reflux over the long term. Himpens et al. observed that incidence of GERD after sleeve gastrectomy is biphasic with peaks at 1 year and 6 years and decreased incidence being found at 3 years after surgery. The addition of a DS procedure was not protective as these patients also developed GERD symptoms.

Parietal cells are present in the body and fundus of the stomach and absent in the pylorus – therefore, parietal cells are found in the body of the stomach after a sleeve gastrectomy.

References:
- Himpens J, Dobbeleir J, Peeters G. Long-term results of laparoscopic sleeve gastrectomy for obesity. Ann Surg 2010; 252(2):319–324.
- Himpens J, Dapri G, Cadière GB. A prospective randomized study between laparoscopic gastric banding and laparoscopic isolated sleeve gastrectomy: results after 1 and 3 years. Obes Surg 2006; 16:1450–1456.
- Chiu S, Birch DW, Shi X, et al. Effect of sleeve gastrectomy on gastroesophageal reflux disease: a systematic review. Surg Obes Relat Dis 2011; 7(4):510–515.

23. **Answer: C.**

OSA is highly prevalent (50–90%) among bariatric candidates, but exceedingly underdiagnosed (only 30% preoperatively). Surgically induced weight loss results in a marked improvement of the apnea-hypopnea index (AHI). However, more than 50% of bariatric recipients with preoperative OSA have residual disease despite weight loss. Reduced AHI after surgery usually corresponds to moderately severe OSA and hence a complete cure of OSA is not to be expected after surgery.

BMI has been correlated with severity of sleep apnea respiratory disturbance index (RDI).

In one study, contrary to what would be expected, nadir oxygen saturation during induction of anesthesia was considerably higher in patients with clinical suspicion of OSA, a significant finding that persisted as a trend after correction for age, gender, and BMI.

References:

- Holty JE, Guilleminault C. Surgical options for the treatment of obstructive sleep apnea. Med Clin North Am 2010; 94(3):479–515.
- Romero-Corral A, Caples SM, Lopez-Jimenez F, et al. Interactions between obesity and obstructive sleep apnea: implications for treatment. Chest 2010; 137 (3):711–719.
- Haines KL, Nelson LG, Gonzalez R, et al. Objective evidence that bariatric surgery improves obesity-related obstructive sleep apnea. Surgery 2007; 141 (3):354–358 [Epub December 8, 2006].
- Aihara K, Oga T, Harada Y, et al. Analysis of anatomical and functional determinants of obstructive sleep apnea. Sleep Breath 2011 May 15 [Epub ahead of print].
- Greenburg DL, Lettieri CJ, Eliasson AH. Effects of surgical weight loss on measures of obstructive sleep apnea: a meta-analysis. Am J Med 2009; 122(6):535–542.
- Eikermann M, Garzon-Serrano J, Kwo J, et al. Do patients with obstructive sleep apnea have an increased risk of desaturation during induction of anesthesia for weight loss surgery? Open Respir Med J 2010; 4:58–62.

24. **Answer: D.**

Hospital stay was not increased in patients with more severe type 2 DM in the study by Schauer et al.

EWL has been shown to be inferior in the more severe forms of diabetes requiring medication usage when compared to those whose diabetes was diet controlled or had only an impaired fasting glucose. Immediate cessation of oral anti-diabetics (OADs) or insulin after surgery was possible in 30% of patients after the surgical treatment, and occurred significantly more often in patients with diabetes durations <10 years and in those treated by OADs rather than insulin. Clinical resolution of diabetes was also significantly less likely to happen in patients with a history of diabetes >10 years and in those with more severe forms of the disease, according to treatment.

Given the gradual loss of β-cell function associated with long-standing type 2 diabetes improvements of glucose control after bariatric surgery in such patients may be expected chiefly as a result of reduced insulin resistance.

References:

- Schauer PR, Burguera B, Ikramuddin S, et al. Effect of laparoscopic Roux-en Y gastric bypass on type 2 diabetes mellitus. Ann Surg 2003; 238(4):467–484; discussion 84–85.
- Renard E. Bariatric surgery in patients with late-stage type 2 diabetes: expected beneficial effects on risk ratio and outcomes. Diabetes Metab 2009; 35(6 pt 2):564–568.

25. **Answer: E.**

Bariatric surgery and other modalities of weight loss have been shown to improve NYHA class, hospital readmission, and ejection fraction in patients with severe systolic failure. Five years after bariatric surgery, the risk of pulmonary edema is significantly reduced.

References:

- Ashrafian H, le Roux CW, Darzi A, et al. Effects of bariatric surgery on cardiovascular function. Circulation 2008; 118(20):2091–2102.
- Ramani GV, McCloskey C, Ramanathan RC, et al. Safety and efficacy of bariatric surgery in morbidly obese patients with severe systolic heart failure. Clin Cardiol 2008; 31(11):516–520.

26. **Answer: B.**

Although the operative costs are greater for the laparoscopic group, the nursing costs and total hospital service costs are lesser for the same when compared to the open surgery patients. Total costs involved in the two approaches are comparable. The evolution of BMI and EWL after the two procedures is also similar. Early postoperative complications are also similar when the two approaches are compared, whereas the late complications are higher with open gastric bypass.

References:

- Luján JA, Frutos MD, Hernández Q, et al. Laparoscopic versus open gastric bypass in the treatment of morbid obesity: a randomized prospective study. Ann Surg 2004; 239(4):433–437.
- Nguyen NT, Goldman C, Rosenquist CJ, et al. Laparoscopic versus open gastric bypass: a randomized study of outcomes, quality of life, and costs. Ann Surg 2001; 234(3):279–289; discussion 289–291.

27. **Answer: B.**

Maximum weight loss is attained by RYGB patients at 12 to 18 months, while the same occurs after 2 to 3 years after LAGB. There is no consensus on the superiority of the weight loss achieved in the long term between RYGB and LAGB though a recent systematic review has shown the weight lost to be comparable in RYGB and LAGB patients in the long term (3–7 years). Sweet eating is not a predictor of weight loss after either RYGB or LAGB. Himpens et al. found that diabetes increased in prevalence in the long term (12 years) after LAGB.

References:

- O'Brien PE, McPhail T, Chaston TB, et al. Systematic review of medium-term weight loss after bariatric operations. Obes Surg 2006; 16(8):1032–1040.
- Himpens J, Cadiere GB, Bazi M, et al. Long-term outcomes of laparoscopic adjustable gastric banding. Arch Surg 2011; 146(7):802–807.
- Mcbride CL, Sugerman H, DeMaria EJ. Outcome of Laparoscopic Gastric Bypass. In: Sugerman HJ, Nguyen N, eds. Management of Morbid Obesity. Boca Raton: CRC Press, 2005.
- Hudson SM, Dixon JB, O'Brien PE. Sweet eating is not a predictor of outcome after lap-band placement. Can we finally bury the myth? Obes Surg 2002; 12 (6):789–794.
- Mallory GN, Macgregor AM, Rand CS. The influence of dumping on weight loss after gastric restrictive surgery for morbid obesity. Obes Surg 1996; 6(6):474–478.

28. **Answer: A.**

Total testosterone and free testosterone both increase after bariatric surgery. Though estrogen was believed to be decreased after weight loss, such a decrease has not been conclusively demonstrated after bariatric surgery. Sex hormone–binding globulin increases after bariatric surgery. It has an inverse correlation with insulin resistance. Bariatric surgery improved sexual quality of life in many studies. Testosterone is inversely related to BMI, diabetes risk, and the risk of having the metabolic syndrome.

Reference:

- Rao RS, Kini S, Tamler R. Sex hormones and bariatric surgery in men. Gend Med 2011; 8(5):300–311.

29. **Answer: A.**

In the case series by Sugerman et al., bariatric surgery (most cases were gastric bypasses) was shown to resolve headache, tinnitus, and cranial nerve dysfunction in almost all patients. Results were reported 1 year after surgery. In fact, resolution of headache and tinnitus was seen just after 4 months of surgery in most patients.

References:

- Sugerman HJ, Felton WL III, Sismanis A, et al. Gastric surgery for pseudotumor cerebri associated with severe obesity. Ann Surg 1999; 229(5):634–640; discussion 640–642.
- Nadkarni T, Rekate HL, Wallace D. Resolution of pseudotumor cerebri after bariatric surgery for related obesity. Case report. J Neurosurg 2004; 101(5):878–880.

30. **Answer: C.**

One year after gastric bypass, mean total cholesterol levels decreased by 16%; triglyceride levels decreased by 63%; low-density lipoprotein (LDL) cholesterol levels decreased by 31%; VLDL cholesterol decreased by 74%; total cholesterol/HDL cholesterol risk ratio decreased by 60%; and HDL cholesterol levels increased by 39%. Also, within 1 year, 23 of 28 (82%) patients requiring lipid-lowering medications preoperatively were able to discontinue their medications. In the study by Woodard et al., total cholesterol decreased by 22% whereas triglycerides decreased by about 40%. They also found an increase in HDL cholesterol.

References:

- Nguyen NT, Varela E, Sabio A, et al. Resolution of hyperlipidemia after laparoscopic Roux-en-Y gastric bypass. J Am Coll Surg 2006; 203(1):24–29.
- Zlabek JA, The effect of laparoscopic gastric bypass surgery on dyslipidemia in severely obese patients. Surg Obes Relat Dis 2005; 1(6):537–542.
- Woodard GA, Peraza J, Bravo S, et al. One year improvements in cardiovascular risk factors: a comparative trial of laparoscopic Roux-en-Y gastric bypass vs. adjustable gastric banding. Obes Surg 2010; 20(5):578–582 [Epub February 26, 2010].

5 | Obesity comorbidities and their management

CHAPTER SUMMARY

- The comorbidities of obesity include diabetes, hypertension (HTN), obstructive sleep apnea (OSA), gastroesophageal reflux disease (GERD), osteoarthritis (OA), polycystic ovary syndrome (PCOS), hypogonadism, and idiopathic intracranial hypertension (IIH).
- Perioperative management of diabetes in a bariatric patient:
  - All oral antidiabetic drugs are stopped before surgery. Metformin is stopped 24 to 48 hours before surgery to avoid lactic acidosis.
  - The IV insulin regimen consists of infusion of glucose, insulin, and potassium (GIK) in the form of a single solution. The initial insulin infusion rate can be estimated as between one-half and three-fourths of the patient's total daily insulin dose expressed as units/hr. Blood glucose is monitored frequently and insulin infusion is adjusted to maintain a blood glucose between 120 and 180 mg/dL.
  - The insulin glargine regimen is better as the former technique is cumbersome. This consists of halving the dose of insulin glargine during the day of surgery and giving short-acting insulin whenever the finger-stick blood glucose is high.
- Diagnosis of OSA in a bariatric surgery patient:
  - The diagnosis of OSA is done by polysomnography. The diagnosis of the OSA syndrome requires the presence of symptoms like excessive daytime somnolence.
  - The pathogenesis is related to loss of dilator muscle tone of the pharynx during sleep. It is exacerbated during REM sleep.
  - OSA is independently related to risk of diabetes. It also predisposes the patient to systemic and pulmonary HTN. Overall, cardiovascular risk is increased in untreated OSAs.
  - The diagnosis of OSA is established by the presence of certain number of events (apnea and hypopnea) per hour of sleep.
  - The definition of apnea is a decrease in airflow on thermistor of at least 75% for at least 10 seconds with evidence of effort (thoracic and abdominal channels). If there is no effort then it is a central apnea. Hypopnea is defined as a decline in airflow on nasal pressure/nasal flow channel of at least 30% with at least 4% desaturation or decline by 50% with at least 3% desaturation or an electrocortical arousal. There should be evidence of continued effort again.
  - Routine polysomnography increases the rate of detection of sleep apnea in a bariatric surgery patient. But at this time it is not recommended.
  - Patients who are already on continuous positive airway pressure (CPAP) are encouraged to continue them before surgery.
  - Role of routine CPAP in a bariatric patient immediately after surgery is also unsettled.
  - CPAP improves systemic and pulmonary arterial blood pressures. It has been shown to reduce cardiovascular mortality in elderly patients with OSA.
- Gastroesophageal reflux disease:
  - Having a body mass index (BMI) > 30 kg/m^2 increases risk of GERD by nearly two times.
  - There is increased risk of Barrett's esophagus and esophageal adenocarcinoma in obese patients.
  - Episodes of GERD are related to transient esophageal sphincter relaxations (TLESR).

- The most important factor related to the pathogenesis of GERD is the function of the lower esophageal sphincter – its total length, intra-abdominal length, and its resting pressure.
- Obese patients also have an increased incidence of hiatal hernia that predisposes to GERD. People with BMI > 25 kg/m^2 have a nearly two times increased risk of developing a hiatal hernia.
- Like lean patients, obese patients also respond to proton pump inhibitors (PPIs).
- Patients with GERD need to undergo preoperative endoscopy.
- Polycystic ovary syndrome:
  - Clinical features include amenorrhea or oligomenorrhea and hirsutism along with obesity.
  - These patients are at an increased risk of metabolic syndrome. They have an increased risk of OSA. Other associated diseases include endometrial hyperplasia and carcinoma.
  - Diagnosis is by measurement of luteinizing hormone (LH), follicle-stimulating hormone (FSH), thyroid-stimulating hormone (TSH) levels, and testosterone and 17-hydroxyprogesterone levels.
  - Treatment includes clomiphene in patients who desire pregnancy. Adding metformin to clomiphene may increase the chances of ovulation. If this fails gonadotropin-releasing hormone agonist (GnRH) or laparoscopic ovarian drilling may be considered. Oral contraceptives or medroxyprogesterone acetate is used in patients who do not desire pregnancy.
  - Bariatric surgery is an option if the patient is morbidly obese.
- Male hypogonadism:
  - Morbid obesity is associated with decreased testosterone and sex hormone–binding globulin (SHBG) levels.
  - This is attributed to increased aromatase activity that causes increased conversion of testosterone to estrogen, thus decreasing testosterone and increasing estrogen levels.
  - Other implicated factors include hypothalamic inflammation, decreased central nervous system (CNS) insulin levels, endogenous opioids, and adipokines like leptin among others.
  - Obese patients have a reduced sexual quality of life.
- Idiopathic intracranial hypertension:
  - Symptoms include headache, tinnitus, and cranial nerve dysfunctions including blindness.
  - Pathogenesis: jugular valve insufficiency along with increased abdominal pressure. Pathogenesis is uncertain.
  - About 70% of patients with IIH are obese. Morbidly obese patients (BMI > 40 kg/m^2) have an increased risk for visual loss.
- Nonalcoholic fatty liver disease (NAFLD):
  - Prevalence of NAFLD in United States is about 30%, while prevalence of nonalcoholic steatohepatitis (NASH) is about 6%.
  - Biopsy is the gold standard for the diagnosis of NAFLD. Liver function tests do not correlate well with severity of NASH.
  - Histologic grading of NASH as well as fibrosis is available.
  - Alcoholic liver disease is a differential diagnosis of NASH.

QUESTIONS

1. **It would be interesting to understand the relation between GERD and its etiological factors. Identify the <u>FALSE</u> statement about the etiological factors of GERD in relation to an obese patient.**
   A. Patients with greater BMI are more likely to have GERD symptoms.
   B. Caucasians show a correlation between abdominal circumference and reflux symptoms.

    C. Abdominal diameter/waist circumference is an independent risk factor for Barrett's esophagus.

    D. An association between esophageal cancer and BMI has not been demonstrated.

2. **OSA is an important perioperative comorbidity. Identify the <u>FALSE</u> statement regarding evaluation of OSA in adults:**

    A. Patient needs to be symptomatic to be diagnosed with OSA.

    B. When a patient has a breathing pause of 10 seconds with evidence of effort, he/she is said to have an apneic episode.

    C. Diagnosis of hypopneic episodes also requires evidence of effort.

    D. Untreated OSA is associated with poor health outcomes (HTN, cardiovascular disease, etc.).

3. **Obesity is known to affect most PCOS women. Identify which of the following is <u>NOT</u> an additional common clinical manifestation of PCOS.**

    A. Acne

    B. Dyslipedemia

    C. OSA

    D. Endometrial hyperplasia and carcinoma

    E. Polymenorrhea

4. **Bariatric surgery is known to cure many of the components of PCOS. Which of the following is <u>NOT</u> consistent with PCOS?**

    A. Decreased leptin levels

    B. Insulin resistance

    C. Increased androgen production from ovary

    D. Increased LH secretion from pituitary

5. **OA is a common comorbid condition associated with obesity. Which of the following statements is <u>FALSE</u> regarding this problem in obese patients undergoing bariatric surgery?**

    A. Obesity is a risk factor for hip OA more than knee OA.

    B. Bariatric surgery resolves OA in more than three out of four patients after surgery in at least one joint.

    C. Obese patients have more severe OA symptoms.

    D. BMI is positively correlated with risk of OA.

6. **Bariatric surgery has been shown to increase testosterone levels. Which of the following hypothetical mechanisms can <u>NOT</u> possibly describe this change?**

    A. Decrease in insulin levels following a decrease in insulin resistance

    B. Decrease in aromatase activity

    C. Decrease in inhibin B levels

    D. Decrease in the inflammatory state

7. **Though bariatric surgery improves sleep apnea, the mechanism is poorly understood. Which of the following statements is <u>FALSE</u> about OSA?**

    A. The volume of parapharyngeal fat contributes to the loss of the retroglossal space during sleep.

    B. Neurological loss of dilator muscle tone in the neck contributes to the sleep apnea.

    C. In obese patients modest weight loss (of about 15–20%) has been shown to improve OSA.

    D. It worsens during nonrapid eye movement (NREM) sleep.

8. **OSA has risk factors which are environmental as well as genetic. Concerning the etiology of OSA, which of the following statements is <u>FALSE</u>?**

A. OSA is twice as common in obese patients compared to nonobese.
B. Adenotonsillar hypertrophy is associated with pediatric OSA.
C. OSA is more common in women.
D. Genetic risk factors for OSA and obesity overlap.

9. **OSA has been closely linked with the metabolic syndrome. Identify the <u>FALSE</u> statement about etiology and associations of OSA.**
   A. OSA is a risk factor for HTN.
   B. OSA is independently associated with a heightened systemic inflammatory state.
   C. Diabetic patients have a higher prevalence of OSA when compared to nondiabetic patients.
   D. Acute sleep fragmentation has not been shown to affect glucose metabolism.

10. **CPAP is the mainstay of therapy for OSA. Identify the <u>FALSE</u> statement concerning the advantages of CPAP for the treatment of OSA.**
    A. The effect of CPAP on insulin resistance is not consistent across studies.
    B. CPAP increases blood pressure.
    C. CPAP lowers pulmonary artery pressure.
    D. CPAP reduces cardiovascular death.

11. **A 48-year-old morbidly obese patient with a BMI of 50 kg/m² presents to the bariatric surgeon after his family physician refers him because he has failed to lose weight with medical treatment for the past 6 months. He has type 2 diabetes, HTN, mild asthma, and OA of both knees. He had a myocardial infarction (MI) 2 years ago. His diabetes and HTN are well controlled with oral hypoglycemics and angiotensin-converting enzyme (ACE) inhibitors, respectively, and he is on adequate statin therapy. He is an ex-smoker who smoked two packs a day for 10 years but stopped 15 years ago. Patient is asymptomatic but reports shortness of breath with usual household activity. Patient agrees to have a Roux-en-Y gastric bypass (RYGB). Preoperative evaluation shows normal chest X ray (CXR) and isolated Q waves in the electrocardiography (EKG). Other routine labs are within normal limits. What is the next best step in management?**
    A. Admit the patient and proceed with the bariatric surgery.
    B. Refer the patient for persantine nuclear stress test.
    C. Refer the patient for an exercise EKG.
    D. Refer the patient for dobutamine stress echocardiogram.
    E. Refer the patient for elective right and left cardiac catheterization and angiography.

12. **A morbidly obese patient is being evaluated preoperatively before performing an RYGB. Tests reveal elevated alanine transaminase (ALT), high normal aspartate transaminase (AST), and normal alkaline phosphatase (ALP) and albumin. Patient consumes alcohol occasionally and hepatitis B surface antigen and anti-HCV antibody are negative. NASH is suspected and a liver biopsy is taken during the surgery. Biopsy reveals prominent hepatocyte ballooning, hepatic steatosis of about 75%, and acinar inflammation in 1 focus per 200x field. Identify the <u>TRUE</u> statement regarding his condition.**
    A. The degree of steatosis is not considered in the pathological diagnosis of steatohepatitis.
    B. Presence of many Mallory-Denk bodies goes in favor of NAFLD.
    C. More steatosis and less inflammation go in favor of NASH while greater degree of inflammation is found in alcoholic liver disease.
    D. Visualization of one portal tract is considered adequate biopsy for evaluation of NASH.

13. **A patient with morbid obesity is being evaluated before bariatric surgery. She is on 40 units insulin glargine, which she takes in the morning, and insulin aspart, which she takes before each meal. Her blood sugar is well controlled as shown by HbA1c level of 6.4%. She is nil per os (NPO) for a laparoscopic gastric bypass scheduled the next day. What is the BEST step in management of this patient as far as her diabetes is concerned?**
    A. Start subcutaneous regular insulin as a "sliding scale," and hold the morning insulin glargine.
    B. Reduce the glargine dose on the day before surgery, and administer rapid-acting insulin based on subsequent blood glucose.
    C. Start IV insulin, and keep blood glucose 80 to 110 mg/dL.
    D. She should continue her insulin regimen during the day of surgery.

14. **Obesity-associated glomerulopathy is a newly recognized entity which is not associated with diabetic or hypertensive renal disease. Identify the FALSE statement about obesity glomerulopathy.**
    A. Pathologically it is focal segmental glomerulosclerosis (FSGS).
    B. It presents with proteinuria.
    C. It is characterized by renal hypoperfusion.
    D. Podocyte lesions and glomerulomegaly are found.

15. **A 35-year-old diabetic female who has a BMI of 45 kg/m^2 presents to the office with psoriatic lesions involving both elbows and forearms. Which of the following does NOT represent the correct pathological state in psoriasis?**
    A. Increased tumor necrosis factor-α (TNF-α)
    B. Increased interleukin-6 (IL-6)
    C. Decreased resistin
    D. Increased C-reactive protein (CRP)

16. **A male patient with a BMI of 50 kg/m^2 presenting with the skin lesion, shown in the image below, undergoes a gastric bypass. The skin lesion completely resolves 12 months after the surgery. Which of the following is TRUE regarding this condition?**

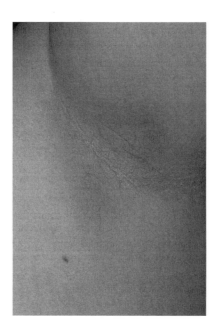

A. This is caused by hyperinsulinemia.

B. This is caused by chronic hyperglycemia.

C. Resolution of this condition after a gastric bypass is extremely rare.

D. This is usually associated with decreased insulin-like growth factor-1 (IGF-1) levels.

17. **Obese patients have an increased susceptibility to fungal and bacterial infections of the skin. Identify the FALSE statement about skin infections in the obese.**

A. Patients with fungal infections must be screened for diabetes if not already diagnosed.

B. Colonization in intertrigo lesions most commonly involves *Candida*.

C. Half of all obese patients have cutaneous infections.

D. Necrotizing fasciitis has no correlation with obesity.

18. **Venous stasis dermatitis is a common problem in obesity, and all surgeons need to be aware of the management of this condition. Identify the FALSE statement about the treatment of stasis dermatitis.**

A. Compression stockings are an effective treatment.

B. Unna boot is useful for management of venous stasis ulcers.

C. Corticosteroids have no role in treatment as this is not an inflammatory disorder.

D. Bariatric surgery resolves venous stasis disease in most patients.

ANSWER KEY

1. D	6. C	11. E	16. A
2. A	7. D	12. C	17. D
3. E	8. C	13. B	18. C
4. A	9. D	14. C	
5. A	10. B	15. C	

ANSWER KEY WITH EXPLANATION

1. **Answer: D.**

   Meta-analyses have found a positive correlation between GERD and increasing BMI. A BMI between 25 and 29 kg/m^2 and a BMI greater than 30 kg/m^2 were associated with an increased risk for GERD symptoms – odds ratios of 1.43 and 1.94, respectively. An independent association between increasing abdominal diameter (independent of BMI) and reflux-type symptoms was seen in whites, but not in blacks or Asians. In a case-control study, abdominal diameter was found to be an independent risk factor for Barrett's esophagus. There is an association between Barrett's esophagus and BMI. There is a well-documented association between BMI and carcinoma of the esophagus and gastric cardia.

   References:
   - Akiyama T, Yoneda M, Maeda S, et al. Visceral obesity and the risk of Barrett's esophagus. Digestion 2011; 83(3):142–145.
   - Anand G, Katz PO. Gastroesophageal reflux disease and obesity. Gastroenterol Clin North Am 2010; 39(1):39–46.

2. **Answer: A.**

   The definition of apnea is a decrease in airflow on thermistor of at least 75% for at least 10 seconds with evidence of effort (thoracic and abdominal channels). If there is no effort then it is a central apnea. Hypopnea is defined as a decline in airflow on nasal pressure/nasal flow channel of at least 30% with at least 4% desaturation or decline by 50% with at least 3% desaturation or an electrocortical arousal. There should be evidence of continued effort again.

There are poor health outcomes (HTN, cardiovascular disease, stroke, etc.) that can be associated with untreated OSAs, and it is especially important to catch those patients that are "asymptomatic."

References:
- Douglas NJ. Chapter 259: Sleep apnea. In: Fauci AS, Braunwald E, Kasper DL, et al., eds. Harrison's Principles of Internal Medicine, 17th ed. New York: McGraw-Hill, 2008.
- Dasheiff RM, Finn R. Clinical foundation for efficient treatment of obstructive sleep apnea. J Oral Maxillofac Surg 2009; 67(10):2171–2182.
- Iber C, Ancoli-Israel S, Chesson AL, et al. The AASM manual for the scoring of sleep and associated events. West Chester, IL: American Academy of Sleep Medicine, 2007.

3. **Answer: E.**

Seventy to eighty percent of the patients have either amenorrhea or oligomenorrhea, and polymenorrhea is highly unusual. In addition, they have insulin resistance and many features of the metabolic syndrome including dyslipidemia and HTN. Acne is also more common in PCOS. OSA has also been found to be higher in PCOS patients when compared to BMI-matched patients without PCOS. Hyperestrogenemia seen in PCOS can lead to endometrial hyperplasia and carcinoma.

References:
- Broekmans FJ, Fauser BC. Diagnostic criteria for polycystic ovarian syndrome. Endocrine 2006; 30(1):3–11.
- Schorge JO, Schaffer JI, Halvorson LM, et al. Chapter 17: Polycystic ovarian syndrome and hyperandrogenism. In: Schorge JO, Schaffer JI, Halvorson LM, et al., eds. Williams Gynecology. New York: McGraw-Hill, 2008. Available at: http://www.accessmedicine.com/content.aspx?aID=3157034.

4. **Answer: A.**

Insulin resistance is considered to be the central cause for PCOS. Increased LH secretion from pituitary and androgen secretion from the ovary are observed in PCOS. Leptin levels are no different compared to women with similar adiposity without PCOS.

Reference:
- Escobar-Morreale HF. Polycystic ovary syndrome: treatment strategies and management. Expert Opin Pharmacother 2008; 9(17):2995–3008.

5. **Answer: A.**

Bariatric surgery has been shown to resolve 89% of OA in at least one joint. The incidence of OA in morbid obesity is about 10% to 20%. A higher incidence has been shown in patients undergoing obesity surgery (about 20%). Every 2 units of increase in BMI increases risk of OA by 36%. The relation between obesity and OA is stronger for women. Obesity has a stronger link with knee OA when compared to hip OA. Obese patients also have more severe OA symptoms.

References:
- Felson DT. Chapter 326: Osteoarthritis. In: Fauci AS, Braunwald E, Kasper DL, et al., eds. Harrison's Principles of Internal Medicine, 17th ed. New York: McGraw-Hill, 2008. Available at: http://www.accessmedicine.com/content.aspx?aID=2897738.
- Howarth D, Inman D, Lingard E, et al. Barriers to weight loss in obese patients with knee osteoarthritis. Ann R Coll Surg Engl 2010; 92(4):338–340.
- Lementowski PW, Zelicof SB. Obesity and osteoarthritis. Am J Orthop (Belle Mead NJ) 2008; 37(3):148–151.
- Scott SK, Rabito FA, Price PD, et al. Comorbidity among the morbidly obese: a comparative study of 2002 U.S. hospital patient discharges. Surg Obes Relat Dis 2006; 2(2):105–111.

- Miller GD, Nicklas BJ, Davis C, et al. Intensive weight loss program improves physical function in older obese adults with knee osteoarthritis. Obesity (Silver Spring) 2006; 14(7):1219–1230.

6. **Answer: C.**

Decrease in insulin resistance can increase SHBG levels. Decrease in aromatase activity can increase testosterone and decrease estrogen levels as testosterone conversion is reduced in the adipose tissue. Hypothalamic inflammation has been shown to decrease GnRH secretion and thus LH secretion. The decrease in this inflammation can thus increase LH levels. Inhibin B levels have been found to be low in obesity and no significant changes have been found after bariatric surgery.

Reference:
- Rao RS, Kini S, Tamler R. Sex hormones and bariatric surgery in men. Gend Med 2011 June 24 [Epub ahead of print]. DOI: 10.1016/j.genm.2011.05.007.

7. **Answer: D.**

The pressure of the parapharyngeal fat pads contributes to the collapse of the retroglossal space during sleep. Fatty deposition results in airway reduction and predisposes to airway collapse, contributed to by neurologic loss of the normal dilator muscle tone in the neck.

In obese patients, weight loss of 18% has been shown to increase upper airway caliber and decrease lateral wall and parapharyngeal fat pad volume. Although not yet confirmed prospectively and thus controversial, meta-analysis of patients undergoing bariatric surgery for morbid obesity has demonstrated resolution of OSA in 86%.

OSA worsens during REM sleep.

References:
- Shahi B, Praglowski B, Deitel M. Sleep-related disorders in the obese. Obes Surg 1992; 2:157–168.
- Eckert DJ, Malhotra A. Pathophysiology of adult obstructive sleep apnea. Proc Am Thorac Soc 2008; 5(2):144–153.
- Welch KC, Foster GD, Ritter CT, et al. A novel volumetric magnetic resonance imaging paradigm to study upper airway anatomy. Sleep 2002; 25:532–542.
- Buchwald H, Avidor Y, Braunwald E, et al. Bariatric surgery: a systematic review and meta-analysis. JAMA 2004; 292(14):1724–1737.

8. **Answer: C.**

The prevalence of OSA is about 4% and 2% in adult men and women, respectively, and occurs twice as much in obese patients. Although obesity is associated with OSA in the pediatric age group, other factors such as adenotonsillar hypertrophy and ethnicity may mediate the association between obesity and OSA. Adenotonsillar hypertrophy is the most common cause of pediatric OSA.

There are data showing substantial overlap in genetic risk factors for OSA and obesity.

References:
- Kohler M. Risk factors and treatment for obstructive sleep apnea amongst obese children and adults. Curr Opin Allergy Clin Immunol 2009; 9:4–9.
- Douglas NJ. Chapter 259: Sleep apnea. In: Fauci AS, Braunwald E, Kasper DL, et al., eds. Harrison's Principles of Internal Medicine, 17th ed. New York: McGraw-Hill, 2008. Available at: http://www.accessmedicine.com/content. aspx?aID=2869549.
- Patel SR. Shared genetic risk factors for obstructive sleep apnea and obesity. J Appl Physiol 2005; 99:1600–1606.

9. **Answer: D.**

Obesity is associated with increased inflammation, and this has been shown to be independent of obesity. Diabetics have been shown to have much higher prevalence of OSA in several population studies. Spiegel and colleagues showed that acute sleep fragmentation, using auditory and mechanical stimulation, decreased insulin sensitivity and glucose effectiveness (the ability of glucose to mobilize itself independent of insulin) the next morning, associated with an increase in the morning levels of cortisol and sympathetic nervous system activity, although not that of systemic inflammation or adipokines. OSA is a well-known cause of systemic HTN.

References:

- Lui MM, Ip MS. Disorders of glucose metabolism in sleep-disordered breathing. Clin Chest Med 2010; 31(2):271–285.
- Botros N, Concato J, Mohsenin V, et al. Obstructive sleep apnea as a risk factor for type 2 diabetes. Am J Med 2009; 122(12):1122–1127.
- Peppard PE, Young T, Palta M, et al. Prospective study of the association between sleep-disordered breathing and hypertension. N Engl J Med 2000; 342(19):1378–1384.

10. **Answer: B.**

CPAP is considered the mainstay of treatment of OSA and has shown benefits in dozens of randomized-controlled trials. These benefits include reducing daytime sleepiness, improving quality of life, and lowering blood pressure. Though data on blood pressure reduction are inconsistent with one meta-analysis reporting a decrease only in the mean arterial pressure but not in systolic blood pressure (SBP) or diastolic blood pressure (DBP) when studies measuring ambulatory blood pressures were analyzed, and decrease in SBP and DBP when studies measuring blood pressures conventionally were analyzed, no study has reported increase in blood pressure with CPAP use. Studies have reported better survival and fewer cardiovascular events in patients treated with CPAP when compared with patients with poor CPAP adherence or those who remained untreated. A recent large-scale prospective study reported a decrease in cardiovascular mortality in elderly patients undergoing CPAP for OSA. CPAP has been shown to reduce pulmonary artery pressure. Data regarding the effect of CPAP on insulin resistance are conflicting.

References:

- Sajkov D, McEvoy RD. Obstructive sleep apnea and pulmonary hypertension. Prog Cardiovasc Dis 2009; 51(5):363–370.
- Sajkov D, Wang T, Saunders NA, et al. Continuous positive airway pressure treatment improves pulmonary hemodynamics in patients with obstructive sleep apnea. Am J Respir Crit Care Med 2002; 165(2):152–158.
- Romero-Corral A, Caples SM, Lopez-Jimenez F, et al. Interactions between obesity and obstructive sleep apnea: implications for treatment. Chest 2010; 137 (3):711–719.
- Steiropoulos P, Tsara V, Nena E, et al. Effect of continuous positive airway pressure treatment on serum cardiovascular risk factors in patients with obstructive sleep apnea-hypopnea syndrome. Chest 2007; 132(3):843–851 [Epub June 15, 2007].
- Robinson GV, Pepperell JC, Segal HC, et al. Circulating cardiovascular risk factors in obstructive sleep apnoea: data from randomised controlled trials. Thorax 2004; 59(9):777–782.
- All-Cause and Cardiovascular Mortality in Elderly Patients with Sleep Apnea. Role of CPAP Treatment. A 6-Year Follow-Up Study (Session A19, Sunday, May 15, 8:15–10:45 a.m., Room 201–203 (Street Level), Colorado Convention Center; Abstract 20052).
- McDaid C, Durée KH, Griffin SC, et al. A systematic review of continuous positive airway pressure for obstructive sleep apnoea-hypopnoea syndrome. Sleep Med Rev 2009; 13(6):427–436.

11. **Answer: E.**

This is a high-risk patient. Certainly, cardiac workup is needed before surgery, but the nature of the cardiac problem is not acute since only isolated Q waves are detected in the EKG. Diabetic patients may sustain silent MI more frequently than other patients. Even mild asthma poses a contraindication for use of persantine in patient with shortness of breath and obesity. Although dobutamine can be used as a stressor for such a patient, echocardiography is an imperfect imaging technique in obese patients due to poor ultrasound penetration through fat tissue and the greater distance between the skin surface and the heart; stress echo test needs to be of particularly high precision. The patient's OA would preclude an exercise EKG. Given that this patient demonstrated shortness of breath, has multiple cardiac risk factors and evidence of old MI on EKG, the best choice would be to perform a right and left cardiac catheterization to obtain information on pulmonary artery pressures (pulmonary HTN is not uncommon with sleep apnea and diastolic left ventricular dysfunction) and ascertain the status of coronary artery patency.

Reference:
- Schirmer BD and Scott JR. Chapter 5: Peri-operative evaluation and assessment of medical problems. In: William BI, Eric JD, Ikramuddin S, eds. Laparoscopic Bariatric Surgery, Vol. 1. Philadelphia, PA, USA: Lippincott Williams & Wilkins, 2005.

12. **Answer: C.**

Biopsy is the gold standard for diagnosis of NASH.
The grading of steatohepatitis is as follows:
Grading of NASH

Score	Steatosis	Hepatocyte ballooning	Acinar inflammation
1	5–33%	Few	<2 foci/200x
2	33–66%	Many/Prominent	2–4 foci/200x
3	>66%		>4 foci/200x

Total score > 4 indicates steatohepatitis. The patient has a score of 6 and hence has steatohepatitis.
The staging of fibrosis is as follows:

Stage 0 None
Stage 1 Perisinusoidal or periportal
Stage 1A Mild zone 3, perisinusoidal
Stage 1B Moderate zone 3, perisinusoidal
Stage 1C Portal/periportal
Stage 2 Perisinusoidal and portal/periportal
Stage 3 Bridging fibrosis
Stage 4 Cirrhosis (even without perisinusoidal fibrosis)

More active inflammation, a higher degree of hepatocellular injury, more frequent Mallory-Denk bodies, the presence of endophlebitis, and a higher degree of perisinusoidal fibrosis may argue more in favor of alcoholic hepatitis, whereas predominating steatosis with less inflammation, as well as the presence of glycogenated nuclei, may argue more in favor of NASH. One important parameter of liver biopsy is length of the biopsy. An adequate liver biopsy needs to be done – usually a minimum length of about 15 to 25 mm and a diameter of 1.2 to 1.8 mm to be representative, as at least 10 portal tracts should be evaluated.

Reference:
- Straub BK, Schirmacher P. Pathology and biopsy assessment of non-alcoholic fatty liver disease. Dig Dis 2010; 28(1):197–202 [Epub May 7, 2010] (review).

13. **Answer: B.**

Since the patient is NPO on the day of surgery, it is advisable to decrease the glargine dose to half the dose on the day of surgery and administer short-acting insulin according to her blood glucose if needed. This method avoids the use of the IV insulin drip, which is cumbersome. This regimen has been shown to be as effective as the IV insulin regimen without any increased incidence of hyperglycemia or hypoglycemia. Though tight control of blood glucose has been shown to be beneficial in the long term, the benefit of tight blood glucose control (80–110 mg%) has not been demonstrated in the hospital setting.

Reference:
- Kang H, Ahn KJ, Choi JY, et al. Efficacy of insulin glargine in perioperative glucose control in type 2 diabetic patients. Eur J Anaesthesiol 2009; 26(8):666–670.

14. **Answer: C.**

The obesity-associated FSGS (obFSGS) is characterized by massive proteinuria and glomerular lesions that are similar to but less pronounced than in idiopathic FSGS, but the long-term prognosis is still dubious. The pathophysiology underlying obesity-associated renal pathology includes insulin resistance and salt sensitivity of blood pressure; more recently, adiponectin deficiency, hyperaldosteronism and many other pathogenetic factors have been identified. The abnormalities of renal structure in obese and morbidly obese individuals include increased kidney weight, glomerulomegaly, disorder of podocytes, mesangial expansion, and more recently also abnormalities of the renal interstitium. This is accompanied by functional abnormalities, that is, renal hyperperfusion, increased filtration fraction and albuminuria. Both obesity and metabolic syndrome have been identified as powerful predictors of chronic kidney disease (CKD) and end-stage renal disease (ESRD). This correlation is not fully explained by associated HTN and prediabetes/diabetes.

Reference:
- Ritz E, Koleganova N, Piecha G. Is there an obesity-metabolic syndrome related glomerulopathy? Curr Opin Nephrol Hypertens 2011; 20(1):44–49.

15. **Answer: C.**

The role of TNF-α in the skin of psoriatic patients has been the basis for therapeutic agents that are generally used to block the effect of TNF-α. TNF-α has also been implicated in obesity-related insulin resistance and shown to hinder insulin receptor signaling.

TNF-α, CRP, IL-6, and resistin are all increased in psoriatic patients. Though CRP has been shown to be reduced after bariatric surgery, the effect of bariatric surgery on other factors is controversial.

References:
- Kaur S, Zilmer K, Kairane C, et al. Clear differences in adiponectin level and glutathione redox status revealed in obese and normal-weight patients with psoriasis. Br J Dermatol 2008; 159(6):1364–1367.
- Johnston A, Arnadottir S, Gudjonsson JE, et al. Obesity in psoriasis: leptin and resistin as mediators of cutaneous inflammation. Br J Dermatol 2008; 159(2):342–350.
- Tobin AM, Kirby B. TNF alpha inhibitors in the treatment of psoriasis and psoriatic arthritis. BioDrugs 2005; 19(1):47–57 (review).
- Hotamisligil GS. Mechanisms of TNF-alpha-induced insulin resistance. Exp Clin Endocrinol Diabetes 1999; 107(2):119–125 (review).

16. **Answer: A.**

The lesion shown is acanthosis nigricans, which is generally caused by hyper-insulinemia. Insulin binds to IGF receptors on keratinocytes and fibroblasts causing their proliferation and the hyperpigmentation of the skin as noted in the image. The decreased insulin resistance associated with gastric bypass is usually accompanied by an improvement of the lesion, due to the normalization of the blood insulin levels. Glucose levels seem to have no role in the pigmentation since the lesion may be seen in hyperinsulinemic-euglycemic patients (prediabetic). Increased TNF-α and increased levels of free IGF-1 are also implicated in the pathogenesis of acanthosis nigricans.

References:

- Menon VU, Kumar KV, Gilchrist A, et al. Acanthosis Nigricans and insulin levels in a south Indian population—(ADEPS paper 2). Obes Res Clin Pract 2008; 2(1):43–50.
- Cruz PD Jr., Hud JA. Excess insulin binding to insulin-like growth factor receptors: proposed mechanism for acanthosis nigricans. J Invest Dermatol 1992; 98(6 suppl):82S–85S.
- Nam SY, Lee EJ, Kim KR, et al. Effect of obesity on total and free insulin-like growth factor (IGF)-1, and their relationship to IGF-binding protein (BP)-1, IGFBP-2, IGFBP-3, insulin, and growth hormone. Int J Obes Relat Metab Disord 1997; 21:355–359.
- Cohen P, Harel C, Bergman R, et al. Insulin resistance and acanthosis nigricans: evidence for a postbinding defect in vivo. Metabolism 1990; 39(10):1006–1011.

17. **Answer: D.**

Necrotizing fasciitis has a strong association with obesity. Diabetes is a predisposing factor for skin infections, and patients with fungal skin infections need to be screened for diabetes. Vaginal candidiasis has no relation to obesity. Half of the obese patients have been found to have cutaneous infections.

Intertrigo is a manifestation of obesity that involves a combination of skin irritation and infection. It is an inflammatory dermatosis involving the body folds. Skin folds are more numerous and deeper in the obese subject. Predisposing factors include friction, maceration, moisture and warmth, sweating, and occlusion. Colonization with bacteria, yeast, and dermatophytes may exacerbate the intertrigo. Colonization most commonly involves candidal infection.

References:

- Scheinfeld NS. Obesity and dermatology. Clin Dermatol 2004; 22(4):303–309.
- Roujeau JC. Necrotizing fasciitis. Clinical criteria and risk factors. Ann Dermatol Venereol 2001; 128:376–381.

18. **Answer: C.**

Venous stasis dermatitis is an inflammatory disorder as leukocytes get trapped in the fibrinous tissue to release cytokines. As such, both topical steroids and calcineurin blockers have been found to be useful for this condition.

Patients have to be advised to keep their leg elevated most of the time. Unna boot is also useful especially for the management of leg ulcers. Compression stockings though reported to be uncomfortable by the patients are also useful treatment modalities.

Bariatric surgery resolves venous stasis disease in more than 90% of the patients.

References:

- Shafritz R, Lamb-Susca L, Graham AM. Comprehensive management for venous stasis ulcers. Surg Technol Int 2008; 17:72–76.
- Sugerman HJ, Kellum JM, DeMaria EJ. Risks and benefits of gastric bypass in morbidly obese patients with severe venous stasis disease. Ann Surg 2001; 234:41–46.
- Felty CL, Rooke TW. Compression therapy for chronic venous insufficiency. Semin Vasc Surg 2005; 18(1):36–40 (review).

6 | Psychiatric issues

CHAPTER SUMMARY

- Multidisciplinary assessment before bariatric surgery must include a consultation with a psychiatrist/psychologist skilled in mental health issues in bariatric patients.
- Though there is no single assessment tool that is universally followed, it is recommended that a comprehensive clinical assessment include the following areas:
  - Assessment of emotional/affective disorders – this includes depression, bipolar disorder, and assessment of coping skills.
  - Assessment of cognitive function – this includes assessment of patient's decisional capacity and knowledge of the surgical intervention and pre- and postoperative management.
  - Assessment of behavioral disorders – this includes screening for eating disorders, substance abuse, the patient's level of participation in exercise and physical activity, and risk of stress eating or emotional eating.
  - Developmental assessment – this includes history of early-life abuse.
  - Motivational assessment – this includes rationale for and expectations after surgery.
  - Assessment of current life situation – this includes stressors and social/family networks.
- There is no single psychiatric condition that is an absolute contraindication for bariatric surgery; however, bariatric surgery should be performed only after psychiatric symptoms are controlled to the point at which the patient is able to comply adequately with pre- and postsurgical activities and expectations.
- The psychiatrist's opinion regarding the impact of the psychiatric disorder on weight loss, and vice versa, and on the ability of the patient to be compliant with medical and surgical demands of the postoperative period should be considered before performing bariatric surgery. Thus, risk assessment is individualized.
- Women in the bariatric population have a higher prevalence than men of psychiatric disorders.
- Weight loss after surgery cannot be related to a single specific psychiatric disorder; however, the number of psychiatric disorders before surgery may influence subsequent weight loss.
- Axis I disorders have a prevalence of 27% to 44% in different studies involving the bariatric population.
- Mood/Affective disorders are the most common axis I disorders and the most common lifetime psychiatric disorder seen in these patients. Major depressive disorder is the most common single lifetime psychiatric diagnosis in different studies.
- Most studies point to anxiety disorders as the most common current psychiatric diagnosis.
- Psychotropic medications can have an impact on a patient's weight after surgery. Extended-release drugs may be less effective after malabsorptional surgery such as gastric bypass.
- Major depressive disorder decreases in incidence immediately after surgery (within 1 year). Over the longer term, the impact of bariatric surgery on depression is not clear. Mood disorders may worsen in the immediate postoperative period.

- Bariatric surgery has been associated with increased suicide rates and increased death rate due to suicide.
- Binge eating disorder (BED) improves with bariatric surgery.
- Vomiting after restrictive surgery and Roux-en-Y gastric bypass (RYGB) is related to binge eating.

QUESTIONS

1. **A 26-year-old female candidate for gastric bypass surgery underwent Lap-Band surgery 4 years earlier but lost no weight, due to consumption of high-caloric liquids. When queried, she stated, "I did the surgery because my mother wanted me to, and I wasn't prepared to lose weight." She now states that she is motivated to lose weight on the basis of physical health risks, such as diabetes. A proper approach to proceeding would be to**
   A. Accept the patient unconditionally as a suitable candidate for surgery due to her enhanced insight.
   B. Accept the patient with the understanding that she participate in psychotherapy before and after surgery to address emotional issues relevant to weight loss.
   C. Reject the patient for surgery due to the failure of her first bariatric surgery.
   D. Reject the patient for surgery due to the presence of unresolved long-term emotional issues.

2. **A 42-year-old male candidate for bariatric surgery has bipolar disorder, for which he takes valproic acid and clonazepam. He is followed monthly by a psychiatrist. The psychiatrist is asked by the patient to write a letter on his behalf to the bariatric team, but declines to do so, stating that he is unfamiliar with psychiatric criteria related to suitability for bariatric surgery. The patient has been psychiatrically stable for several years. Which of the following course is appropriate?**
   A. The patient should be rejected for surgery as his mental health treater is unwilling to write a letter of support.
   B. The patient should be rejected as bipolar disorder is an absolute contraindication to bariatric surgery.
   C. The patient should be accepted as he has been psychiatrically stable.
   D. The patient should be referred to a psychiatrist or psychologist skilled in the assessment of psychiatric suitability for bariatric surgery.

3. **A 37-year-old female seeking bariatric surgery reports a history of "stress eating," which she relates to history of generalized anxiety disorder and depression. She currently is taking buspirone 5 mg twice daily and sertraline 75 mg daily, but states that she still is symptomatic. Both agents are prescribed by her primary care physician. Which of the following course is appropriate?**
   A. The bariatric surgeon should perform the surgery and increase the dosages of the psychotropic agents postoperatively for better control of the patient's psychiatric symptoms.
   B. The patient should not be offered bariatric surgery because "stress eating" tendencies have the potential to undermine the patient's success and satisfaction with such surgery.
   C. Before bariatric surgery is undertaken, the patient should be referred to a psychiatrist for better control of her symptoms.
   D. The patient should be accepted for surgery unconditionally, as she has good insight into the psychological factors contributing to "stress eating" tendencies.

4. **A 63-year-old female legal secretary seeking bariatric surgery indicates that her primary reason for seeking weight loss is the desire to improve her appearance. She indicates that her ability to be competitive in the job market will depend on**

her ability to be more physically attractive. The patient has had several cosmetic surgeries, including a face lift at age 57 and an abdominoplasty at age 60. Which of the following is <u>TRUE</u>?

A. Bariatric surgery is suitable because it will complement cosmetic surgeries previously performed.
B. Bariatric surgery is unsuitable because the patient's primary motivation is not related to anticipated improvement in her physical health status.
C. Bariatric surgery is unsuitable because the patient likely has a personality disorder not susceptible to improvement through surgery.
D. The suitability of bariatric surgery should be based on a mental health professional's appraisal of the patient's psychiatric stability and the reasonableness of her expectations regarding surgical outcome.

5. **Several months after Lap-Band surgery, a 39-year-old male with a remote history of alcohol and marijuana abuse reports that he has resumed alcohol use as a means of dealing with stress previously relieved by overeating. The bariatric surgeon should**

A. Reassure the patient that alcohol use likely will subside as he gradually develops other means for coping with stress.
B. Recommend that Lap-Band surgery be reversed since alcohol use is likely to escalate.
C. Administer disulfiram to promote a return to alcohol abstinence.
D. Refer the patient to a substance use expert familiar with bariatric surgery.

6. **Which of the following is appropriate in the management of a 27-year-old female with borderline personality disorder and cocaine abuse, in stable remission, seeking bariatric surgery?**

A. Due to the seriousness of these disorders and the challenges posed by them to ongoing collaboration with the bariatric team, the patient should be rejected for surgery.
B. If the patient signs a treatment contract to participate in regular mental health and substance care, she is a suitable candidate for surgery.
C. Risk assessment must be individualized and no statement about psychiatric suitability for surgery can be made on these diagnostic grounds alone.
D. If the patient agrees to a trial of mood stabilizer medication and has insight into her psychiatric issues, she is a suitable candidate for bariatric surgery.

7. **A 34-year-old female with recurrent unipolar depression, diabetes mellitus, back pain, and hypertension reports that her mood has worsened since gastric bypass was performed 2 months ago. Since then, she has lost 24 lb. Psychotropic medications, identical to those taken before surgery, include clonazepam 1 mg twice daily, venlafaxine extended-release 225 mg daily, and zolpidem 10 mg at bedtime. Which of the following may explain the patient's deterioration in mood?**

A. The patient's blood level of venlafaxine may have dropped due to inadequate absorption postoperatively of the extended-release version of this antidepressant agent.
B. The patient may be undergoing an adjustment reaction related to body image changes related to rapid weight loss.
C. Medical problems that the patient anticipated would subside after bariatric surgery may not yet have done so.
D. Mood disorders typically worsen in the immediate postoperative period and stabilize within 6 months of bariatric surgery.
E. A, B, and C are true.
F. A, B, C, and D are true.

8. **Which of the following need <u>NOT</u> be considered in the preoperative psychiatric screening of bariatric surgery candidates?**
   A. The adequacy of the patient's reasons for wishing bariatric surgery.
   B. The patient's ability to tolerate change as impacted by past psychiatric history.
   C. The role of "emotional eating" in the patient's overweight status.
   D. The patient's capacity to rationally manipulate risks and benefits regarding bariatric surgery.
   E. The degree to which a family consensus exists regarding the patient's desire to have bariatric surgery.

9. **Which of the following is an absolute psychiatric contraindication to bariatric surgery?**
   A. Cocaine dependence, in stable remission
   B. Chronic paranoid schizophrenia
   C. Narcissistic personality disorder
   D. Bulimia nervosa, in stable remission
   E. None of the above

10. **Identify the <u>FALSE</u> statement about the prevalence of psychiatric disorders in bariatric surgery candidates.**
    A. Women compared to men have a higher lifetime prevalence of psychiatric disorders.
    B. Avoidant personality disorder is the most common personality disorder in bariatric surgery candidates.
    C. Mood disorders are the most common lifetime psychiatric disorders in bariatric surgery patients.
    D. Drug abuse is the most common type of substance abuse seen.

11. **Identify the <u>TRUE</u> statement about the connection between early-life sexual abuse and obesity.**
    A. Risk of obesity is heightened only in female, not male, victims of sexual abuse.
    B. Sexual abuse impacts weight only if the patient meets formal criteria for posttraumatic stress disorder related to that abuse.
    C. Risk of obesity is directly proportional to severity of sexual abuse.
    D. Sexual abuse has no impact on psychological adjustment to bariatric surgery.

12. **Major depression is a common psychiatric disorder in obese patients, which has the potential to influence outcomes after surgery. Identify the <u>TRUE</u> statement about obesity and depression.**
    A. The lifetime prevalence of major depression is <10% in patients presenting for bariatric surgery.
    B. Depressive symptoms improve after bariatric surgery during the first year.
    C. Men presenting for bariatric surgery are more likely to have a diagnosis of major depression than women.
    D. Bariatric surgery has been definitively shown to decrease suicide rate in morbidly obese patients.

13. **Investigators have suspected that psychiatric disorders that present before bariatric surgery may impact the degree of weight loss after surgery. Which of the following statements is definitely <u>TRUE</u>?**
    A. The number of disorders preoperatively has been shown to have a correlation with weight loss after surgery.
    B. Anxiety disorders before surgery influence weight loss after surgery.
    C. Eating disorders before surgery influence weight loss after surgery.
    D. Weight loss cannot be clearly related to any specific psychiatric disorder present prior to surgery.
    E. Depression before surgery influences weight loss after surgery.

14. **BED is a common comorbidity in obese patients presenting for bariatric surgery. Which of the following statements is <u>TRUE</u> regarding BED and bariatric surgery?**
   A. Patients with BED tend to have more vomiting postoperatively after either restrictive surgery or RYGB.
   B. Biliopancreatic diversion causes an increase in vomiting postoperatively in BED patients.
   C. BED does not improve after any type of bariatric surgery.
   D. There are no standardized instruments to assess BED.

ANSWER KEY

1. B	5. D	9. E	13. D
2. D	6. C	10. D	14. A
3. C	7. F	11. C	
4. D	8. E	12. B	

ANSWER KEY WITH EXPLANATION

1. **Answer: B.**

   Patients who fail bariatric surgery on emotional grounds must be carefully reappraised for psychiatric suitability in order to avert failure after subsequent surgery. If the patient shows insight into the causes of the first failure and is motivated to address emotional issues, repeat surgery may be undertaken. A period of observation for compliance with psychotherapy may be advisable before an operative date is established.

   References:
   • Vallis TM, Ross MA. The role of psychological factors in bariatric surgery for morbid obesity: identification of psychological predictors of success. Obes Surg 1993; 3:346–359.
   • Wadden TA, Sarwer DB, Fabricatore AN, et al. Psychosocial and behavioral status of patients undergoing bariatric surgery: what to expect before and after surgery. Med Clin North Am 2007; 91:451–469.

2. **Answer: D.**

   Mental health screening of candidates for bariatric surgery should be undertaken by clinicians skilled in the assessment of emotional suitability for this surgery. Many patients experience improved mood after such surgery, but, for some, especially those with extensive "stress eating" and difficulty with life transitions, a period of psychiatric instability may follow surgery, requiring increased psychiatric attention. Well-managed bipolar disorder is not a contraindication to bariatric surgery.

   References:
   • Norris L. Psychiatric issues in bariatric surgery. Psychiatr Clin North Am 2007; 30:717–738.
   • Bauchowitz AU, Gonder-Frederic LA, Olbrisch ME, et al. Psychosocial evaluation of bariatric surgery candidates: a survey of present practices. Psychosom Med 2005; 67:825–832.

3. **Answer: C.**

   Many candidates for bariatric surgery are receiving psychiatric medications but continue to experience symptoms that may promote overeating tendencies. Such patients should be referred to mental health providers familiar with the emotional aspects of bariatric surgery. Improved symptom management may enhance outcome and patient satisfaction with bariatric surgery.

   Reference:
   • Walfish S, Vance D, Fabricatore AN. Psychological evaluation of bariatric surgery applicants: procedures and reasons for delay or denial of surgery. Obes Surg 2007; 17:1578–1583.

4. **Answer: D.**

Candidates for bariatric surgery should have reasonable expectations with regard to cosmetic appearance and physical health after surgery. Ideally, motivation to improve physical health will predominate.

References:
- Marcus MD, Kalarchian MA, Courcoulas AP. Psychiatric evaluation and follow-up of bariatric surgery patients. Am J Psychiatry 2009; 166:285–291.
- van Hout GC, Verschure SK, van Heck GL. Psychosocial predictors of success following bariatric surgery. Obes Surg 2005; 15:552–560.

5. **Answer: D.**

Patients with substance histories occasionally may relapse as they seek to find a substitute for food "addiction" that preceded bariatric surgery. Assessment by a trained professional is appropriate in order to appraise the seriousness of the relapse, and commence appropriate interventions.

Reference:
- Ertelt TW, Mitchell JE, Lancaster K, et al. Alcohol abuse and dependence before and after bariatric surgery: a review of the literature and report of a new data set. Surg Obes Relat Dis 2008; 4:647–650.

6. **Answer: C.**

Neither of these conditions is an absolute contraindication to bariatric surgery, but both present risks in the postoperative period. Risk assessment must be individualized.

Reference:
- Ruelaz AR. Psychiatric involvement in obesity treatment. Focus 2009; 7:311–316.

7. **Answer: F.**

Factors A through D are directly relevant to a patient's success and satisfaction with bariatric surgery. While family consensus may be helpful, it is not an essential ingredient in the psychiatric screening process.

References:
- Marcus MD, Kalarchian MA, Courcoulas AP. Psychiatric evaluation and follow-up of bariatric surgery patients. Am J Psychiatry 2009; 166:285–291.
- Pull CD. Current psychological assessment practices in obesity surgery programs: what to assess and why. Curr Opin Psychiatry 2010; 23(1):30–36.

8. **Answer: E.**

Psychiatric suitability for bariatric surgery is not diagnosis dependent, but instead relies on the degree to which the disorder is under adequate management and impacts on the patient's ability to work cooperatively with the bariatric surgery team and mental health providers.

References:
- Marcus MD, Kalarchian MA, Courcoulas AP. Psychiatric evaluation and follow-up of bariatric surgery patients. Am J Psychiatry 2009; 166:285–291.
- Walfish S, Vance D, Fabricatore AN. Psychological evaluation of bariatric surgery applicants: procedures and reasons for delay or denial of surgery. Obes Surg 2007; 16:567–573.

9. **Answer: E.**

Psychiatric suitability for bariatric surgery is not diagnosis dependent, but instead relies on the degree to which the disorder is under adequate management and impacts on the patient's ability to work cooperatively with the bariatric surgery team and mental health providers.

References:
- Marcus MD, Kalarchian MA, Courcoulas AP. Psychiatric evaluation and follow-up of bariatric surgery patients. Am J Psychiatry 2009; 166:285–291.

- Walfish S, Vance D, Fabricatore AN. Psychological evaluation of bariatric surgery applicants: procedures and reasons for delay or denial of surgery. Obes Surg 2007; 16:567–573.

10. **Answer: D.**

Women presenting for bariatric surgery have a higher lifetime prevalence of psychiatric disorders. The most common of lifetime diagnosis in patients presenting for bariatric surgery is mood disorder (45.5%), whereas the most common class of disorder at the time of preoperative evaluation is anxiety disorder (24.0%). However, there is no consensus on the latter (current diagnosis).

Alcohol abuse is the most common type of substance abuse seen in patients presenting for bariatric surgery.

There is also no consensus on the most common type of eating disorder seen in bariatric patients with most studies pointing to BED.

Avoidant personality disorder is the most common personality disorder in bariatric surgery candidates and is present in about 17% of such patients.

References:
- Rosenberger PH, Henderson KE, Grilo CM. Psychiatric disorder comorbidity and association with eating disorders in bariatric surgery patients: A cross-sectional study using structured interview-based diagnosis. J Clin Psychiatry 2006; 67 (7):1080–1085.
- Powers PS, Perez A, Boyd F, et al. Eating pathology before and after bariatric surgery: a prospective study. Int J Eat Disord 1999; 25(3):293–300.
- Kalarchian MA, Marcus MD, Levine MD, et al. Psychiatric disorders among bariatric surgery candidates: relationship to obesity and functional health status. Am J Psychiatry 2007; 164:328–334.
- Mühlhans B, Horbach T, de Zwaan M. Psychiatric disorders in bariatric surgery candidates: a review of the literature and results of a German prebariatric surgery sample. Gen Hosp Psychiatry 2009; 31:414–421.

11. **Answer: C.**

Sexual abuse in adolescence and teenage years may increase risk of obesity, in both males and females, as added weight is used as a "shield" by victims against sexual interactions. Overweight patients may see themselves as less sexually appealing than normal weight individuals; therefore, emotional challenges may arise after bariatric surgery. Sexual abuse victims need not have a formal diagnosis of posttraumatic stress disorder for their weight to be influenced by the sexual abuse. Risk of obesity increases with increased severity of abuse.

References:
- Midei AJ, Matthews KA. Interpersonal violence in childhood as a risk factor for obesity: a systematic review of the literature and proposed pathways. Obes Rev 2011; 12(5):e159–e172.
- Gustafson TB, Sarwer DB. Childhood sexual abuse and obesity. Obes Rev 2004; 5(3):129–135.

12. **Answer: B.**

Depressive symptoms improve after bariatric surgery during the first year although this may not be maintained in the long term. The course of major depression in the longer term (2–3 years) is not clear, with one study reporting a decreasing prevalence of depressive disorder at 2 to 3 years, while another study in adolescents reported a slight increase in depressive symptoms during the second year after surgery. The Swedish obese subjects (SOS) study reported a beneficial effect of surgery on depression for up to 10 years. The suicide rates after bariatric surgery in such patients have not been found to be increased in most studies involving groups. However, in studies focusing on individual patients, increased suicide rates have been found.

The lifetime prevalence of major depression in patients presenting for bariatric surgery varies from 26% to 42% in various studies. Women presenting for bariatric surgery are more likely to have a history of affective disorder, particularly major depressive disorder.

Diagnosis of depression is more difficult in the morbidly obese as many of the vegetative symptoms of depression can be confused with those of obesity (e.g., sleep apnea–related fatigue and joint pain–related psychomotor retardation).

References:
- Karlsson J, Taft C, Rydén A, et al. Ten-year trends in health-related quality of life after surgical and conventional treatment for severe obesity: the SOS intervention study. Int J Obes (Lond) 2007; 31(8):1248–1261 [Epub March 13, 2007].
- Adams TD, Gress RE, Smith SC, et al. Long-term mortality after gastric bypass surgery. N Engl J Med 2007; 357:753–761.
- De Zwann M, Enderle J, Wagner S, et al. Anxiety and depression in bariatric surgery patients: a prospective, follow-up study using structured clinical interviews. J Affect Disord. 2011 Sep; 133(1–2):61–68.
- Zeller MH, Reiter-Purtill J, Ratcliff MB, et al. Two-year trends in psychosocial functioning after adolescent Roux-en-Y gastric bypass. Surg Obes Relat Dis. 2011 Nov; 7(6):727–732.
- Rosenberger PH, Henderson KE, Grilo CM. Psychiatric disorder comorbidity and association with eating disorders in bariatric surgery patients: a cross-sectional study using structured interview-based diagnosis. J Clin Psychiatry 2006; 67(7):1080–1085.
- Assimakopoulos K, Karaivazoglou K, Panayiotopoulos S, et al. Bariatric surgery is associated with reduced depressive symptoms and better sexual function in obese female patients: a one-year follow-up study. Obes Surg 2011; 21(3):362–366.
- Norris L. Psychiatric issues in bariatric surgery. Psychiatr Clin North Am 2007; 30:717–738.

13. **Answer: D.**

Weight loss cannot be clearly related to any specific psychiatric disorder present prior to surgery, but the presence of more than one psychiatric condition might play a role. However, older systematic reviews have found that causes of psychological distress like depression and anxiety were predictors of weight loss.

Reference:
- Pataky Z, Carrard I, Golay A. Psychological factors and weight loss in bariatric surgery. Curr Opin Gastroenterol 2011; 27:167–173.

14. **Answer: A.**

There are various instruments to assess BED, one of the most popular being the Three-Factor Eating Questionnaire (TFEQ). Studies utilizing such questionnaires like the SOS study have reported improvement in scores in patients with BED. Such improvement is seen for both restrictive and malabsorptive surgery, including biliopancreatic diversion. BED patients have an increased incidence of vomiting postoperatively, and this is seen with restrictive surgery and RYGB, but not biliopancreatic diversion. Binge eating becomes almost impossible for bariatric patients due to restriction of the stomach. Hence they may resort to other maladaptive eating behaviors like grazing.

Reference:
- Herpertz S, Kielmann R, Wolf AM, et al. Does obesity surgery improve psychosocial functioning? A systematic review. Int J Obes Relat Metab Disord 2003; 27:1300–1314.

7 | Surgical techniques

CHAPTER SUMMARY

- Technique of insertion of an adjustable gastric band:
  - The pars flaccida technique is the preferred approach – this involves placing the band above the lesser sac, including the fat and the vagus nerve branch within the band. The hepatic branch of the vagus may be injured during this step.
  - An opening is made in the pars flaccida. Blunt dissection is done to create a retrogastric tunnel.
  - A blunt instrument is passed under visualization through the retrogastric tunnel toward the angle of His.
  - The band is introduced through a large port and placed in the retrogastric tunnel. Gastrogastric sutures are used to secure the band.
  - The "buckle" of the band is positioned on the lesser curvature.
  - The port is usually fixed on the anterior rectus sheath with sutures.
  - The band is NOT filled during its insertion. Priming of the band can be done.
  - Belachew et al. proposed certain guidelines for learning the Lap-Band technique nearly 10 years ago that are valid even today.
  - Perigastric (PG) technique is largely abandoned due to high incidence of erosion and slippage when compared to the pars flaccida technique.
- Technique of adjusting a Lap-Band:
  - The first adjustment is made 6 weeks postoperatively.
  - The initial adjustment consists of adding about 2 to 3 mL of fluid. Patient is then followed every 4 to 6 weeks. An optimal weight loss would be 0.5 to 1 kg/wk. If less weight loss is observed, about 1 mL of fluid is added at the next adjustment.
  - The Center of Obesity of the Monash Medical School in Australia has come with an easy-to-use diagram that can help in office adjustment of the Lap-Band.

Add Fluid	Optimal Zone	Remove Fluid
Hungry	Early and prolonged satiety	Dysphagia
Big meals	Small meals satisfy	Reflux/heartburn
Looking for food	Satisfactory weight loss/ maintenance	Night cough
		Regurgitation
		Maladaptive eating

  - The access port can be identified either radiologically or by simple palpation.
  - The needle must be inserted perpendicular to the access port septum and must not be moved once it is in the port.
  - Only noncoring deflected tip needles must be used.
  - Access port should be entered with a syringe connected to the needle.
  - The needle is pushed until the needle hits the bottom of the portal chamber. Then some saline is drawn to confirm its position.
  - If fluid has been added to the band, the patient is asked to drink water to make sure that there is no overrestriction.
- Technique of Roux-en-Y gastric bypass (RYGB):
  - Creation of the gastric pouch: window created near the lesser curvature about 5 cm from the gastroesophageal junction. Blunt dissection continued along the posterior wall of the stomach until the greater curvature. Green load

staples are fired horizontally and then vertically in the line of the angle of His.

- Jejunum is transected about 40 to 50 cm from the ligament of Treitz.
- The Roux limb used is generally 100 to 150 cm.
- The Roux limb can be positioned in various ways relative to the colon and the stomach remnant. An antecolic approach is known to increase the tension of the gastrojejunostomy (GJ) anastomosis but decrease the incidence of internal hernia.
- The gastrojejunostomy can be done using a circular stapler, linear stapler, or by hand-sewn method.
- A side-to-side (functional end-to-side) jejunojejunostomy is performed by using a linear cutting stapler.
- All the mesenteric defects are meticulously closed.
- The gastrojejunal anastomosis is usually tested by injecting methylene blue through an orogastric tube, by insufflating air and placing the anastomosis under saline, or by an intraoperative endoscopy.

- Technique of sleeve gastrectomy:
  - The vascular supply of the greater curvature is divided by dividing the greater omentum.
  - Some adhesions of the stomach to the pancreas separated as well.
  - Usually a blunt-tipped 32- to 40-Fr bougie is introduced transorally and placed along the lesser curvature to calibrate the size of the sleeve gastrectomy.
  - The stomach is stapled close to the bougie starting around 5 cm from the pylorus and terminating at the angle of His. Thick tissue staples are used for the thicker antrum and the cardia. Regular sized staples can be used for the thinner mid-stomach and fundus.
  - The specimen is retrieved with or without a bag.
  - Either a part of the staple line or the whole staple line can be reinforced by continuous absorbable sutures.
  - Use of reinforced staples decreases blood loss but not leakage rates.
  - The staple line is tested by injecting methylene blue, by insufflating air, or by an intraoperative endoscopy (and placing the stomach under saline). The duodenum is compressed with atraumatic instruments.

- Technique of biliopancreatic diversion–duodenal switch (BPD-DS):
  - It is technically challenging and accounts for only 2% to 3% of the bariatric operations in the United States.
  - The greater curvature of the stomach is freed from the greater omentum.
  - The duodenum and pylorus are dissected posteriorly and separated from the vasculature.
  - A 50- to 60-Fr bougie is introduced transorally and a sleeve gastrectomy is completed starting 1 cm proximal to the pylorus and proceeding till the lateral side of the angle of His. Continuous seroserosal sutures are placed along the staple line.
  - The common limb is measured 50 to 100 cm from the ileocecal valve. The alimentary limb is measured about 300 cm from the ileocecal valve. These points are marked off. Thus, the length of the common channel (CC) is about 50 to 100 cm and that of the alimentary limb (AL) is about 200 to 300 cm. The bowel is divided at this point.
  - The biliopancreatic limb is joined to the common limb by a side-to-side (functional end-to-side) anastomosis.
  - The duodenoileostomy is performed as a functional end-to-end anastomosis.
  - The sleeve gastrectomy specimen is removed.
  - The BPD procedure differs only in that a distal gastrectomy is performed and the pouch has a volume of about 200 mL.

QUESTIONS

1. One of the features that appeals to patients is that the degree of restriction can be altered by adjusting the band. About the process of adjusting a band, identify the FALSE statement.
   A. The port should be punctured by the needle at a 90° angle.
   B. After performing a band adjustment, the patient's ability to swallow should be tested by asking the patient to drink water.
   C. The port should be accessed with the needle alone first; then a prefilled syringe is attached to perform a fill.
   D. The regular hypodermic needle cannot be used.

2. The saying "see 1, do 1, teach 1" no longer holds true for preparing oneself for a newer procedure. Bariatric surgery has a learning curve even for experienced laparoscopic surgeons. Which of the following regarding learning the laparoscopic adjustable gastric band (LAGB) insertion is TRUE?
   A. The ideal patient during learning is a female patient who is super-obese and with android obesity.
   B. The ideal patient during learning is a male patient who is super-obese and has a gynecoid obesity.
   C. The ideal patient during learning is a female with a body mass index (BMI) of 40 to 50 kg/m^2 and has gynecoid obesity.
   D. It is better not to have the company advisor to be present during the procedure.

3. Performing the laparoscopic BPD-DS (LBPD-DS) in two stages has many advantages. Which of the following is a FALSE statement?
   A. Operative times are reduced and thus ventilation may be less compromised in obese patients.
   B. A significant percentage of patients intended for a two-stage procedure may achieve enough weight loss and remission/improvement of comorbidities that they do not require the second stage.
   C. Many of the comorbidities have resolved by the time of the second procedure.
   D. The two-stage procedure has never been shown to have decreased morbidity and mortality when compared to the single-stage procedure.

4. Which one of the following is NOT true regarding the operative technique for a sleeve gastrectomy?
   A. Devascularization of the stomach distal to a point that is 2 cm proximal to the pylorus should be avoided.
   B. Normal tissue thickness staples (e.g., blue staples) should be used for the fundus as these are known to cause lesser staple line hemorrhage when compared to thick tissue staples (e.g., green staples).
   C. One should stay close to the serosa of the stomach while dividing the short gastric vessels.
   D. An ultrasonic shears is better than Ligasure in sealing of blood vessels.

5. The adjustable gastric band has proven to be an effective modality of weight loss in the long term. Identify the FALSE statement about the protocol followed for adjustment of a band.
   A. The first adjustment is usually done 6 weeks postoperatively and not at the time of the band placement.
   B. The initial adjustment is a larger amount (2–3 mL) and subsequent adjustments are about 1 mL.
   C. The weight loss should be around 2 to 3 kg/wk.
   D. The band should be loosened if the patient develops acid reflux or vomiting.

6. **A 35-year-old woman comes for her sixth adjustment 1 year after an adjustable gastric band was inserted. Her last adjustment was 1 month ago. Which of the following does <u>NOT</u> indicate a state of optimal restriction?**
   A. The patient feels full after eating about half of the food that she used to eat before placement of the Lap-Band.
   B. Patient does not feel hungry like before and does not snack between meals anymore.
   C. She has lost 6 lb since her last adjustment.
   D. She has vomited twice since her last adjustment.
   E. She has not been able to tolerate soft food for the past 2 weeks and is now on a liquid diet.

7. **There are two methods of placing a gastric band – pars flaccida technique and PG technique. Identify the <u>TRUE</u> statement about the pars flaccida technique.**
   A. It has a longer operative time when compared with the PG technique.
   B. In the pars flaccida technique, the band is placed behind the posterior aspect of the stomach through the lesser sac.
   C. The pars flaccida technique has reduced the incidence of Band erosion.
   D. The pars flaccida technique has increased incidence of vascular injury and conversion to laparotomy.

8. **Gastric band insertion is learnt more easily by surgeons who have some experience in esophageal/upper gut surgery. Identify the <u>FALSE</u> statement about the surgical technique of insertion of gastric band.**
   A. The surgeon needs to watch out for the hepatic branch of the vagus nerve when he/she begins the dissection of the pars flaccida.
   B. The surgeon needs to dissect carefully to the left of the right crus where he/she may encounter the inferior vena cava (IVC).
   C. The PG band placement is associated with a higher rate of band slippage.
   D. The band should be oriented with the lateral side at the angle of His.

9. **Identify the <u>FALSE</u> statement about fixation of the access port and tubing after placement of an adjustable gastric band.**
   A. Care should be taken to prevent acute kinking of the tubing.
   B. A part of the silastic tube needs to be excised to prevent intra-abdominal complications of excess free tube.
   C. A noncoring Huber needle should be used to prime the port with saline at the time of Band insertion.
   D. The Lap-Band should not be filled at the time of placement of band.

10. **Identify which of the following is a contraindication to adjustable gastric band placement.**
    A. Duodenal ulcer
    B. Esophageal varices
    C. Patient on long-term steroid treatment
    D. All of the above

11. **A bariatric surgeon is performing LRYGB on a patient with BMI of 60 kg/m^2. Which of the following is a <u>FALSE</u> statement about the technique that he should employ?**
    A. Close mesenteric defect at jejunojejunostomy.
    B. Construct a 75-cm-long Roux limb.
    C. Close Petersen's defect.
    D. Create a gastric pouch based on the upper lesser curvature of the stomach.

12. **LBPD is a technically challenging and a not so commonly performed bariatric procedure. About the surgical technique of BPD, identify the <u>FALSE</u> statement.**
    A. The common channel has a length of 50 to 100 cm.

    B. The alimentary limb has a length of 200 to 300 cm.

    C. The point of ileal transection is identified by measuring from the ligament of Treitz.

    D. The distal cut end of the ileum is anastomosed to the posterior aspect of the gastric pouch in an end-to-side fashion.

    E. A common channel of 150 cm results in less weight loss when compared with a common channel of 100 cm.

13. **One of the crucial steps during a band placement is the creation of a retrogastric tunnel. About the creation of a retrogastric tunnel during gastric band placement, identify the <u>FALSE</u> statement.**

    A. Electrocautery should be avoided if possible.

    B. The opening should not be enlarged too much.

    C. The band can be placed through the same retrogastric tunnel during replacement/repositioning of the band.

    D. The spleen may be injured during passage of an instrument behind the gastroesophageal junction.

14. **A bariatric surgeon encounters increased difficulty in maintaining the pneumo-peritoneum intraoperatively. The pressure monitor indicates an intra-abdominal pressure of 18 mmHg. What is his immediate next step?**

    A. Connect another insufflator to one of the trocars.

    B. Convert to open procedure.

    C. Ask anesthetist if muscle relaxation is adequate.

    D. Increase CO_2 in flow.

15. **Sleeve gastrectomy is a relatively new surgical procedure that was initially designed as the first stage of a two-stage procedure. Identify the <u>FALSE</u> statement about the steps involved in doing a sleeve gastrectomy.**

    A. A blunt bougie is usually used.

    B. The gastroepiploic vascular branches are divided starting around 5 cm from the pylorus till angle of His.

    C. 60-Fr bougie is the most commonly used bougie size.

    D. Detachment of the omentum and stapling of the stomach can be done in any order.

16. **Identify the <u>TRUE</u> statement about the technical details of a sleeve gastrectomy.**

    A. The distal end of the staple line can be started at 0.5 cm from the pylorus.

    B. The pouch created usually has a volume of 250 mL.

    C. Staple line reinforcement has been shown to decrease blood loss.

    D. A tapered (Maloney) bougie is preferred to a blunt-tipped (Hurst) bougie while performing a sleeve gastrectomy.

17. **There are various methods to create the gastrojejunal anastomosis during an RYGB. About the creation of a gastrojejunostomy, identify the <u>FALSE</u> statement.**

    A. Anastomotic bleeding rates are more with hand-sewn gastrojejunostomy.

    B. Antecolic approach is more commonly used than a retrocolic approach.

    C. Robotic technology can be utilized for hand-sewn anastomosis.

    D. A circular stapled anastomosis can be facilitated by passing the stapler anvil either transorally or through a distal gastrostomy.

18. **Identify the <u>TRUE</u> meaning of the "1 centimeter rule" that is used in creating a gastrojejunostomy.**

    A. Always create a stoma greater than 1 cm.

    B. Gastric and gastrojejunal anastomotic staple lines should always be less than 1 cm from each other.

C. The gastrojejunostomy should not be more than 1 cm from the lesser curvature.

D. The gastrojejunostomy and gastric transection staple line can cross at right angles but if they are parallel, as in a linear stapled anastomosis, they should be more than 1 cm from each other.

19. **Creation of a gastric pouch is a critical step during an RYGB. Identify the <u>FALSE</u> statement about creation of the gastric pouch in laparoscopic gastric bypass.**

A. The pouch size is usually 30 to 50 cc.

B. The pouch is created 5 cm from the gastroesophageal junction.

C. A 50-Fr bougie may be used to create the pouch by placing it along the lesser curvature.

D. The vagal nerve is invariably injured during creation of the pouch.

20. **All bariatric procedures are technically challenging, and surgeons need to perform a critical number of procedures before obtaining the ideal outcomes. This has been termed the learning curve. Identify which of the following is most influenced by the learning curve for a bariatric operation.**

A. Operative time

B. Blood loss

C. Hospital stay

D. All of the above

21. **Given that most bariatric surgeries are now performed laparoscopically, it is important to understand the equipment and specific equipment-related parameters related to laparoscopic bariatric surgery. Identify the <u>FALSE</u> statement about laparoscopic equipment used during bariatric surgery.**

A. Both CRT and LCD monitors can provide high-resolution images.

B. Bariatric patients sometimes require higher intra-abdominal pressure (about 20 cm of H_2O) compared to nonobese patients.

C. Some bariatric surgeries need a high flow rate of CO_2.

D. Warming the insufflated air alone without humidification can prevent hypothermia during a lengthy bariatric procedure.

22. **Laparoendoscopic single-site (LESS) surgery for gastric banding is still novel, but has been shown to be feasible. Regarding single-incision laparoscopic banding, all of the following are true, <u>EXCEPT</u>.**

A. Early single-center experiences have suggested that patients may use less narcotics following a single-incision gastric banding than following a traditional 5-trocar band.

B. LESS gastric banding is significantly quicker to perform (shorter operative times), especially as only one port needs to be placed.

C. There are no large-volume randomized, prospective studies that demonstrate significant advantages of LESS surgery for gastric banding over traditional LAGB.

D. Overall costs are about equal between a single-incision band and a traditional adjustable gastric band procedure.

23. **The DaVinci robotic surgical system has been utilized in bariatric surgery usually as robotically assisted surgeries that have been performed at various centers. Identify the <u>FALSE</u> statement about the use of surgical robots in bariatric surgery.**

A. Robotic surgery has significantly decreased the time from the start of the case to establishment of the pneumoperitoneum.

B. Robotic surgery has significantly higher procedural cost.

C. BPD has been shown to be feasible using robotic assistance.

D. Robotic surgery reduces operative time in higher BMI patients.

24. **Robotically assisted bariatric surgery has not come into widespread clinical practice even though the first robotic gastric bypass was performed nearly a**

decade ago. Identify the <u>TRUE</u> statement about the potential advantage of robotically assisted bariatric surgery over conventional laparoscopic surgery.
A. The 3D view facilitates better vision.
B. The articulating wrists increase degrees of freedom.
C. Motion scaling allows precise hand movement.
D. Mechanical forces can counteract the abdominal wall torque.
E. All of the above.

ANSWER KEY

1. C	7. C	13. C	19. D
2. C	8. B	14. C	20. A
3. D	9. B	15. C	21. D
4. D	10. D	16. C	22. B
5. C	11. B	17. A	23. A
6. E	12. C	18. D	24. E

ANSWER KEY WITH EXPLANATION

1. **Answer: C.**

   The port should be accessed with a Huber needle attached to the syringe, otherwise saline will leak out. The amount of saline in the band is confirmed by drawing the entire amount of saline in the band. This is then reinjected along with additional saline.

   The port should be punctured by the needle at a $90°$ angle. Moving the syringe when in the port may damage the septum. After injecting saline, adjustment can be checked by asking the patient to drink water.

   Reference:
   - Lap band training manual from Allergan Academy. Available at: http://www.allergan.com/assets/pdf/lapband_dfu.pdf. Accessed April 30, 2011.

2. **Answer: C.**

   Belachew et al. provided 10 rules for anybody wishing to learn the Lap-Band technique. They are to be followed for at least the first 10 procedures a surgeon performs and are as follows.
   1. Good patient selection. The ideal patient during the learning curve is a female with BMI 40 to 45 kg/m² with gynecoid-type obesity.
   2. Know all the details of the operation. Study again and again the real-time video of the procedure. Follow the protocol strictly.
   3. Go back to the animal lab if necessary to improve your laparoscopic skill.
   4. Train your surgical assistant, anesthesiologists, and nurses who are working with you in the OR.
   5. Be sure to have adequate instrumentation – a good liver retractor, good cautery hook, and a good suction-irrigation.
   6. Make sure that a company's advisor is present. They know the technical details of the operation, and can be of help.
   7. Do not take any unreasonable risk by persisting in the laparoscopic approach when there is danger; convert to laparotomy.
   8. If the dissection of the retrogastric space has been very difficult and if you have any doubt concerning gastric integrity, ask the anesthesiologist to inject methylene blue through the nasogastric tube.
   9. In the early postoperative days, if a patient complains of abnormal abdominal pain or respiratory problems or if the chart shows moderate fever and/or tachycardia, suspect gastric perforation.
   10. Do not leave the balloon of the silicone band overinflated at the operation, because this may result in early food intolerance due to postoperative edema.

Reference:
- Belachew M, Legrand MJ, Vincent V. History of Lap-band: from dream to reality. Obes Surg 2001; 11(3):297–302.

3. **Answer: D.**

The two-stage procedure has been shown to have decreased morbidity and mortality rate in super-super-obese patients.

For the surgeons, LBPD-DS is technically difficult, physically demanding, and requires advanced laparoscopic skills. For the super-super-obese patients who carry much of their weight in the neck, torso, and abdomen, the various positions of the operative table to facilitate exposure may compromise their ventilation and preclude them from extended anesthesia. At times, increased pneumoperitoneum to 20 mmHg may be necessary to counter the excessive weight of the abdominal wall. A large, fatty liver – as well as heavily laden omentum and mesentery – also could jeopardize the anastomosis. The above technical difficulties may also increase the operative time. Tremendous and sustainable weight loss is desirable, but should not compromise patient safety. With this intention the two-stage procedure was initially designed. Many comorbidities may resolve after the sleeve gastrectomy making the patient a better candidate for the DS procedure. The patient may not need the second procedure as the sleeve gastrectomy may itself cause good weight loss and resolution of comorbidities.

References:
- Camilo B, Michel G. Chapter 30: Two-stage approach for high-risk patients. In: Pitombo C, Jones K, Higa K, et al., eds. Obesity Surgery: Principles and Practice. 1st ed. New York: McGraw-Hill, 2007.
- William BI, Eric JD, Ikramuddin S, eds. Laparoscopic Bariatric Surgery, Vol. 1. Philadelphia, PA, USA: Lippincott Williams & Wilkins, 2005.

4. **Answer: D.**

One should elevate the stomach to divide the short gastrics at the level of the left posterior crus. Dissection should not be started near the left gastric nodes as it may lead to inadvertent injury to the left gastric vessels. The anterior fad pad at the angle of His will need to be carefully dissected as there is a vessel supplying this part which needs to be ligated. Devascularizing the stomach beyond 2 cm proximal to the pylorus may lead to damage to the right gastric vessels. The stomach again needs to be lifted up so that the right gastric may be divided perpendicularly.

The staples of lesser height lead to lesser bleeding. They can be used for thinner regions of the stomach like the mid-fundus. Green load needs to be applied near the cardia and the antrum that have a thicker wall.

One needs to stay close to the serosa of the stomach while coagulating the short gastrics to prevent injury to the splenic hilum.

Though the harmonic device produces faster sealing of blood vessels, it has not been shown to be superior to the Ligasure device in terms of the quality of sealing of the vessel and the burst pressure of the sealed vessel.

References:
- Jossart GH. Complications of sleeve gastrectomy: bleeding and prevention. Surg Laparosc Endosc Percutan Tech 2010; 20(3):146–147.
- Noble EJ, Smart NJ, Challand C, et al. Experimental comparison of mesenteric vessel sealing and thermal damage between one bipolar and two ultrasonic shears devices. Br J Surg 2011; 98(6):797–800.

5. **Answer: C.**

The initial weight loss aimed at is about 0.5 to 1 kg/wk, and the band is tightened if the weight loss is less than this. Fluid is not added at the time of band placement as it may cause discomfort to the patient due to postoperative edema. The first adjustment is done at 6 weeks when 2 to 3 mL of fluid is added. Later the patient is followed up every 4 to 6 weeks, and about 1 mL of fluid is added if desired weight loss is not seen. The band is loosened if the patient develops vomiting or reflux. It is also useful to loosen the band in pregnancy if the patient is symptomatic, if the patient is acutely ill, and if the patient is planning to visit a remote place where adjustment of the band will not be possible.

6. **Answer: E.**

The Centre for Obesity Research and Education (CORE), Monash Medical School, Melbourne, Australia, effectively describes this optimal adjustment state as the "Green Zone," or the point at which the LAP-BAND AP™ System is most effective for a particular patient. The three zones defined by the same institution are as follows:

> The yellow zone: This is an underfilled state that is manifested as excessive hunger, eating big meals, and seeking for food.
> The green zone: This is the zone of optimal restriction that is manifested by satiety and satisfaction attained due to small meals.
> The red zone: This is an overfilled state characterized by dysphagia, reflux, and maladaptive eating.

Choices A to D are considered normal in a Lap-Band patient as they indicate optimal restriction and do not need adjustment of band.

Reference:
- http://www.lapbandcentral.com/local/files/documentlibrary/AP_ART_ OF_ADJUSTMENT_Guide.pdf. Accessed April 30, 2011

7. **Answer: C.**

In the pars flaccida technique, the dissection is started in the lesser omentum between the stomach and the caudate lobe, and an avascular tunnel is created posterior to the stomach in the direction of the angle of His. The band is placed above the free lesser sac.

The results of a study that compared the PG and the pars flaccida techniques are as follows:
- Operative time was significantly longer in the PG technique.
- Hospital stay was similar in the two groups.
- Laparotomic conversion was significantly higher in the PG group.
- Gastric pouch dilation and intragastric migration were significantly more frequent in the PG group.
- The excess weight loss was similar in both groups.

Reference:
- Di Lorenzo N, Furbetta F, Favretti F, et al. Laparoscopic adjustable gastric banding via pars flaccida versus perigastric positioning: technique, complications, and results in 2,549 patients. Surg Endosc 2010; 24(7):1519–1523 [Epub March 31, 2010].

8. **Answer: B.**

The IVC does not pass in between the two crura, but through the caval opening situated anterior to it. The IVC is present to the right of the right crus.

The surgeon may encounter the hepatic branch of the vagus and the aberrant left hepatic artery during initial incision of the pars flaccida.

The band should be placed with the lateral side at the angle of His.

The pars flaccida technique has a slippage rate of 1.4% compared to 25% slippage rate seen in the perigastric technique.

References:
- Fielding GA, Allen JW. A step-by-step guide to placement of the LAP-BAND adjustable gastric banding system. Am J Surg 2002; 184:S26–S30.
- Schirmer B, Schauer PR. Chapter 27: The surgical management of obesity. In: Brunicardi FC, Andersen DK, Billiar TR, et al., eds. Schwartz's Principles of Surgery. 9th ed. New York: McGraw-Hill, 2010. Available at: http://www. accessmedicine.com/content.aspx?aID=5032782.

- Di Lorenzo N, Furbetta F, Favretti F, et al. Laparoscopic adjustable gastric banding via pars flaccida versus perigastric positioning: technique, complications, and results in 2,549 patients. Surg Endosc 2010; 24(7):1519–1523 [Epub March 31, 2010].

9. **Answer: B.**

A noncoring Huber needle can be used to prime the Lap-Band in order to remove air from the system before placing the band.

The tubing is left free in the abdomen and not fixed. The 15-mm port incision is extended lateral and deep down to the rectus sheath. Narrow Deaver retractors facilitate this, as the sheath is often farther down than anticipated. The anterior fascia is incised approximately 2 cm lateral to the fascial defect. The tubing is connected to the access port, and, in turn, the access port is affixed to the fascia. This is accomplished by placing an Ethibond suture in each corner of the incised fascia and placing these into the four holes on the access port. The access port is then parachuted down onto the rectus sheath. The sutures are tied. The tubing is simply slid back into the abdomen, and the wounds are closed. Care is taken to prevent any acute kinking of the tubing. The band is left empty. An upper gastrointestinal (GI) radiograph using water-soluble contrast is performed the next morning to exclude gastric perforation, malposition, and obstruction. Once this is reviewed, the patient can be discharged.

A port fixation device by Ethicon Endo-Surgery, Inc. (Ohio, U.S.) has proved very useful for fixation of the port.

References:

- http://www.allergan.com.au/userfiles/file/LAP-BAND_AP_IFU.pdf. Accessed April 30, 2011.
- Fielding GA, Allen JW. A step-by-step guide to placement of the LAP-BAND adjustable gastric banding system. Am J Surg 2002; 184:S26–S30.

10. **Answer: D.**

The LAP-BAND AP System is contraindicated in the following:

1. Patients with inflammatory diseases of the GI tract, such as Crohn's disease.
2. Patients who are poor surgical candidates.
3. Patients with potential upper GI bleeding conditions such as esophageal or gastric varices or congenital or acquired intestinal telangiectasias.
4. Patients with portal hypertension.
5. Patients with congenital or acquired anomalies of the GI tract such as atresias or stenoses.
6. Patients who have/experience an intraoperative gastric injury during the implantation procedure, such as a gastric perforation at or near the location of the intended band placement.
7. Patients with cirrhosis.
8. Patients with chronic pancreatitis.
9. Patients who are addicted to alcohol and/or drugs.
10. Patients under 18 years of age.
11. Patients who have an infection anywhere in their body or where the possibility of contamination prior to or during the surgery exists.
12. Patients on chronic, long-term steroid treatment.
13. Patients who are unable or unwilling to comply with dietary restrictions.
14. Patients who are known to have, or suspected to have, an allergic reaction to materials contained in the system or who have exhibited pain intolerance to implanted devices.
15. Patients or family members with a known diagnosis or preexisting symptoms of autoimmune connective-tissue disease such as systemic lupus erythematosus or scleroderma.

16. Pregnancy: Placement of the LAP-BAND AP System is contraindicated for patients who currently are or may be pregnant. Patients who become pregnant after band placement may require deflation of their bands.

Reference:

- http://www.allergan.com.au/userfiles/file/LAP-BAND_AP_IFU.pdf. Accessed April 30, 2011.

11. **Answer: B.**

The usual length of the Roux limb is about 100 to 150 cm. For a super-obese patient, a longer Roux limb (about 200 cm) is used. Creating a gastric pouch based on the lesser curvature will minimize its dilation. It is beneficial to close all potential spaces that can lead to internal hernias including the defect at the jejunojejunostomy and the Petersen's defect in the retrocolic gastric bypass.

References:

- William BI, Eric JD, Ikramuddin S, eds. Laparoscopic Bariatric Surgery. Vol. 1. Philadelphia: Lippincott Williams & Wilkins, 2005.
- Quebbemann BB, Dallal RM. The orientation of the antecolic Roux limb markedly affects the incidence of internal hernias after laparoscopic gastric bypass. Obes Surg 2005; 15(6):766–770; discussion 770.

12. **Answer: C.**

The lengths of various limbs while doing a BPD are measured from the ileocecal valve.

The length of the common channel is about 50 to 100 cm. The alimentary channel has a length of 200 to 300 cm. A common channel of 100 cm is commonly used and has been shown to result in greater weight loss when compared to common channel of 150 cm.

In Scopinaro's BPD the distal cut end of the ileum is anastomosed to the posterior aspect of gastric pouch in an end-to-side fashion.

References:

- McConnell DB, O'rourke RW, Deveney CW. Common channel length predicts outcomes of biliopancreatic diversion alone and with the duodenal switch surgery. Am J Surg 2005; 189(5):536–540; discussion 540.
- Schirmer B, Schauer PR. Chapter 27: The surgical management of obesity. In: Brunicardi FC, Andersen DK, Billiar TR, et al., eds. Schwartz's Principles of Surgery. 9th ed. New York: McGraw-Hill, 2010. Available at: http://www.accessmedicine.com/content.aspx?aID=5032782.

13. **Answer: C.**

During insertion of a Lap-Band, electrocautery should be avoided in creating a retrogastric tunnel, and the retrogastric opening should not be enlarged much. Passage of the blunt instrument behind the stomach should be done without much effort as if "being passed through butter." Avoidance of force also avoids injury to the spleen during this step. Failure to create a new tunnel for the band during repositioning may lead to further slipping.

Reference:

- http://www.allergan.com.au/userfiles/file/LAP-BAND_AP_IFU.pdf. Accessed April 30, 2011.

14. **Answer: C.**

Adequate muscle relaxation is important in maintaining the pneumoperitoneum. This has to be checked by the anesthetist before an increase in CO_2 flow is done or another insufflator is connected to one of the trocars. Conversion to an open procedure would be a last resort.

15. **Answer: C.**

Since the introduction of the sleeve gastrectomy as a stand-alone bariatric procedure, the bougie size has been gradually reduced to 32 to 36 Fr. A tapered bougie should be avoided to prevent narrowing at the antrum. The gastroepiploic vascular branches are divided starting 4 to 6 cm from the pylorus till angle of His. Either detaching the greater omentum followed by gastric stapling or stapling the stomach first may be done.

Reference:
- Braghetto I, Korn O, Valladares H, et al. Laparoscopic sleeve gastrectomy: surgical technique, indications and clinical results. Obes Surg 2009; 17: 1442–1450.

16. **Answer: C.**

The staple line is begun 4 to 6 cm from the pylorus during a sleeve gastrectomy. Blunt-tipped bougie is preferred to a tapered bougie in order to prevent outlet obstruction due to distal narrowing of the sleeve. A vertical subtotal, sleeve gastrectomy is then fashioned along the lesser curvature alongside bougie toward the esophagogastric junction. This procedure is performed with multiple firings of a linear cutting stapler.

Staple line reinforcement can be used. Though it has been shown to decrease blood loss which is statistically significant, this has not been shown to decrease leak rates.

The volume of the gastric pouch is usually about 125 mL.

References:
- Consten EC, Gagner M, Pomp A, et al. Decreased bleeding after laparoscopic sleeve gastrectomy with or without duodenal switch for morbid obesity using a stapled buttressed absorbable polymer membrane. Obes Surg 2004; 14(10): 1360–1366.
- Yehoshua RT, Eidelman LA, Stein M, et al. Laparoscopic sleeve gastrectomy— volume and pressure assessment. Obes Surg 2008; 18:1083–1088.

17. **Answer: A.**

Though one study reported a greater stricture rate with circular stapled anastomosis (CSA), lesser time taken for linear stapled anastomosis (LSA) and hand-sewn anastomosis (HSA), and greater infection rate for CSA, these may be due to learning curve associated with the use of staples. No difference was noted in the anastomotic bleeding/leak rates in the same study. Most surgeons practice an antecolic antegastric approach.

The CSA can be performed by passing the stapler either transorally or through a gastrostomy. Robotic technology can be utilized for HSA.

References:
- Tinoco RC, Tinoco AC. Chapter 20: Laparoscopic gastric bypass: trans-oral circular stapling. In: Pitombo C, Jones K, Higa K, et al., eds. Obesity Surgery: Principles and Practice. 1st ed. New York: McGraw-Hill, 2007. Available at: http://www.accesssurgery.com/content.aspx?aID=142746.
- Gonzalez R, Lin E, Venkatesh KR, et al. Gastrojejunostomy during laparoscopic gastric bypass: analysis of 3 techniques. Arch Surg 2003; 138(2):181–184.

18. **Answer: D.**

If staple lines are crossed at approximately $90°$ angle, the risk of ischemia will be less, and if staple lines are parallel and less than 1 cm apart (the "1 centimeter rule"), or as the crossing staple lines approach parallel, there will be a higher risk of leakage.

Reference:
- Jones Jr., Kenneth B. Chapter 4: Current role of open bariatric surgery. In: Pitombo C, Jones K, Higa K, et al., eds. Obesity Surgery: Principles and Practice. 1st ed. New York: McGraw-Hill, 2007. Available at: http://www.accesssurgery.com/content.aspx?aID=145011.

19. **Answer: D.**

When a vertically oriented pouch is created, a 50-Fr blunt-tipped bougie may be placed along the lesser curvature and placed against the horizontal staple line. The stapler is repositioned in a vertical position along the bougie and fired to create a vertically oriented pouch. The use of an endoscopic ruler to measure a 5-cm pouch length results in a consistent pouch size of about 30 to 50 cc. The vagal nerve is usually spared during the creation of the gastric pouch.

Reference:
- Williams MD, Champion JK. Chapter 23: Laparoscopic gastric bypass: linear technique. In: Pitombo C, Jones K, Higa K, et al., eds. Obesity Surgery: Principles and Practice. 1st ed. New York: McGraw-Hill, 2007. Available at: http://www.accesssurgery.com/content.aspx?aID=142972.

20. **Answer: A.**

Laparoscopic bariatric surgery has a long learning curve. The learning curve seems to flatten after 100 procedures. Only operative times have been found to be an indicator of the learning curve in all studies so far. Schauer et al. showed that wound infection rates and leak rates decreased as the surgeon gained increasing experience. They did not find length of hospital stay or blood loss to be an indicator of learning curve. However, morbidity/reoperation/readmission were not found to be indicators of learning curve by Søvik et al. In another study, reoperations and complications were greater early in the learning curve. Mortality has also not been found to vary as a surgeon progresses through the learning curve. There is no consensus on how the learning curve influences outcomes in laparoscopic bariatric surgery. A systematic review did find a decrease in morbidity and mortality with formal training in laparoscopic bariatric surgery. However, the hospital stay did not change.

References:
- Sánchez-Santos R, Estévez S, Tomé C, et al. Training programs influence in the learning curve of laparoscopic gastric bypass for morbid obesity: a systematic review. Obes Surg 2011 Apr 1 [Epub ahead of print].
- Zacharoulis D, Sioka E, Papamargaritis D, et al. Influence of the learning curve on safety and efficiency of laparoscopic sleeve gastrectomy. Obes Surg 2011 May 12 [Epub ahead of print].
- Søvik TT, Aasheim ET, Kristinsson J, et al. Establishing laparoscopic Roux-en-Y gastric bypass: perioperative outcome and characteristics of the learning curve. Obes Surg 2009; 19(2):158–165 [Epub June 20, 2008].
- Schauer P, Ikramuddin S, Hamad G, et al. The learning curve for laparoscopic Roux-en-Y gastric bypass is 100 cases. Surg Endosc 2003; 17(2):212–215 [Epub December 4, 2002].
- Pournaras DJ, Jafferbhoy S, Titcomb DR, et al. Three hundred laparoscopic Roux-en-Y gastric bypasses: managing the learning curve in higher risk patients. Obes Surg 2010; 20(3):290–294 [Epub July 23, 2009].

21. **Answer: D.**

The CRT monitors provide the best resolution as of today although the LCD monitors are fast catching up.

It is not unusual to measure initial pressures (just after the gas is turned on) as high as 15 cm H_2O in morbidly obese patients. Thus, the insufflation apparatus has to function with high-pressure levels; 20 cm H_2O is enough for most bariatric operations carried out by laparoscopy, and this can be increased with the advice of an anesthesiologist. As surgical exposition depends on sustained abdominal distension, the flow capacity has to be high too (20–30 L/min maximum flow rate), since the amount of gas required to propel into a larger abdominal cavity to reach a fixed pressure is bigger.

Though warming of the injected gas may prevent endoscope fogging, there is no evidence, however, that it helps to avoid hypothermia unless the gas is humidified too. There is no consensus on the benefits of warm and humidified

CO_2 in laparoscopy as far as preventing hypothermia or reducing postoperative pain is concerned.

References:

- Milcent M, Loss A, Manso JE. Chapter 8: Intraoperative issues. In: Pitombo C, Jones K, Higa K, et al., eds. Obesity Surgery: Principles and Practice. 1st ed. New York: McGraw-Hill, 2007. Available at: http://www.accesssurgery.com/content.aspx?aID=147213.
- Hamza MA, Schneider BE, White PF, et al. Heated and humidified insufflation during laparoscopic gastric bypass surgery: effect on temperature, postoperative pain, and recovery outcomes. J Laparoendosc Adv Surg Tech A 2005; 15 (1):6–12.
- Champion JK, Williams M. Prospective randomized trial of heated humidified versus cold dry carbon dioxide insufflation during laparoscopic gastric bypass. Surg Obes Relat Dis 2006; 2(4):445–449; discussion 449–450.
- Sammour T, Kahokehr A, Hayes J, et al. Warming and humidification of insufflation carbon dioxide in laparoscopic colonic surgery: a double-blinded randomized controlled trial. Ann Surg 2010; 251(6):1024–1033.

22. **Answer: B.**

Recently, LESS surgery has been proposed to minimize the invasiveness of laparoscopic surgery. Some reports suggest a decreased pain medicine requirement following single-incision banding; however, to date, no randomized prospective trials have been completed to support any clear statistically significant advantages. The results of a comparative study have been summarized:

- There were no statistical differences for operative time, blood loss, pain score, or complication rates. Perioperative outcomes of LESS gastric banding are comparable with those of the standard LAGB procedure.
- Length of stay was shorter for the LESS.
- The mean operative cost for the LESS banding was $20,502/case versus $20,346/case for the standard LAGB, with no statistically significant difference between the approaches.

As a result, LESS surgery can be proposed as a valid alternative to the standard procedure with cosmetic advantage and comparable complication rate.

References:

- Ayloo SM, Buchs NC, Addeo P, et al. Traditional versus single-site placement of adjustable gastric banding: a comparative study and cost analysis. Obes Surg 2010 Aug 31 [Epub ahead of print].
- Raman SR, Franco D, Holover S, et al. Does transumbilical single incision laparoscopic adjustable gastric banding result in decreased pain medicine use? A case-matched study. Surg Obes Relat Dis 2011; 7(2):129–133.

23. **Answer: A.**

Most studies have shown an overall increased operative time and higher procedural cost. It takes some time to set up a robot and thus the time from start of the case to establishment of the pneumoperitoneum is increased. Robotically assisted BPD-DS has been found to be feasible, though time-consuming, by Sudan et al. who performed a robotically assisted duodenoileostomy. Robotic surgery has been shown to reduce operative time/BMI ratio.

References:

- Mühlmann G, Klaus A, Kirchmayr W, et al. DaVinci robotic-assisted laparoscopic bariatric surgery: is it justified in a routine setting? Obes Surg 2003; 13(6):848–854.
- Mohr CJ, Nadzam GS, Curet MJ. Totally robotic Roux-en-Y gastric bypass. Arch Surg 2005; 140(8):779–786.
- Sudan R, Puri V, Sudan D. Robotically assisted biliary pancreatic diversion with a duodenal switch: a new technique. Surg Endosc 2007; 21(5):729–733.

24. **Answer: E.**

The advantages of robotic surgery include articulating wrists, 3D view, motion scaling for precise hand movement, and mechanical forces to counteract the abdominal wall torque. Operative times have not been proven to be lower than conventional laparoscopic surgery.

References:
- Scozzari G, Rebecchi F, Millo P, et al. Robot-assisted gastrojejunal anastomosis does not improve the results of the laparoscopic Roux-en-Y gastric bypass. Surg Endosc 2011; 25(2):597–603 [Epub July 13, 2010].
- Ayloo SM, Addeo P, Buchs NC, et al. Robot-assisted versus laparoscopic Roux-en-Y gastric bypass: is there a difference in outcomes? World J Surg 2011; 35 (3):637–642.

8 | Complications

CHAPTER SUMMARY

- Roux-en-Y gastric bypass (RYGB):
  - Internal hernia:
    - The incidence of internal hernia after retrocolic laparoscopic RYGB is in the range of 3% to 5% in large series. The most common site of herniation is the transmesocolic defect.
    - Laparoscopic gastric bypass is believed to have a higher incidence of internal hernias when compared to open gastric bypass.
    - A retrocolic approach increases the risk for developing an internal hernia.
    - Nausea, emesis, and postprandial abdominal pain are the most common symptoms.
    - CT scan is the diagnostic method of choice. The CT film should also be reviewed by the surgeon who is more aware of the postoperative anatomy.
    - Signs on CT include small bowel loops in the left or right upper quadrant, evidence of small bowel mesentery traversing the transverse colon mesentery, and/or location of the jejunojejunostomy superior to the transverse colon, crowding, stretching, and engorgement of the main mesenteric trunk to the right. The "swirl sign" of the mesentery has a sensitivity between 60% and 83% for an internal hernia.
    - Prevention is by meticulous closure of the mesenteric defects.
    - Most internal hernias can be managed laparoscopically.
    - A Richter's hernia occurs at the port site and cannot be easily diagnosed without the use of oral contrast.
  - Leaks:
    - The incidence of leakage in various series is about 1% to 2%. The rate is higher with revisional surgery.
    - The majority of the leaks occur at the gastrojejunal anastomosis when compared to the jejunojejunal anastomosis.
    - Presentation can vary from peritonitis with vascular collapse to an insidious presentation with fever, malaise, and abdominal pain.
    - The upper GI contrast study does not diagnose distal leaks.
    - If a prophylactic drainage is placed, a leak can be detected by a change in the nature of the effluent. Prophylactic drains are recommended patients at high risk for a leak (e.g., revisional surgery).
    - Those who present with rapid deterioration require a laparotomy whereas patients presenting with an insidious presentation can usually be managed by percutaneous drainage.
    - A leak at the jejunojejunal anastomosis usually requires surgery.
    - Stenting (using self-expanding stents) a gastrojejunostomy (GJ) leak is also an option, with the advantage of continued intake by mouth.
  - Marginal ulcers:
    - Occurs in about 1% to 2% of RYGB patients.
    - Most common symptom is epigastric pain radiating to the back, and pain is the only symptom in about half of the patients. Bleeding occurs in about 20% of patients.
    - Can present with perforation.

- Patients who have *Helicobacter pylori* preoperatively are more likely to have marginal ulcers postoperatively. Treatment, however, reduces the incidence of marginal ulcers.
- Smoking and nonsteroidal anti-inflammatory drugs (NSAIDs) are important contributing factors. Others include alcohol use steroids and breakdown of the staple line in nondivided gastric pouch.
- Other etiological factors are controversial and include ischemia of the pouch, hand sewn versus stapled anastomosis, large gastric pouches, open approach to primary surgery, etc.
- The use of absorbable sutures decreases incidence of marginal ulcers.
- Gastrogastric fistula has to be suspected in the presence of a nonhealing marginal ulcer [one which does not respond to proton pump inhibitors (PPIs) for 3 to 6 months].
- Diagnosis is by endoscopy. Marginal ulcers are found on the jejunal side of the anastomosis.
- Bleeding ulcers can be cauterized.
- Dumping syndrome:
  - It has two forms: early dumping syndrome, occurring immediately after meal intake, and late dumping syndrome, occurring 1 to 3 hours after meal intake.
  - Early dumping syndrome is due to release of water into the duodenum after entry of hyperosmolar chyme. Late dumping is due to increased release of insulin.
  - Symptoms include nausea, bloating (gastrointestinal symptoms) and flushing, perspiration, lightheadedness, hypotension, fainting (vasomotor symptoms), etc.; symptoms of hypoglycemia are seen with late dumping.
  - Prevention is by intake of smaller meals and avoidance of water intake till 30 minutes after meal intake.
  - Medical treatment options include acarbose, somatostatin analogues, and diazoxide. Surgical treatment options include reversal of the RYGB or continuous enteral feeding in severe cases.
- Noninsulinoma pancreatogenous hypoglycemia syndrome:
  - β-cell hyperplasia in the pancreas that occurs after RYGB. GLP-1 is implicated.
  - Causes postprandial hypoglycemia and can be confused with dumping syndrome.
  - Insulinoma has to be ruled out first. Diagnosis can be confirmed by invasive test – celiac artery cannulation and selective arterial calcium stimulation test.
  - Treatment is by somatostatin analogues or calcium channel blockers. Total or subtotal pancreatectomy or reversal of RYGB is reserved for intractable cases.
- Gallstone disease:
  - According to a population-based study, the risk of gallstone disease is five times higher in bariatric patients when compared to the general population.
  - CT is more useful than ultrasound in bariatric patients for the diagnosis of gallstone disease.
  - The incidence of gallstones increases in the first few months after bariatric surgery due to rapid weight loss.
  - Postoperative ursodeoxycholic acid for 6 months decreases incidence of gallstones.
  - There is no consensus regarding the role of routine prophylactic cholecystectomy during a RYGB.

- Lap-Band:
  - Prolapse/slippage of band:
    - The rate of slippage with pars flaccida approach is around 1% to 2% and 13% to 14% for the perigastric technique.
    - Anterior slippage: Etiological factors include lack of anterior gastrogastric sutures, premature band inflation, hiatal hernia, and recurrent vomiting. On erect X ray, the band appears horizontal and the pouch eccentric and anterior to the band.
    - Posterior slippage: It is more common with perigastric approach that increases posterior mobility of the band, when compared to the pars flaccida approach. Erect X ray shows a vertically positioned band with an eccentric pouch posterior to the band.
        The first step is to deflate the band. This is followed by either repositioning of the band, which is associated with a high incidence of recurrence, or replacement of the band, or conversion to another bariatric procedure.
  - Erosion of Lap-Band:
    - Reported incidence is around 1%.
    - Usually presents within the first year.
    - Commonly presents with port-site infection (about 40% of cases). Other symptoms include epigastric pain and failure of weight loss. It can also be asymptomatic.
    - Upper GI contrast study can detect only late erosions. Endoscopy can detect early erosions too. CT scan can detect abscess.
    - Total intragastric migration can be treated by endoscopy by using a gastric band cutter.
    - Usual line of management is removal of the band with gastrorrhaphy. Replacement of the band or another bariatric procedure can be performed during the procedure although most surgeons prefer to do it after a few months.
- Sleeve gastrectomy:
  - Leaks:
    - The overall incidence of leaks is about 1% to 2%.
    - Leakage is more in the upper part of the staple line when compared to the lower part.
    - Tachycardia is the most important clinical sign.
    - Diagnosis is by upper GI contrast study or CT scan.
    - Management:
      - Enteral nutrition by jejunostomy or nasojejunal tube.
      - Proximal leaks should be managed by stenting and insertion of a drain.
      - Distal staple line leaks should be managed by suturing and insertion of drain.
  - Bleeding:
    - The rate of clinically significant bleeding is about 1%.
    - Reinforcement of the staples used for creating the sleeve has been shown to decrease postoperative bleeding.
    - Diagnosis is by CT scan.
    - Can present as intra-abdominal septic collections within a week after surgery.
    - Treatment: blood transfusion, CT-guided drainage, rarely surgery.
  - Stricture/Obstruction of the sleeve:
    - Stricture after sleeve gastrectomy is related to oversewing the staple lines.
    - It can present either immediately after surgery or later.

- Common symptoms include intolerance to food and vomiting but can also present as gastroesophageal reflux.
- Diagnosis is made by upper GI contrast study or by endoscopy. There is no standardized definition, but inability to pass a 9.8-mm endoscope is generally considered a stricture.
- Obstruction during the immediate postoperative period is usually due to mucosal edema. Kinking of the sleeve can also result in obstruction – kinking has been related to oversewing of the sleeve.
- Ischemia of the pouch with scarring has been implicated in chronic strictures.
- Technical steps to avoid strictures: keep the bougie in place while oversewing, preserve the left gastric artery branches to avoid ischemia, maintain an even staple line thus avoiding twisting of the sleeve.
- Pneumatic dilation and use of covered stents have been shown to be feasible for strictures. For obstruction presenting in the early postoperative period, laparoscopy with cutting of the sutures or removal of hematoma should be done depending on the suspected cause. Seromyotomy has been described for long strictures. Strictureplasty has also been proposed as an option for intractable strictures of the sleeve.
- Biliopancreatic diversion
- Wound infection:
  - Wound is the most common site of infection in the post–bariatric surgery patient.
  - Antibiotic prophylaxis should be given only before incision.
- Pulmonary venous thromboembolism in bariatric surgery:
  - There is no good evidence regarding the efficacy of prophylactic anti-coagulation in bariatric surgery patients.
  - The use of sequential compression devices with or without pharmacologic methods is recommended in bariatric surgery patients.
  - The role of inferior vena cava (IVC) filters in high-risk bariatric patients is not clear.
  - It is reasonable to continue anticoagulation in high-risk patients after discharge as thromboembolic events have been reported as late as 1 month after discharge.
  - Higher doses of unfractionated heparin or low–molecular weight heparin (LMWH) may be necessary in bariatric patients for more effective anti-coagulation.
  - Laparoscopic bariatric surgery has a lesser incidence of venous thromboembolism when compared to open surgery.
  - Pulmonary embolism (PE) is one of the most common cause of mortality after bariatric surgery.
- Mortality due to bariatric surgery:
  - The mortality of laparoscopic restrictive procedures is about 0.1%.
  - The mortality rate of laparoscopic RYGB is about 0.2%.
  - The mortality rate of open RYGB is about 0.5%.
  - Mortality rate for laparoscopic biliopancreatic diversion (BPD) (or duodenal switch, DS) is 1% to 2%.

QUESTIONS

1. Sleeve gastrectomy is a relatively novel surgical procedure and ways of minimizing its complications and managing them are still under study. Identify the <u>TRUE</u> statement about complications after sleeve gastrectomy.
   A. Oversewing of staple line is related to increased incidence of strictures.
   B. Decreasing bougie size from 60 Fr to 36 Fr increases the number of strictures.
   C. Buttressing of the staple line decreases leakage.
   D. A leak can easily be managed by stenting in most cases.
   E. The leakage occurs equally commonly in the two ends of the staple line.

2. Internal hernias are very difficult to diagnose in a patient status post gastric bypass. Which of the following items does <u>NOT</u> support the diagnosis of internal hernia?
   A. A history if intermittent, severe epigastric pain
   B. A "swirl sign" on CT scan
   C. Pain out of proportion to physical examination
   D. Hematemesis

3. Identify the <u>FALSE</u> statement about internal hernias occurring after RYGB.
   A. Mesenteric hernia at the Petersen's defect is more common when compared to hernia at the jejunojejunostomy after retrocolic gastric bypass.
   B. Transmesocolic hernia is more common than a Petersen's hernia after retrocolic gastric bypass.
   C. Surgeon's review of radiological films may be more accurate than the radiologist's report in the diagnosis of internal hernia.
   D. Antecolic RYGB has a lower incidence of internal hernia when compared with a retrocolic RYGB.

4. A patient wants information regarding anastomotic leakage after RYGB. Identify the <u>TRUE</u> statement about anastomotic leakage after RYGB.
   A. The jejunojejunostomy accounts for half the incidence of anastomotic leakage after RYGB.
   B. Hand-sewn anastomosis has a lower incidence of anastomotic leakage compared to stapled anastomosis.
   C. A hypotensive patient with leakage should be taken to the OR to try to control sepsis.
   D. Leaks after RYGB have a high (90%) mortality irrespective of timely management.

5. A 45-year-old woman comes to the emergency room with severe central chest pain. EKG and enzyme levels are not suggestive of cardiac ischemia. On further probing, the patient reveals history of food intolerance in the recent past and history of gastric banding surgery 5 months ago. Examination shows left upper quadrant tenderness but no frank signs of peritonitis. An emergency UGI study showed that there was a fairly large portion of the stomach above the band and the band was in a vertical position. Identify the <u>TRUE</u> statement about the diagnosis:
   A. The patient has a posterior prolapse and needs emergent surgery after decompression of the band.
   B. The patient has an anterior prolapse and needs emergent surgery after decompression of the band.
   C. The patient has an anterior prolapse and can be initially managed conservatively.
   D. The patient has a pouch dilation and needs revision after decompression of the band.

6. **A 45-year-old white female presents 10 months s/p LAGB with pain, redness, and tenderness at the port site. A small portion of the band is visible in the stomach on upper GI endoscopy. Which of the following is <u>TRUE</u> regarding this complication of gastric banding?**
   A. The patient usually rapidly deteriorates.
   B. Endoscopy is not only useful for diagnosis but can also be therapeutic.
   C. It never presents as intra-abdominal abscess.
   D. Both upper GI contrast study and upper endoscopy are equally effective in detecting early erosions.

7. **A 35-year-old female presents to the surgeon for a routine checkup 2 years after a LRYGB. She complains of chronic abdominal pain and postprandial vomiting for the past 6 months. She was also diagnosed with marginal ulcers by endoscopy 6 months ago. Examination reveals pale mucous membranes. Patient complains that the pain is not improved despite PPI treatment for the past 6 months. Patient is also a chronic smoker and is trying to quit. Patient refuses a barium swallow study as she has severe nausea and vomiting during two previous attempts at the same. Esophagogastroduodenoscopy (EGD) shows marginal ulcers with an isolated raised red spot high on the fundus. Nevertheless, she has had good weight loss over the past year. Which of the following is the <u>NEXT</u> best step in management?**
   A. Continue PPI, ask her to stop smoking and add *H. pylori* treatment
   B. Remnant gastrectomy
   C. Endoscopic treatment
   D. Redo gastrojejunostomy

8. **The longitudinal assessment of bariatric surgery is an NIH-funded multicenter study that has been designed with the aim of elucidating the short- as well as the long-term outcomes of bariatric surgery. Though an ongoing study, some results with regard to the short-term outcomes have been recently published. Identify the <u>FALSE</u> statement about short-term complications of bariatric surgery.**
   A. Open gastric bypass has a higher mortality when compared to the laparoscopic gastric bypass.
   B. Laparoscopic gastric bypass has a lower incidence of tracheal reintubation or tracheostomy postoperatively.
   C. Sleep apnea is associated with an overall higher complication rate at 30 days.
   D. Laparoscopic gastric bypass has a higher incidence of PE or deep venous thrombosis (DVT).

9. **Dumping syndrome is well described after RYGB and many patients mistakenly think that "dumping" refers to diarrhea. Which symptom is highly suggestive of dumping syndrome?**
   A. Nausea
   B. Headache
   C. Abdominal fullness
   D. Fainting

10. **A 45-year-old African-American male presents 6 months after a gastric bypass with faintness, abdominal fullness, breathlessness, and weakness a few minutes after a meal. Which of the following is <u>FALSE</u> about the pathogenesis of his condition?**
   A. Rapid emptying of undigested food into the duodenum with fluid shift causing hemoconcentration and decreased intravascular volume.
   B. Increased release of GLP-1.
   C. There is a strong association between this condition and the release of neurotensin.
   D. There is a strong association between this condition and the release of vasoactive intestinal polypeptide (VIP).

11. **A 50-year-old woman presents 2 years post RYGB having lost a significant amount of weight and her BMI now is 30. She complains of dizziness and sweating 2 hours after eating a meal. The surgeon suspects late dumping syndrome and confirms it with a very low postprandial blood glucose 2 hours after ingestion of 75 g glucose. He asks her to undertake dietary modifications. She fails to respond to this and the surgeon starts her on subcutaneous octreotide t.i.d. and increases the dose appropriately. She fails to respond to this regimen even after 3 months. Insulin and c-peptide levels are normal. Imaging studies are unrevealing. What is the MOST APPROPRIATE next step?**
    A. Exploration for an insulinoma
    B. Selective arterial calcium stimulation test
    C. Reversal of RYGB
    D. Somatostatin scintigraphy

12. **Identify the TRUE statement about the treatment of dumping syndrome.**
    A. Long-acting octreotide unlike short-acting octreotide is not useful for dumping syndrome.
    B. Acarbose helps mostly late dumping but not early dumping symptoms.
    C. Octreotide is effective in ameliorating early but not late dumping syndrome.
    D. Plenty of liquid intake during a meal will prevent dumping symptoms.

13. **The gastric band erosion is a complication that is difficult to diagnose. Identify the TRUE statement about the problem of gastric band erosion.**
    A. It has an incidence of about 15%.
    B. The etiology is mostly related to patient-associated factors.
    C. It can be asymptomatic.
    D. Diagnosis of band erosion is usually made after 2 years.

14. **A 46-year-old male, whose BMI is 52, with no past medical history, undergoes a gastric bypass. On the second postoperative day, on morning rounds, appears to be anxious and is complaining of left shoulder pain and has difficulty catching his breath. Vital signs recorded by the nurse 2 hours ago were as follows: heart rate 100/min, BP 130/70 mmHg, respiratory rate 16/min, and oxygen saturation 98% on room air. Now his heart rate is 124/min, BP is 100/70 mmHg, respiratory rate is 28/min, and oxygen saturation is 88% despite 4 L nasal oxygen supplementation. Abdominal examination reveals tenderness mostly around the port sites but no distension or guarding. EKG is normal. Which of the following is the NEXT best step?**
    A. Immediate surgical exploration
    B. Upper GI series
    C. Obstructive series (chest film, KUB, upright abdomen)
    D. CT angiogram of chest, with abdomen, pelvis
    E. Reassurance of patient and medication with benzodiazepines

15. **In the same patient as above, a CT angiogram of the chest was performed that showed no PE but did reveal a left-sided pleural effusion. Free air was noted on abdominal CT scan. An upper GI contrast series was ordered and was negative. The tachycardia and tachypnea persist and the BP now is 90/50 mmHg. Otherwise, the exam is unchanged but the patient is becoming increasingly worried. In addition to resuscitating the patient with fluids after placing a central venous access and starting broad spectrum antibiotics, what is the IMMEDIATE NEXT step?**
    A. Immediate surgical exploration
    B. Reassurance of patient and medication with benzodiazepines
    C. Placement of left chest tube
    D. Get a GI consult for a possible stenting of the leak
    E. Placement of a percutaneous abdominal drain

16. **A 45-year-old female patient has vomiting 5 days post RYGB. She visits her bariatric surgeon and complains that she has been vomiting continuously over the past 24 hours. On examination she appears dehydrated and has normal vitals. What should the surgeon do initially?**
    A. Admit her and give IV fluids
    B. Do endoscopy
    C. UGI series
    D. Give metoclopramide
    E. Reoperate

17. **Diagnosing a small bowel obstruction (SBO) in a post-RYGB patient is a challenge. This leads to delayed intervention and associated morbidity. Identify the FALSE statement about SBO occurring after RYGB.**
    A. Bilious vomiting is never seen in a post-RYGB patient.
    B. Presence of air fluid levels on abdominal radiograph is not required to diagnose SBO.
    C. Internal hernia is the most common cause of SBO in retrocolic gastric bypass.
    D. CT scan is the first line of investigation.

18. **A 55-year-old patient is seen by his bariatric surgeon for regain of weight and epigastric discomfort 4 years after a RYGB. The surgeon does an endoscopy and finds a stomal diameter of 30 mm. What is TRUE about his next step in management?**
    A. Do a revision surgery as it is the only choice available.
    B. The plicating device has been shown to cause loss of >50% of the weight regained as a result of stomal dilation (at 6 months).
    C. Use of sclerotherapy does not produce weight loss but the weight gain stabilizes.
    D. Transoral sutured revision has been shown to reduce stomal diameter.

19. **A patient presents status post RYGB with vomiting. Upper GI contrast study reveals delayed emptying of the gastric pouch. Stomal stenosis is suspected. Identify the TRUE statement about stomal stenosis occurring after RYGB.**
    A. It has maximum incidence about 3 years after gastric bypass.
    B. Its most common symptom is vomiting.
    C. The incidence of stomal stenosis is about 1%.
    D. The stenosed stoma is dilated up to 20 mm.

20. **A 36-year-old Latin American patient comes to the clinic complaining of epigastric pain and nausea a year after a gastric bypass. An upper endoscopy finds marginal ulcers at the GJ. No physical cause for the ulcer was identified at endoscopy. The patient's history is significant for osteoarthritis. Labs reveal Hb of 14 and normal liver and renal function tests. What is the NEXT best step in management?**
    A. Revise the gastrojejunal anastomosis.
    B. Place patient on PPI.
    C. Repeat endoscopy in 3 months.
    D. Enquire about the patient's lifestyle and drug intake and put her on PPI.

21. **A patient who underwent a gastric bypass 2 years ago and has been treated for a marginal ulcer for 3 months presents to the office for follow-up. She has been successful in quitting smoking. On further questioning she confides that she has had black stools for the past 3 weeks. Routine labs reveal a hemoglobin of 7. Her stool test is positive for fecal occult blood. Endoscopy reveals marginal ulcer with stigmata of recent hemorrhage at the same site as seen previously. What is the NEXT step in the management?**
    A. Evaluate the bypassed stomach.
    B. Revise the GJ.

    C. Do endoscopy and cauterize the ulcer.

    D. Proceed to arteriographic embolization.

22. **A 35-year-old patient who is 2 years post RYGB presents with black tarry stools. An upper endoscopy and colonoscopy do not reveal any source of bleeding. The next day this progresses to bright red bleeding per rectum. Bleeding from stomach remnant is suspected but percutaneous access fails due to overlying bowel loops. Shortly later, the patient deteriorates with vitals reveal HR 120 and BP 80/60 despite aggressive fluid resuscitation with normal saline and cross-matched packed RBCs. What is the <u>NEXT</u> step in management?**

    A. Perform a laparotomy.

    B. Perform a laparoscopy and resect as much of the gastric remnant as possible.

    C. Perform a diagnostic laparoscopy and pass an endoscope through a gastrostomy.

    D. Carry out a virtual gastroscopy using CT scan.

    E. Proceed to arteriography and embolization.

23. **Prophylactic IVC filter insertion is sometimes used in high-risk bariatric surgical patients, though the practice is not evidence based. Identify the <u>FALSE</u> statement about IVC filter insertion as a prophylaxis in bariatric surgery patients.**

    A. The groin approach is a more successful approach in bariatric surgery patients.

    B. Only retrievable filters are recommended to be used.

    C. There is no clear data to date to convincingly recommend prophylactic IVC filters in any patient without a contraindication to anticoagulation.

    D. IVC thrombosis is a known complication of the filter.

24. **Marginal ulcer is one of the commoner complications that occur after a RYGB. Identify the <u>FALSE</u> statement regarding marginal ulcers after RYGB.**

    A. Smoking is an important risk factor.

    B. Hand-sewn anastomoses are associated with an increased incidence of marginal ulcers.

    C. Nonabsorbable sutures have the same incidence of stomal ulcers when compared to absorbable sutures.

    D. Patients who test positive for *H. pylori* preoperatively and are treated have a decreased incidence of marginal ulcers when compared to those who are not treated.

25. **Hiatal hernia is commonly seen at time of placement of gastric band. Identify the <u>FALSE</u> statement about the problem associated with performing a gastric band in a patient with hiatal hernia/gastroesophageal reflux disease (GERD).**

    A. Hiatal hernia has higher risk of gastric prolapse and pouch dilation in a post-LAGB patient.

    B. Hiatal hernia if repaired at the time of band insertion decreases the overall rate of reoperation.

    C. Pouch formation is related to development of reflux symptoms after LAGB.

    D. Overall, LAGB does not improve reflux.

26. **The risk of gallstone formation increases after bariatric surgery. Which of the following about gall stones is <u>TRUE</u>?**

    A. The risk of cholecystitis rises after bariatric surgery.

    B. Concomitant cholecystectomy is not recommended due to greater morbidity of the combined procedure.

    C. CT cholecystography is as sensitive as ultrasonography (USG) to detect gall stones in bariatric surgery patients.

    D. About 90% of the patients who develop problems due to gallstones present with within 3 months after surgery.

27. **A 55-year-old patient who had undergone RYGB 4 months ago comes to the clinic with bloating, epigastric fullness, and occasional pain over upper abdomen associated with meals. A suspicion of gall stones is made and confirmed with USG. Which of the following statements about gall stones after bariatric surgery is FALSE?**
    A. Weight loss more than 25% is the most important predictor of development of gall stones after bariatric surgery.
    B. Prophylactic cholecystectomy increases incidence of postoperative complications after gastric bypass.
    C. There is no consensus on the rate of symptomatic gallstone disease after bariatric surgery.
    D. The usual duration of prophylactic ursodioxycholic acid (UDCA) therapy in postbariatric patients is about 6 months.

28. **A patient with BMI 50 kg/m² is scheduled for laparoscopic gastric bypass. He reports occasional epigastric pain with meals along with bloating. He also had an episode of severe pain about 3 days ago, which lasted intermittently for about 3 hours and radiated to the interscapular area and was associated with nausea and vomiting. Gallstones are suspected and are confirmed by an ultrasound that shows a 2 cm gallstone. What would be the best line of management?**
    A. Perform a laparoscopic cholecystectomy first.
    B. Perform the gastric bypass first and do laparoscopic cholecystectomy after 6 months.
    C. Do a cholecystectomy during gastric bypass.
    D. Perform a gastric bypass and place the patient on ursodiol postoperatively.

29. **A patient who has undergone laparoscopic gastric banding calls your office. She ate a hot dog and was throwing up a day ago but also casually tells you her port incision was red and her primary care physician opened the wound to reveal pus. She is now packing this and is taking amoxicillin–clavulanic acid. On visit to the office, the bariatric surgeon notices severe inflammation at the port site. He deflates the band. What should be done as a part of IMMEDIATE management of this condition?**
    A. Remove the access port.
    B. Get a CT scan of abdomen.
    C. Continue broad spectrum antibiotics.
    D. Perform an upper GI endoscopy to rule out band erosion.
    E. All of the above.

30. **There are several types of adjustable gastric bands available. The two leading brands are the Lap-Band® and the Realize® band. They differ in the technical aspects. Which is TRUE regarding the differences between these band systems?**
    A. Swedish adjustable gastric band is a low-pressure, low-volume device.
    B. The 10-cm version of the Lap-Band was a high-pressure, low-volume device.
    C. A higher incidence of gastric erosion is seen in Lap-Band.
    D. A lower incidence of band slippage is seen in Realize band.

31. **Obese patients are known to be more predisposed to postoperative wound infection, which is a major problem with open bariatric surgery. Identify the FALSE statement about postoperative wound infection in bariatric surgery.**
    A. There is no evidence to give postoperative antibiotics.
    B. Use of circular staplers can enhance rate of port-site infection if adequate precautions are not taken.
    C. The operative wound site is the most common site of infection in bariatric surgery patients.
    D. Diabetes has been definitively shown as an independent predictor for risk of infection after bariatric surgery.

32. **Wound infection is an important cause of morbidity after bariatric surgery. Identify the <u>TRUE</u> statement about the same issue.**
   A. *Staphylococcous aureus* is the most frequently isolated organism.
   B. It is most likely to occur 2 days after surgery.
   C. The incidence of wound infection after open bariatric surgery is <1%.
   D. Wound infection has no influence on rate of formation of incisional hernia in bariatric surgery patients.

33. **Prevention of wound infection in a bariatric surgical patient is very important. Identify the <u>FALSE</u> statement about prophylaxis of wound infection in bariatric surgery.**
   A. If vancomycin is used, its dosage should be calculated based on actual body weight.
   B. Therapeutic concentrations of the antibiotic will not be obtained by usual doses of cefazolin in super obese patients.
   C. Topical antibiotics used along with intravenous antibiotics are the standard of care in prevention of wound infection after bariatric surgery.
   D. Prophylactic antibiotics prevent not only wound infections but also other infections in open bariatric surgery patients.

34. **A patient presents to the bariatric surgeon 5 months status post LRYGB. He now has a BMI of 34. He complains of right upper quadrant abdominal pain and vomiting for the past 3 days. USG shows stones in the common bile duct (CBD) and none in the gallbladder. Erect X ray shows multiple air fluid levels and no free air under the diaphragm. Labs show elevated direct bilirubin and alkaline phosphatase (ALP) of 300. Which of the following is <u>NOT</u> appropriate?**
   A. Do a CT scan as internal hernia is also suspected.
   B. Use a laparoscopic approach to treat this patient's problems.
   C. Do endoscopic retrograde cholangiopancreatography (ERCP) first as his obstruction can be treated conservatively for 24 hours.
   D. Do a magnetic resonance cholangiopancreatography (MRCP) with concomitant MRI of abdomen.

35. **DVT and PE are important problems in obese patients undergoing any major surgery. Identify the <u>TRUE</u> statement about venous thromboembolism after bariatric surgery in the current era of use of antithrombotic drugs and laparoscopic techniques.**
   A. The incidence of DVT/PE in bariatric surgery patients is about 10%.
   B. Lower doses of unfractionated heparin should be used in obese patients.
   C. Venous thromboembolic events may occur even a month after discharge.
   D. There is good evidence about the efficacy of prophylactic anticoagulation from several randomized controlled trials in bariatric surgery.

36. **The increased incidence of urinary stones after bariatric surgery has been well recognized. Identify the <u>FALSE</u> statement about urinary stone formation after bariatric surgery.**
   A. Gastric banding does not result in an increase in the incidence of oxalate stones.
   B. Hyperoxaluria is common in malabsorptive bariatric surgery patients.
   C. High fat diet is recommended to prevent oxalate stones.
   D. The use of certain bacteria has been shown as a promising strategy for the prevention of oxalate stones in patients with hyperoxaluria.

37. **There are various causes of SBO after RYGB; internal hernias are considered an important cause. Identify the <u>TRUE</u> statement about SBO occurring after RYGB.**
   A. Laparoscopic gastric bypass has a decreased incidence of internal hernia when compared to open gastric bypass.

    B. Conservative management is not considered ideal in a patient with obstruction after laparoscopic gastric bypass.

    C. Obstruction due to internal hernias usually present within 30 days after LRYGB.

    D. Internal hernias always present as intermittent obstruction, not complete obstruction.

38. **Occurrence of Richter hernias at port sites after bariatric surgery is a concern. Identify the <u>TRUE</u> statement about Richter hernia.**
    A. It usually does not strangulate.
    B. It can be diagnosed easily without the use of oral contrast.
    C. It has an incidence of 10% after LRYGB.
    D. It presents early in the postoperative period.

39. **Postoperative bleeding is a complication that can occur after any surgery including RYGB. Identify the <u>TRUE</u> statement about a hematoma/bleeding occurring after RYGB.**
    A. Hematoma and infected collection can be distinguished from each other easily radiologically.
    B. Staple lines are the source of hemorrhage in most cases.
    C. It is not known to be a cause of bowel obstruction after RYGB.
    D. Angiography with embolization is a definitive treatment.

40. **Though NASH usually improves after bariatric surgery, it is known to worsen after malabsorptive procedures and especially with jejunoileal bypass. Which of the following has <u>NOT</u> been proposed as a factor underlying such worsening of hepatic function/histology?**
    A. Bacterial overgrowth in bypassed segment
    B. Malabsorption of nutrients
    C. Injury to the intestinal mucosal barrier
    D. Portal vein thrombosis (PVT)

41. **Venous stasis is a major problem in laparoscopic bariatric surgery patients as it can predispose to DVT. Identify the <u>FALSE</u> statement about the same.**
    A. The reverse Trendelenberg position has been shown to decrease femoral venous flow.
    B. The increased abdominal pressure has been shown to decrease femoral venous flow.
    C. Sequential compression devices are relatively ineffective in obese compared to nonobese patients.
    D. Sequential compression devices alone are not effective in preventing venous thomboembolism in obese patients undergoing bariatric surgery.

42. **A patient presents 5 years post biliopancreatic diversion with severe diarrhea and is found to have a decreased serum albumin. The primary care physician prescribes metronidazole for the diarrhea and gives him some dietary advice. He comes back 15 days later to say that he took the metronidazole tablets thrice a day for the past 2 weeks and now his diarrhea has resolved. On measuring serum albumin it was found to have normalized. What is the most likely mechanism behind this finding?**
    A. The patient had endogenous protein loss.
    B. Metronidazole stimulates protein synthesis in the liver.
    C. The patient probably decreased fat intake during the last 2 weeks.
    D. This is a laboratory error.

43. **Lateral femoral cutaneous nerve injury is common in bariatric surgery patients owing to the position on the operating table and the pressure exerted by their body. Identify the FALSE statement about the etiology and clinical presentation of meralgia paraesthetica.**
    A. Pain is aggravated by palpation lateral and superior to mid-inguinal point.
    B. It can be aggravated by flexion of thigh.
    C. It occurs because the nerve passes through the inguinal ligament rather than beneath it.
    D. It occurs because sometimes the nerve passes through the Sartorius muscle.

44. **Identify the FALSE statement about management/prevention of meralgia paraesthetica.**
    A. Conservative management is enough in most cases.
    B. Neurectomy is not a surgical option.
    C. Release and transposition is an option if a single nerve trunk is involved.
    D. Proper patient positioning during surgery can help prevent the condition.

45. **A 40-year-old female who had a retrocolic laparoscopic gastric bypass 12 months ago presents to the emergency room with intermittent crampy abdominal pain in the mid-abdomen, which is exacerbated by meals. She also has nausea and nonbilious vomiting. She is unable to tolerate liquids. On physical exam, she is afebrile, normotensive, and not tachycardic. She had 115-lb weight loss and now weighs 126 lb. Her mucous membranes are dry and she is mildly tender in the mid-abdomen. There are no peritoneal signs. Labs are all normal. A CT scan of the abdomen and pelvis demonstrates dilated loops of small intestine and a dilated excluded stomach. She is being hydrated with intravenous fluids. What is the NEXT best step in management?**
    A. Observation
    B. Diagnostic laparoscopy
    C. Upper GI endoscopy
    D. Upper GI contrast study

46. **Where is the problem most likely to be found?**
    A. Petersen's defect
    B. At a 12-mm port site
    C. Transverse mesocolon
    D. Jejunojejunostomy

47. **BPD-DS is not commonly performed partly owing to its high incidence of protein malnutrition, when compared with in a standard RYGB. Which of the following statements is FALSE regarding outcomes/complications of BPD-DS when compared to a BPD?**
    A. Heartburn is more prevalent in BPD-DS patients when compared to BPD patients.
    B. BPD-DS patients have a greater incidence of postoperative vomiting.
    C. BPD has a higher revision rate when compared to BPD-DS.
    D. Rate of inadequate weight loss is equal in both procedures.

48. **Duodenal switch was initially proposed as an improvement over BPD. Which of the following is NOT an advantage of the BPD-DS over the BPD?**
    A. Lower incidence of stomal ulcer
    B. Lower revision rate due to malnutrition
    C. Reduced incidence of dumping syndrome
    D. Lower mortality

ANSWER KEY

1. A	13. C	25. D	37. B
2. D	14. D	26. A	38. D
3. A	15. A	27. B	39. B
4. C	16. A	28. C	40. D
5. A	17. A	29. E	41. D
6. B	18. D	30. B	42. A
7. B	19. B	31. D	43. A
8. D	20. D	32. A	44. B
9. D	21. C	33. C	45. B
10. B	22. A	34. C	46. C
11. B	23. A	35. C	47. B
12. B	24. C	36. C	48. D

ANSWER KEY WITH EXPLANATION

1. **Answer: A.**

   Staple line oversewing rather than bougie size has been related to strictures. Staple line oversewing has been related to kinking of the sleeve.

   Buttressing a staple line with Gore Seamguard decreases only hemorrhage during stapling but not leakage. It has no effect on the operative time.

   The leakage rates are more common on the upper aspect of the staple line near the esophagogastric junction.

   Gastric leaks are more difficult to manage post sleeve gastrectomy compared to RYGB due to larger intragastric pressure and bile reflux in the former. Stenting of staple line leaks in gastric remnant after sleeve gastrectomy is tougher than RYGB as there is a greater incidence of stent migration. Stent migration occurs in about 42% of sleeve gastrectomy patients who have been stented after a staple line complication. The latter can be explained by the fact that a sleeve does not ensure proper containment of prosthesis.

   References:
   - Casella G, Soricelli E, Rizzello M, et al. Nonsurgical treatment of staple line leaks after laparoscopic sleeve gastrectomy. Obes Surg 2009; 19(7):821–826.
   - Dapri G, Cadiere GB, Himpens J. Reinforcing the staple line during laparoscopic sleeve gastrectomy: prospective randomized clinical study comparing three different techniques. Obes Surg 2010; 20(4):462–467.
   - Zundel N, Hernandez JD, Galvao Neto M, et al. Strictures after laparoscopic sleeve gastrectomy. Surg Laparosc Endosc Percutan Tech 2010; 20(3):154–158.
   - Casella G, Soricelli E, Rizzello M, et al. Nonsurgical treatment of staple line leaks after laparoscopic sleeve gastrectomy. Obes Surg 2009; 19:821–826.

2. **Answer: D.**

   The most common clinical symptom of internal hernia include intermittent, postprandial abdominal pain and/or nausea/vomiting (86%), although 20% have no abdominal tenderness. Classic SBO is only present in about 50% of cases. CT findings suggestive of internal hernia include small bowel loops in the left upper quadrant and evidence of small bowel mesentery traversing the transverse colon mesentery. The swirl sign of the mesentery is very suggestive of an internal hernia. Most repairs of the internal hernias can be performed laparoscopically without significant complications. Internal hernia is difficult to diagnose and hence patients have a long time to intervention after the onset of symptoms, which emphasizes that one needs to maintain a high index of suspicion for this complication.

References:

- Garza E Jr., Kuhn J, Arnold D, et al. Internal hernias after laparoscopic Roux-en-Y gastric bypass. Am J Surg 2004; 188(6):796–800.
- Higa KD, Ho T, Boone KB. Internal hernias after laparoscopic Roux-en-Y gastric bypass: incidence, treatment and prevention. Obes Surg 2003; 13(3):350–354.

3. **Answer: A.**

The most common sites of internal hernia after retrocolic gastric bypass include the transmesolic defect, jejunojejunostomy, and the Petersen's defect in the decreasing order of incidence. Surgeon's review of contrast-enhanced CT scans detected 100% of internal hernias whereas the radiologist was successful in detecting only about 40% in one series. This may be attributed to the surgeon's knowledge of altered anatomy after bariatric surgery. Antecolic roux limbs are associated with a lesser incidence of internal hernia due to avoidance of a defect in the transverse mesocolon.

References:

- Garza E Jr., Kuhn J, Arnold D, et al. Internal hernias after laparoscopic Roux-en-Y gastric bypass. Am J Surg 2004; 188:796–800.
- Morgan H, Chastanet R, Lucha PA Jr. Internal hernia after laparoscopic gastric bypass surgery: a case report and literature review. Postgrad Med 2008; 120(2): E01–E05.
- Patel RY, Baer JW, Texeira J, et al. Internal hernia complications of gastric bypass surgery in the acute setting: spectrum of imaging findings. Emerg Radiol 2009; 16 (4):283–289 [Epub December 17, 2008].
- Higa KD, Ho T, Boone KB. Internal hernias after laparoscopic Roux-en-Y gastric bypass: incidence, treatment and prevention. Obes Surg 2003; 13(3):350–354.
- Taylor JD, Leitman IM, Rosser JB, et al. Does the position of the alimentary limb in Roux-en-Y gastric bypass surgery make a difference? J Gastrointest Surg 2006; 10(10):1397–1399.

4. **Answer: C.**

In the series by Marshall et al., 62% of the patients developed leak at the GJ and 16% at the jejunojejunostomy. Gonzalez et al. reported similar incidence of leak rates as Marshall et al.

Stapled anastomosis has been shown to be similar to hand-sewn anastomosis as far as leaks are concerned, though stapled anastomosis has been associated with higher rates of other complications like marginal ulcers.

The management of a leak is based on the condition of the patient. An unstable sick patient needs to undergo emergent laparotomy. If the onset of leakage has been insidious, a percutaneous drain can be placed. If a drain is already in place and the patient is stable, he/she can just be treated on an outpatient basis.

The mortality of a leak is between 10% and 20%.

References:

- Almahmeed T, Gonzalez R, Nelson LG, et al. Morbidity of anastomotic leaks in patients undergoing Roux-en-Y gastric bypass. Arch Surg 2007; 142(10):954–957.
- Marshall JS, Srivastava A, Gupta SK, et al. Roux-en-Y gastric bypass leak complications. Arch Surg 2003; 138(5):520–523; discussion 523–524.
- Gonzalez R, Sarr MG, Smith CD, et al. Diagnosis and contemporary management of anastomotic leaks after gastric bypass for obesity. J Am Coll Surg 2007; 204 (1):47–55 [Epub November 17, 2006].
- Yurcisin BM, DeMaria EJ. Management of leak in the bariatric gastric bypass patient: reoperate, drain and feed distally. J Gastrointest Surg 2009; 13(9):1564– 1566 [Epub March 20, 2009].

5. **Answer: A.**

The first investigation usually ordered when a patient s/p gastric band surgery presents with food intolerance is a barium meal contrast X ray.

When a prolapse is diagnosed the band is decompressed.

In an anterior prolapse the band appears to be in the horizontal position or with the left side of the band lower than the right. It should be initially managed by decompression of the band. If conservative management fails, the band needs to be removed, replaced, or the slippage needs to be repaired.

In a posterior prolapse, the band appears to be in the vertical position. It has to be managed surgically by removal of the old band and reinsertion of a new one (replacement). As adhesions are common, reinsertion of a band may be very difficult. The patient also needs to be informed preoperatively that an alternative procedure like a RYGB or a sleeve gastrectomy will need to be considered depending on the intraoperative findings.

References:

- Sherwinter DA, Powers CJ, Geiss AC, et al. Posterior prolapse: an important entity even in the modern age of the pars flaccida approach to lap-band placement. Obes Surg 2006; 16(10):1312–1317.
- Abuzeid AW, Banerjea A, Timmis B, et al. Gastric slippage as an emergency: diagnosis and management. Obes Surg 2007; 17(4):559–561.

6. **Answer: B.**

Gastric band erosion usually presents with mild pain in abdomen or no symptoms. Other symptoms include weight regain, failure of weight loss, or a port-site infection (40%). It can also present as intra-abdominal abscess and liver abscess.

But a barium meal being noninvasive is performed first (as in this case). However, upper GI endoscopy can diagnose only late erosions. The diagnosis can be confirmed by endoscopy and band can also be removed by endoscopy in case of a total intragastric erosion. The operative approach is debated though laparoscopy has been shown to be feasible. Conversion to laparotomy may be necessary if dense adhesions are present. If the band is removed, the patient will have to undergo another bariatric procedure 6 to 8 months later. High leakage rates and infection may be seen if a bariatric procedure is attempted during the same operation. Some surgeons, however, have reported good results for another bariatric operation or insertion of a new band done at the time of band removal.

References:

- Cherian PT, Goussous G, Ashori F, et al. Band erosion after laparoscopic gastric banding: a retrospective analysis of 865 patients over 5 years. Surg Endosc 2010; 24(8):2031–2038 [Epub February 23, 2010].
- Hainaux B, Agneessens E, Rubesova E, et al. Intragastric band erosion after laparoscopic adjustable gastric banding for morbid obesity: imaging characteristics of an underreported complication. AJR Am J Roentgenol 2005; 184(1): 109–112.
- Rao RS, Kini SU. Gastric band erosion presenting as fibrinous exudative idiopathic pleuritis. Surg Obes Relat Dis 2011; Apr 13. [Epub ahead of print].
- Lattuada E, Zappa MA, Mozzi E, et al. Band erosion following gastric banding: how to treat it. Obes Surg 2007; 17(3):329–333.

7. **Answer: B.**

The patient most likely has a nonhealing marginal ulcer due to gastrogastric fistula. The patient needs an excision of the gastrogastric fistula with remnant gastrectomy. A nonhealing ulcer by definition does not respond to acid suppression for 3 to 6 months (which is the case here). It is standard practice to screen and eradicate *H. pylori* preoperatively. Hence, *H. pylori* is unlikely to cause marginal ulcers in this case. Asking her to stop smoking, though important, does not address gastrogastric fistula, which is the cause of a nonhealing marginal ulcer here.

Conservative management would be indicated in a patient with good weight loss if the symptoms resolve and marginal ulcer heals with PPI therapy, in which case long-term PPI treatment should be considered. Any patient with poor weight loss and gastrogastric fistula should undergo surgery.

A gastrogastric fistula is present more frequently on the lateral wall of the pouch and a redo of the GJ is usually not necessary. Endoscopic closure of a gastrogastric fistula by tissue apposition system has not met with much success. Other modalities like fibrin glue injection are also considered investigational at this point.

References:

- Stanczyk M, Deveney CW, Traxler SA, et al. Gastro-gastric fistula in the era of divided Roux-en-Y gastric bypass: strategies for prevention, diagnosis, and management. Obes Surg 2006; 16(3):359–364.
- Carrodeguas L, Szomstein S, Soto F, et al. Management of gastrogastric fistulas after divided Roux-en-Y gastric bypass surgery for morbid obesity: analysis of 1,292 consecutive patients and review of literature. Surg Obes Relat Dis 2005; 1 (5):467–474 [Epub August 31, 2005].
- Spaun GO, Martinec DV, Kennedy TJ, et al. Endoscopic closure of gastrogastric fistulas by using a tissue apposition system (with videos). Gastrointest Endosc 2010; 71(3):606–611 [Epub December 16, 2009].
- Salimath J, Rosenthal RJ, Szomstein S. Laparoscopic remnant gastrectomy as a novel approach for treatment of gastrogastric fistula. Surg Endosc 2009; 23 (11):2591–2595 [Epub May 22, 2009].

8. **Answer: D.**

Open gastric bypass has a 30-day mortality of 2.1% while that of laparoscopic gastric bypass is 0.2%. Laparoscopic gastric bypass has a tracheal reintubation rate of 0.4% and open bypass has a reintubation rate of 1.4%. Tracheostomies were needed more often with open gastric bypass when compared to the laparoscopic technique. Extremes of BMI, an inability to walk 200 ft, a history of deep vein thrombosis or venous thromboembolism, and a history of obstructive sleep apnea are independently associated with an increased rate of complications including death 30 days after surgery. Patients with BMI < 53 are associated with a higher probability of the composite end point (defined as death, deep vein thrombosis or venous thromboembolism, reintervention, or failure to be discharged by 30 days), although the confidence interval for this was found to be large. Laparoscopic gastric bypass has a lower incidence of PE and DVT when compared to open gastric bypass.

Reference:

- Longitudinal Assessment of Bariatric Surgery (LABS) Consortium; Flum DR, Belle SH, King WC, et al. Perioperative safety in the longitudinal assessment of bariatric surgery. N Engl J Med 2009; 361(5):445–454.

9. **Answer: D.**

Fainting or shock (hypotension) after an RYGB is the most suggestive of dumping syndrome. Other symptoms may include desire to sit down, breathlessness, weakness, sleepiness, palpitation, dizziness, headaches, restlessness, feeling of warmth, nausea, abdominal fullness, and borborygmus.

Reference:

- Sigstad H. A clinical diagnostic index in the diagnosis of the dumping syndrome. Changes in plasma volume and blood sugar after a test meal. Acta Med Scand 1970; 188(6):479–486.

10. **Answer: B.**

The scenario described is consistent with early dumping syndrome. Dumping syndrome has been attributed to entry of hyperosmolar food contents into the small bowel with resulting fluid shift into the small bowel. This causes symptoms like bloating, distension, borborygmi, and symptoms due to loss of intravascular volume (like dizziness and syncope). Since these symptoms are not relieved by administration of fluid, it is not known whether fluid sequestration is a cause or consequence of dumping syndrome.

It may also be due to splanchnic vasodilation and hypotension caused by release of neurotensin and VIP. These hormones also cause changes in GI motility and secretion.

Increased release of GLP-1 and thus insulin is responsible for late dumping syndrome that occurs 1 to 3 hours after a meal.

References:
- Tack J, Arts J, Caenepeel P, et al. Pathophysiology, diagnosis and management of postoperative dumping syndrome. Nat Rev Gastroenterol Hepatol 2009; 6:583–590.
- Eagon JC, Miedema BW, Kelly KA. Postgastrectomy syndromes. Surg Clin North Am 1992; 72(2):445–465 (review).

11. **Answer: B.**

RYGB is known to cause increased release of GLP-1. This is postulated to cause a proliferation of the β cells, which causes an increased release of insulin upon eating.

Nesidioblastosis or noninsulinoma pancreatogenous hypoglycemia syndrome is a differential diagnosis for late dumping syndrome after RYGB. One has to suspect this when dumping syndrome does not respond to standard treatment. After ruling out insulinoma, the diagnosis of nesidioblastosis can be confirmed only by invasive tests – celiac artery cannulation and calcium infusion. Increased insulin level in the hepatic venous blood confirms the diagnosis of nesidioblastosis. Venous insulin levels are found to be increased when multiple pancreatic arterial branches are stimulated individually, unlike in an insulinoma.

An insulinoma produces fasting not postprandial hypoglycemia. It has been ruled out by normal levels of insulin and c-peptide and negative imaging. Further management in this direction is not appropriate. Reversal of RYGB may be considered as an option after confirmation of nesidioblastosis.

References:
- Service GJ, Thompson GB, Service FJ, et al. Hyperinsulinemic hypoglycemia with nesidioblastosis after gastric-bypass surgery. N Engl J Med 2005; 353(3):249–254.
- Cummings DE. Gastric bypass and nesidioblastosis—too much of a good thing for islets? N Engl J Med 2005; 353(3):300–302.

12. **Answer: B.**

Somatostatin analogs like octreotide can retard the gastric emptying rate, retard transit through the small bowel, inhibit the release of gastrointestinal hormones, inhibit insulin secretion, and inhibit postprandial vasodilation. As such, these analogs show a broad range of activity against the full spectrum of symptoms of dumping syndrome. Both short- and long-acting octreotide are effective for preventing dumping symptoms. Short-acting octreotide may be more efficacious in preventing hypoglycemia. However, the long-acting form is more acceptable to patients. Acarbose prevents absorption of carbohydrates by inhibiting α-glucosidase enzyme on the mucosal brush border and as such would be effective only for late dumping syndrome. Liquid intake is not recommended until 30 minutes after a meal in order to avoid dumping symptoms in post-RYGB patients.

Reference:
- Tack J, Arts J, Caenepeel P, et al. Pathophysiology, diagnosis and management of postoperative dumping syndrome. Nat Rev Gastroenterol Hepatol 2009; 6: 583–590.

13. **Answer: C.**

Gastric erosion has an incidence of about 1%, occurring after a mean period of 1 to 1½ years. A systematic review reported an incidence of 1.46%. Though the exact etiology is not known, it is suspected to be related to surgeon-associated factors.

These include undetected stomach wall damage or microperforation during the initial LAGB operation, cautery injuries, instruments passing through the stomach, and the tension created from the gastrogastric sutures. Patients most often present with cessation of weight loss, weight regain, increased hunger, and/or decreased satiety, frequently combined with abdominal pain. It can also be asymptomatic though it is relatively rare (0.03% in a systematic review). Up to 90% of the Band erosions present within 2 years of insertion.

References:
- Egberts K, Brown WA, O'Brien PE. Systematic review of erosion after laparoscopic adjustable gastric banding. Obes Surg 2011; 21(8):1272–1279.
- Cherian PT, Goussous G, Ashori F, et al. Band erosion after laparoscopic gastric banding: a retrospective analysis of 865 patients over 5 years. Surg Endosc 2010; 24(8):2031–2038.
- Neto MP, Ramos AC, Campos JM, et al. Endoscopic removal of eroded adjustable gastric band: lessons learned after 5 years and 78 cases. Surg Obes Relat Dis 2010; 6(4):423–427.

14. **Answer: D.**

The patient can have a pulmonary embolus or an anastomotic leak. A CT scan of the chest with pulmonary angiography is done and the CT is extended to the abdomen and pelvis. The latter can help diagnose a leak. Upper GI series is not sensitive for detection of a leak. Moreover, the diagnosis of pulmonary embolus as well as leak can be made with a CT scan.

References:
- Carter JT, Tafreshian S, Campos GM, et al. Routine upper GI series after gastric bypass does not reliably identify anastomotic leaks or predict stricture formation. Surg Endosc 2007; 21(12):2172–2177.
- Arteaga JR, Huerta S, Livingston EH. Management of gastrojejunal anastomotic leaks after Roux-en-Y gastric bypass. Am Surg 2002; 68(12):1061–1065.
- Kendrick ML, Dakin GF. Surgical approaches to obesity. Mayo Clin Proc 2006; 81 (10 suppl):S18–S24.

15. **Answer: A.**

The patient has a leak at the GJ with accompanying sepsis. Therefore, the patient needs surgical exploration. Nonoperative management with percutaneous abdominal drain or chest tube is not advisable for a hypotensive patient. Stenting has a place in a stable patient especially presenting later in the postoperative period. An upper GI contrast is not sensitive for leaks. This is a surgical emergency and reassurance of the patient should not be done.

References:
- Carter JT, Tafreshian S, Campos GM, et al. Routine upper GI series after gastric bypass does not reliably identify anastomotic leaks or predict stricture formation. Surg Endosc 2007; 21(12):2172–2177.
- Arteaga JR, Huerta S, Livingston EH. Management of gastrojejunal anastomotic leaks after Roux-en-Y gastric bypass. Am Surg 2002; 68(12):1061–1065.
- Kendrick ML, Dakin GF. Surgical approaches to obesity. Mayo Clin Proc 2006; 81 (10 suppl):S18–S24.

16. **Answer: A.**

Most cases of intractable vomiting after RYGB are due to stomal edema and will resolve with conservative management with IV fluids. Further investigation is indicated if the vomiting does not subside.

17. **Answer: A.**

Air fluid levels may not be seen when the obstruction is in the bypassed segment. Hence, a CT is done. The patient with a Roux limb obstruction will typically report nausea, fullness, and midepigastric abdominal pain that is temporarily relieved by emesis. A biliopancreatic limb obstruction occurs only rarely, and will result in gastric distention with nausea, fullness, tachycardia, hiccoughs, and shoulder and back pain. Obstruction of the common limb can present with bilious emesis. Adhesions are the most common cause of SBO after open RYGB. The most common SBO seen after LRYGB is internal hernia as was seen in a very large series. On dividing their group into retrocolic and antecolic cohorts, Koppman et al. found that jejunojejunostomy stenosis was the most common cause of obstruction in antecolic LRYGB, while internal hernia remained the most common cause in retrocolic LRYGB. The incidence of internal hernia was three times higher in the retrocolic group when compared to the antecolic group.

References:
- Nelson LG, Gonzalez R, Haines K, et al. Spectrum and treatment of small bowel obstruction after Roux-en-Y gastric bypass. Surg Obes Relat Dis 2006; 2(3):377–383; discussion 383.
- Felsher J, Brodsky J, Brody F. Small bowel obstruction after laparoscopic Roux-en-Y gastric bypass. Surgery 2003; 134:501–505.
- Koppman JS, Li C, Gandsas A. Small bowel obstruction after laparoscopic Roux-en-Y gastric bypass: a review of 9,527 patients. J Am Coll Surg 2008; 206(3):571–584.

18. **Answer: D.**

Various options are available (none are well established, though) in addition to revisional surgery. Incisionless revision (plicating device) in patients with stomal stenosis has been shown to cause loss of 32% of weight regained at 6 months. After treatment with sclerotherapy, at ≥12 months, about 56% of patients lose weight, 34% have their weight stabilize, and 9% continue to gain weight. Transoral sutured revision has been shown to be effective in reducing stomal diameter. It also has been shown to cause some weight loss up to 16 months and only 50% of patients had a weight above their baseline weight at that time point. Overall, such approaches have not been found to be effective in producing durable weight loss.

References:
- Horgan S, Jacobsen G, Weiss GD, et al. Incisionless revision of post-Roux-en-Y bypass stomal and pouch dilation: multicenter registry results. Surg Obes Relat Dis 2010; 6(3):290–295 [Epub February 13, 2010].
- Spaulding L, Osler T, Patlak J. Long-term results of sclerotherapy for dilated gastrojejunostomy after gastric bypass. Surg Obes Relat Dis 2007; 3(6):623–626 [Epub October 23, 2007].
- Catalano M, Rudic G, Anderson A, et al. Weight gain after bariatric surgery as a result of a large gastric stoma: endotherapy with sodium morrhuate may prevent the need for surgical revision. Gastrointest Endosc 2007; 66(2):240–245.
- Ryou MK, Yu S, Greenwalt IT, et al. Transoral sutured revision of dilated gastrojejunostomy for treatment of weight regain in Roux-en-Y gastric bypass patients: a retrospective review of 243 procedures in 186 consecutive patients with 2 year Kaplan-Meier. Gastroenterology 2010; 138(5 suppl 1):S-511.
- Thompson CC, Slattery J, Bundga ME, et al. Peroral endoscopic reduction of dilated gastrojejunal anastomosis after Roux-en-Y gastric bypass: a possible new option for patients with weight regain. Surg Endosc 2006; 20:1744–1748.

19. **Answer: B.**

Stomal stenosis is a relatively common complication of RYGB occurring in up to 15% of the patients. Its most common symptom is vomiting. The mean postoperative incidence is about 2 months (range 1–6 months).

The stenosed GJ is dilated only to 12 to 15 mm in order prevent weight regain and dumping symptoms.

References:
- Ukleja A, Afonso BB, Pimentel R, et al. Outcome of endoscopic balloon dilation of strictures after laparoscopic gastric bypass. Surg Endosc 2008; 22(8):1746–1750.

- Pratt JSA. Chapter 25: Roux-en-Y Gastric Bypass: Stomal Stenosis. In: Nguyen NT, DeMaria EJ, Ikramuddin S, et al., eds. The Sages Manual. Vol. 4. New York: Springer, 2008:211–212.

20. **Answer: D.**

Before embarking on surgical treatment of marginal ulcers, the patient needs to be on PPIs + sucralfate for 3 months and all risk factors (smoking, alcohol, NSAIDs, etc.) have to be eliminated.

Reference:

- Shikora SA, Claros L, Kim JJ, et al. Chapter 38: Late complications: ulcers, stenosis, and fistula. In: Pitombo C, Jones K, Higa K, et al., eds. Obesity Surgery: Principles and Practice. Available at: http://www.accesssurgery.com/content. aspx?aID=144793.

21. **Answer: C.**

The patient's anemia stems from a chronic marginal ulcer refractory to medical management. Revision of the gastrojejunal anastomosis will ultimately be necessary, but cauterizing the ulcer as the next step will help stem further blood loss, and will allow time to optimize this patient for a complex operation. Although other sites of bleeding should be ruled out, angiographic embolization is indicated only for an acute and hemodynamically significant bleed. Evaluation of the bypassed stomach can be performed during the revisional operation.

References:

- Rasmussen JJ, Fuller W, Ali MR. Marginal ulceration after laparoscopic gastric bypass: an analysis of predisposing factors in 260 patients. Surg Endosc 2007; 21 (7):1090–1094.
- Carrodeguas L, Szomstein S, Soto F, et al. Management of gastrogastric fistulas after divided Roux-en-Y gastric bypass surgery for morbid obesity: analysis of 1,292 consecutive patients and review of literature. Surg Obes Relat Dis 2005; 1 (5):467–474.

22. **Answer: A.**

She is unstable and requires a laparotomy.

References:

- Ceppa FA, Gagné DJ, Papasavas PK, et al. Laparoscopic transgastric endoscopy after Roux-en-Y gastric bypass. Surg Obes Relat Dis 2007; 3(1):21–24.
- Silecchia G, Catalano C, Gentileschi P, et al. Virtual gastroduodenoscopy: a new look at the bypassed stomach and duodenum after laparoscopic Roux-en-Y gastric bypass for morbid obesity. Obes Surg 2002; 12(1):39–48.

23. **Answer: A.**

Neck approach may be easier in bariatric surgery patients as redundant folds of skin in the groin may pose a problem. Only retrievable filters are recommended to be used and with accumulating new data regarding retrievable filters, the use of permanent filters seems less favorable. According to American College of Chest Physicians, there is no clear data to date to convincingly recommend prophylactic IVC filters in any patient without a contraindication to anticoagulation.

Inferior vena cava thrombosis is a known complication of IVC filters.

References:

- Lee L, Taylor J, Munneke G, et al. Radiology-led follow-up system for IVC filters: effects on retrieval rates and times. Cardiovasc Intervent Radiol 2011 Jun 4 [Epub ahead of print].
- Geerts WH, Bergqvist D, Pineo GF, et al.; American College of Chest Physicians. Prevention of venous thromboembolism: American College of Chest Physicians Evidence-Based Clinical Practice Guidelines (8th Edition). Chest 2008; 133(6 suppl):381S–453S.
- Abou-Nukta F, Alkhoury F, Arroyo K, et al. Clinical pulmonary embolus after gastric bypass surgery. Surg Obes Relat Dis 2006; 2(1):24–28; discussion 29.

- Ingber S, Geerts WH. Vena caval filters: current knowledge, uncertainties and practical approaches. Curr Opin Hematol 2009; 16(5):402–406.
- http://www.guidelines.gov/content.aspx?id=15730. Accessed Jul 6, 2011.
- Proctor MC, Greenfield LJ. Form and function of vena cava filters: how do optional filters measure up? Vascular 2008; 16(1):10–16 (review).

24. **Answer: C.**

The etiology of marginal ulcers after RYGB has not been definitively identified. Hand-sewn anastomoses are associated with an increased incidence of mariginal ulcers. This is thought to be secondary to the submucosa becoming "bunched up" and resulting in ischemia.

Nonabsorbable sutures have a higher incidence of stomal ulcers when compared to absorbable sutures as was seen in a large study. Use of absorbable sutures for both layers of anastomosis further decreases the ulcer rate when compared to use of absorbable sutures for only the inner layer. Patients who test positive for *H. pylori* preoperatively and are treated have a decreased incidence of marginal ulcers when compared to those who are not treated. Smoking is a well-known risk factor for marginal ulcers.

References:
- Rasmussen JJ, Fuller W, Ali MR. Marginal ulceration after laparoscopic gastric bypass: an analysis of predisposing factors in 260 patients. Surg Endosc 2007; 21 (7):1090–1094 [Epub May 19, 2007].
- Sapala JA, Wood MH, Sapala MA, et al. Marginal ulcer after gastric bypass: a prospective 3-year study of 173 patients. Obes Surg 1998; 8(5):505–516.
- Capella JF, Capella RF. Gastro-gastric fistulas and marginal ulcers in gastric bypass procedures for weight reduction. Obes Surg 1999; 9(1):22–27; discussion 28.

25. **Answer: D.**

Overall, LAGB is accepted as an effective anti-reflux operation though long-term data are awaited. Some authors advised caution when performing gastric banding in the presence of a hiatal hernia as patients with a hiatal hernia have a higher risk of developing a pouch dilatation and band slippage that leads to a greater reoperation rate. Hiatal hernia repair added to a LAGB reduces the number of reoperations and causes a significant reduction in GERD symptoms. Pouch formation has been shown to be related to development of GERD symptoms after LAGB.

References:
- Angrisani L, Lovino P, Lorenzo M, et al. Treatment of morbid obesity and gastroesophageal reflux with hiatal hernia by Lap-band. Obes Surg 1999; 9 (4):396–398.
- de Jong JR, van Ramshorst B, Timmer R, et al. The influence of laparoscopic adjustable gastric banding on gastroesophageal reflux. Obes Surg 2004; 14(3): 399–406.
- Gulkarov I, Wetterau M, Ren CJ, et al. Hiatal hernia repair at the initial laparoscopic adjustable gastric band operation reduces the need for reoperation. Surg Endosc 2008; 22(4):1035–1041.

26. **Answer: A.**

It has been well established that gallstones are more prevalent among overweight people. In addition, the risk of cholecystitis is relatively high in patients after bariatric surgery as their rapid weight loss causes them to be stone formers. Cholecystitis in this setting is much more difficult to treat, and the morbidity and mortality are higher. Patients tend to develop gallstones within 6 months after surgery, the period of rapid weight loss. In one study, no cholecystectomies for gallstones were required in the first 3 months after surgery.

If concomitant cholecystectomy is decided, it has to be performed first as alteration of the gastric and intestinal anatomy may make management of any biliary complication more difficult.

Ultrasound has 50% sensitivity in diagnosing gallstones in the obese population. CT cholecystography has a sensitivity of 100% for gallstones, and a specificity of 100%.

References:
- Neitlich T, Neitlich J. The imaging evaluation of cholelithiasis in the obese patient-ultrasound vs CT cholecystography: our experience with the bariatric surgery population. Obes Surg 2009; 19(2):207–210.
- Colquitt JL, Picot J, Loveman E, et al. Surgery for obesity. Cochrane Database Syst Rev 2009; (2):CD003641.
- Caruana J, McCabe M, Smith A, et al. Incidence of symptomatic gallstones after gastric bypass: is prophylactic treatment really necessary? Surg Obes Relat Dis 2005; 1(6):564–567.

27. **Answer: B.**

The known risk factors for gallstone formation in the general population, such as age and female gender, may not help with the selection of post–bariatric surgery patients who require screening for gall stones. In a study by Vicki Ka Ming Li et al., only the postoperative factor of weight loss of more than 25% of original weight was found to be associated with symptomatic gallstone formation. Yang et al. also found the same factor was found to be the only risk factor for symptomatic gallstones after rapid weight loss using very low calorie diet.

The incidence of symptomatic gallstones after gastric bypass was about 8% in one study. Hence, some authorities argue that it would not be advisable to do a prophylactic cholecystectomy when 92/100 of them would have been unnecessary. Other reports put the rate of symptomatic gallstones at 5% to 40%. Since there is no consensus on the rate of symptomatic gallstone disease postoperatively, it is difficult to comment on the usefulness of prophylactic cholecystectomy. UDCA therapy is indicated during the period of rapid weight loss, which is the first 6 months after bariatric surgery, as this is the time the patients are at highest risk of gallstone formation. Prophylactic cholecystectomy, though increases the operative time and hospital stay, does not increase the postoperative complication rate. Thus, some authorities advocate routine prophylactic cholecystectomy.

References:
- Li VKM, Pulido N, Fajnwaks P. Predictors of gallstone formation after bariatric surgery: a multi variate analysis of risk factors comparing gastric bypass, gastric banding and sleeve gastrectomy. Surg Endosc 2009; 23:1640–1644.
- Escalona A, Boza C, Muñoz R, et al. Routine preoperative ultrasonography and selective cholecystectomy in laparoscopic Roux-en-Y gastric bypass. Why not? Obes Surg 2008; 18(1):47–51 [Epub December 15, 2007].
- Caruana JA, McCabe MN, Smith AD, et al. Incidence of symptomatic gallstones after gastric bypass: is prophylactic treatment really necessary? Surg Obes Relat Dis 2005; 1(6):564–567; discussion 567–568.
- Desbeaux A, Hec F, Andrieux S, et al. Risk of biliary complications in bariatric surgery. J Visc Surg 2010; 147(4):e217–e220.
- Inabnet WB, DeMaria EJ, Ikramuddin S. Laparoscopic Bariatric Surgery. Vol. 1. Philadelphia: Lippincott Williams & Wilkins, 2004.
- Yang H, Peterson GM, Roth MP, et al. Risk factors for gallstones formation during rapid loss of weight. Dig Dis Sci 1992; 37:912–918.

28. **Answer: C.**

The patient has symptomatic gallstones and hence should undergo a cholecystectomy during the gastric bypass. Some also advocate prophylactic cholecystectomy for asymptomatic stones detected preoperatively in a gastric bypass patient. Prophylactic cholecystectomy is usually not done in a patient undergoing restrictive surgery.

References:

- Sugerman HJ, Brewer WH, Shiffman ML, et al. A multicenter, placebo-controlled, randomized, double-blind, prospective trial of prophylactic ursodiol for the prevention of gallstone formation following gastric-bypass-induced rapid weight loss. Am J Surg 1995; 169:91–96.
- Worobetz LJ, Inglis FG, Shaffer EA. The effect of ursodeoxycholic acid therapy on gallstone formation in the morbidly obese patient during rapid weight loss. Am J Gastroenterol 1993; 88:1705–1710.
- Miller K, Hell E, Lang B, et al. Gallstone formation prophylaxis after gastric restrictive procedures for weight loss: a randomized double-blind placebo-controlled trial. Ann Surg 2003; 238:697–702.

29. **Answer: E.**

Port-site infection can manifest as port-site abscess or induration and uncommonly as cutaneous port erosion or port-cutaneous sinus. The abscess must be drained. In all cases, gastroscopy should be performed to rule out the possibility of band erosion. In addition, a CT scan of abdomen can diagnose intra-abdominal sepsis. The port will need to be removed when recurrent infection occurs. At operation, the tubing is cut as far from the site of infection as possible and the port is implanted in another area. If the infection is very severe, the port has to be removed and the tube is sealed, pushed into the abdomen, and sutured to the fascia to prevent it from lying free in the abdominal cavity. If gastric band erosion is diagnosed, the band has to be removed. Even if band erosion is diagnosed, the band can be removed by laparoscopy, although conversion to laparotomy may be required in the presence of dense adhesions.

References:

- Keidar A, Carmon E, Szold A, et al. Port complications following laparoscopic adjustable gastric banding. Obes Surg 2005; 15(3):361–365.
- bu-Abeid S, Bar ZD, Sagie B, et al. Treatment of intra-gastric band migration following laparoscopic banding: safety and feasibility of simultaneous laparoscopic band removal and replacement. Obes Surg 2005; 15(6):849–852.

30. **Answer: B.**

There is no difference in the complications between the two band systems. The old Lap-Band® was a high-pressure, low-volume device (though this has been changed to a higher-volume, lower-pressure system with the AP Lap-Band) and the Realize® band is a low-pressure, high-volume device.

References:

- Cunneen SA, Phillips E, Fielding G, et al. Studies of Swedish adjustable gastric band and Lap-Band: systematic review and meta-analysis. Surg Obes Relat Dis 2008; 4(2):174–185.
- Gravante G, Araco A, Araco F, et al. Laparoscopic adjustable gastric bandings: a prospective randomized study of 400 operations performed with 2 different devices. Arch Surg 2007; 142(10):958–961.

31. **Answer: D.**

Several studies have looked into factors predicting the risk of wound infection after bariatric surgery. BMI, diabetes, duration of surgery, and gender have been investigated as such predictive factors. However, there is no consensus on such predictive factors.

Circular staplers can lead to increased incidence of port-site infection. Hence, they need to be covered while withdrawing it from the abdomen and the wound needs to be irrigated. Wound is the most common site of infection followed by abdominal collections and urinary tract infections. There is no evidence to give postoperative antibiotics.

References:

- Christou NV, Jarand J, Sylvestre JL, et al. Analysis of the incidence and risk factors for wound infections in open bariatric surgery. Obes Surg 2004; 14(1): 16–22.
- Alasfar F, Sabnis A, Liu R, Chand B, et al. Reduction of circular stapler-related wound infection in patients undergoing laparoscopic Roux-en-Y gastric bypass, Cleveland clinic technique. Obes Surg 2010; 20(2):168–172 [Epub October 7, 2008].
- Ribeireiro T, Swain J, Sarr M, et al. NAFLD and insulin resistance do not increase the risk of postoperative complications among patients undergoing bariatric surgery-a prospective analysis. Obes Surg 2011; 21(3):310–315.

32. **Answer: A.**

Christou et al. found that the actual incidence of wound infection was 20%. Incidence of wound infection in other studies has ranged from 2% to 17%. Wound infection after bariatric surgery typically occurs 5 to 10 days after surgery and hence is not seen at the time of discharge.

   S. aureus is the most common pathogen and was seen in about 40% of infections. There is a high correlation between wound infection and subsequent incisional hernia formation.

References:

- Ferraz ÁA, Ferraz EM. Chapter 36: Infection in obesity surgery. In: Pitombo C, Jones K, Higa K, et al., eds. Obesity Surgery: Principles and Practice. Available at: http://www.accesssurgery.com/content.aspx?aID=144306.
- Christou NV, Jarand J, Sylvestre JL, et al. Analysis of the incidence and risk factors for wound infections in open bariatric surgery. Obes Surg 2004; 14 (1):16–22.

33. **Answer: C.**

Evaluating the cefazolin concentration in its action place, it was observed that therapeutic levels were obtained in less than 30% of the patients with BMI between 50 and 59 kg/m^2 and in only 10.2% of the patients with BMI equal or superior to 60 kg/m^2. The dosage of antibiotic prophylaxis in bariatric surgery patients needs further study, but one study found a decrease in infection rates with doubling of the cefazolin dosage. When used along with intravenous antibiotics, topical antibiotics do not further decrease wound infection rates in bariatric surgery patients. Vancomycin is used for prophylaxis, the appropriate dose should be calculated using actual bodyweight rather than lean bodyweight in accordance with Infectious Disease Society of America recommendations. In one study, use of vancomycin resulted in higher rate of wound infection. The only prospective study examining the prophylactic administration of antibiotics before bariatric surgery was performed in 1981 by Pories et al. in a double-blind prospective analysis of 53 consecutive patients undergoing open RYGB. Their study demonstrated that a perioperative regimen of cefazolin decreased wound infections from 21% to 4% ($P < 0.05$) in this high-risk group of patients, and the incidence of urinary tract infection or pneumonia from 17% to 0% ($P < 0.05$). More dramatic were the results in diabetic patients.

References:

- Freeman JT, Anderson DJ, Hartwig MG, et al. Surgical site infections following bariatric surgery in community hospitals: a weighty concern? Obes Surg. 2011 Jul;21(7):836–840.
- Forse RA, Karam B, MacLean LD, et al. Antibiotic prophylaxis for surgery in morbidly obese patients. Surgery 1989; 106(4):750–756.
- Edmiston CE, Krepel C, Kelly H, et al. Perioperative antibiotic prophylaxis in the gastric bypass patient: Do we achieve therapeutic levels? Surgery 2004; 136 (4):738–747.
- Christou NV, Jarand J, Sylvestre JL, et al. Analysis of the incidence and risk factors for wound infections in open bariatric surgery. Obes Surg 2004; 14(1): 16–22.

- Rybak MJ, Lomaestro BM, Rotschafer JC, et al. Vancomycin therapeutic guidelines: a summary of consensus recommendations from the infectious diseases Society of America, the American Society of Health-System Pharmacists, and the Society of Infectious Diseases Pharmacists. Clin Infect Dis 2009; 49(3): 325–327.
- Pories WJ, van Rij AM, Burlingham BT, et al. Prophylactic cefazolin in gastric bypass. Surgery 1981; 90:426–432.

34. **Answer: C.**

The best option for a patient suspected to have an internal hernia along with choledocholithiasis is probably a laparoscopic management viz a repair of the internal hernia and a laparoscopic CBD exploration or laparoscopic-assisted ERCP.

The other option is an open approach with bile duct exploration. Also, choledocholithiasis may be managed by a double-balloon ERCP or a percutaneous transhepatic cholangiography (PTC) and an internal/external drain followed by a more elective double-balloon ERCP and a laparoscopic cholecystectomy.

Conservative management is never an option for internal hernia. MRCP is a well-established tool to evaluate for CBD stones. MRI has been found to be useful to diagnose internal hernias and may be the preferred option in pregnant patients.

References:
- Lopes TL, Wilcox CM. Endoscopic retrograde cholangiopancreatography in patients with Roux-en-Y anatomy. Gastroenterol Clin North Am 2010; 39(1):99–107.
- Lygidakis NJ. Acute suppurative cholangitis: comparison of internal and external biliary drainage. Am J Surg 1982; 143(3):304–306.
- Rosenkrantz AB, Kurian M, Kim D. MRI appearance of internal hernia following Roux-en-Y gastric bypass surgery in the pregnant patient. Clin Radiol 2010; 65 (3):246–249 [Epub January 15, 2010].
- Emmett DS, Mallat DB. Double-balloon ERCP in patients who have undergone Roux-en-Y surgery: a case series. Gastrointest Endosc 2007; 66(5):1038–1041.

35. **Answer: C.**

The incidence of PE and DVT after bariatric surgery, especially with the current use of thromboprophylaxis, is very low (about 2–3% in various studies for PE as well as DVT). Venous thromboembolism can occur after discharge and hence thromboprophylaxis can be continued after discharge in selected high-risk patients. A systematic review found only one RCT in bariatric surgery thromboprophylaxis and most of the other nonrandomized studies did not have a control group. Higher-dose unfractionated heparin may be required in obese patients, although the risks and benefits of the same are to be further investigated.

References:
- Agarwal R, Hecht TE, Lazo MC, et al. Venous thromboembolism prophylaxis for patients undergoing bariatric surgery: a systematic review. Surg Obes Relat Dis 2010; 6(2):213–220.
- Geerts WH, Bergqvist D, Pineo GF, et al.; American College of Chest Physicians. Prevention of venous thromboembolism: American College of Chest Physicians Evidence-Based Clinical Practice Guidelines (8th Edition). Chest 2008; 133(6 suppl):381S–453S.

36. **Answer: C.**

Various theories have been proposed to explain the enteric hyperoxaluria after RYGB. Whether increased oxalate absorption is caused by fat malabsorption, a reduction in intestinal oxalate secretion secondary to diversion of normal gut traffic, alterations in oxalate-degrading intestinal flora, or some other process is not known. However, hyperoxaluria and hypocitraturia are commonly seen in malabsorptive bariatric surgery patients including jejunoileal bypass. Typical treatment strategies for enteric hyperoxaluria are prescription of a low-fat, low-oxalate diet, generous fluid intake, use of oral oxalate binders such as calcium, and potassium citrate as a crystallization inhibitor. Oral administration of *Oxalobacter formigenes* and lactic acid bacteria may represent a promising treatment strategy because their oxalate-degrading enzymes may reduce plasma oxalate levels as well as urinary oxalate excretions.

Gastric banding, being just a restrictive procedure, does not increase incidence of oxalate urinary stones.

References:
- Cooper CS, Joudi FN, Williams RD. Chapter 38: Urology. Doherty Gerard M.: CURRENT Diagnosis & Treatment: Surgery, 13th Edition. Available at: http://www.accesssurgery.com/content.aspx?aID=5312459.
- Asplin JR. Obesity and urolithiasis. Adv Chronic Kidney Dis 2009; 16(1):11–20.
- Lieske JC, Kumar R, Collazo-Clavell ML. Nephrolithiasis after bariatric surgery for obesity. Semin Nephrol 2008; 28(2):163–173.
- Semins MJ, Asplin JR, Steele K, et al. The effect of restrictive bariatric surgery on urinary stone risk factors. Urology 2010; 76(4):826–829.

37. **Answer: B.**

SBO after LRYGB can present early (<30 days) or late. Early obstructions are more likely due to technical problems with the Roux limb, whereas SBO presenting later is mostly due to internal hernias or adhesions.

Laparoscopic gastric bypass has been shown to have increased the incidence of SBO when compared to open surgery according to one study. Other observations show that the incidence of SBO in the open and laparoscopic approaches is similar. These discrepancies are likely related to different operative techniques. The incidence of internal hernias is also higher after laparoscopic gastric bypass when compared to open gastric bypass. All patients who present with obstruction after RYGB should undergo exploration, preferably laparoscopically. Conservative management should not be done in a patient presenting with obstruction after laparoscopic gastric bypass, as is done in the general postsurgical patient.

Most internal hernias after RYGB (>50%) present as complete obstructions.

References:
- Sunnapwar A, Sandrasegaran K, Menias CO, et al. Taxonomy and imaging spectrum of small bowel obstruction after Roux-en-Y gastric bypass surgery. AJR Am J Roentgenol 2010; 194(1):120–128.
- Nelson LG, Gonzalez R, Haines K, et al. Spectrum and treatment of small bowel obstruction after Roux-en-Y gastric bypass. Surg Obes Relat Dis 2006; 2(3):377–383; discussion 383.
- Thodiyil PA, Rogula T, Mattar SG, et al. Management of complications after laparoscopic gastric bypass. In: Inabnet WB, DeMaria EJ, Ikramuddin S, eds. Laparoscopic Bariatric Surgery. Philadelphia: Lippincott Williams & Wilkins, 2005:229–232.

38. **Answer: D.**

In morbidly obese patients, a thick preperitoneum has been thought to predispose to the development of Richter hernia. Richter hernia usually presents early during the postoperative period and is uncommon, with a reported incidence of 0.02% in one series of laparoscopic gastric bypass. In one systematic review, it was found that about half of the cases of trocar site hernias presenting early were Richter's hernias. It was, however, rare with hernias presenting late. SBO resulting from Richter hernia may be confused for adhesions because the herniated bowel loop is very small and may easily be overlooked. Differentiation is very important because Richter hernia has a high risk of strangulation. Optimal opacification of bowel loops with oral contrast material is important for this purpose.

References:

- Tonouchi H, Ohmori Y, Kobayashi M, et al. Trocar site hernia. Arch Surg 2004; 139(11):1248–1256.
- Sunnapwar A, Sandrasegaran K, Menias CO, et al. Taxonomy and imaging spectrum of small bowel obstruction after Roux-en-Y gastric bypass surgery. AJR Am J Roentgenol 2010; 194(1):120–128.
- Rao RS, Gentileschi P, Kini SU. Management of ventral hernias in bariatric surgery. Surg Obes Relat Dis 2011; 7(1):110–116.

39. **Answer: B.**

The reported incidence of postoperative hematoma in one series was 3.2%, with a higher incidence noted after laparoscopic RYGB (5.1% vs. 2.4%). The hematoma may be intraluminal, intramural, or extrinsic to the bowel. Tachycardia and a sense of "impending doom" is one of the common presentations of intraluminal hematoma, which causes obstruction at the jejunojejunostomy site. A mesocolic hematoma may cause acute obstruction of the alimentary limb and results when the surgeon fails to identify a small bleeding vessel. The staple lines are the source of hemorrhage in most cases. CT is definitive in most cases and shows high-density hematoma, either intrinsic or extrinsic. It is sometimes difficult to diagnose a hematoma and an infected collection radiologically (both present as high-attenuation foci on CT scan) and the diagnosis of hematoma may be made only in the absence of signs of infection. Angiography/embolization is generally not an option due to multiple arterial supply to the stomach. Laparotomy may be required if the patient is unstable.

References:

- Nguyen NT, Goldman C, Rosenquist CJ, et al. Laparoscopic versus open gastric bypass: a randomized study of outcomes, quality of life, and costs. Ann Surg 2001; 234(3):279–289.
- Thodiyil PA, Rogula T, Mattar SG, et al. Management of complications after laparoscopic gastric bypass. In: Inabnet WB, DeMaria EJ, Ikramuddin S, eds. Laparoscopic Bariatric Surgery. Philadelphia: Lippincott Williams & Wilkins, 2005:229–232.
- Sunnapwar A, Sandrasegaran K, Menias CO, et al. Taxonomy and imaging spectrum of small bowel obstruction after Roux-en-Y gastric bypass surgery. AJR Am J Roentgenol 2010; 194(1):120–128.

40. **Answer: D.**

The long jejunoileal excluded loop after a jejunoileal bypass can lead to impaired function of the mucosal barrier that may facilitate the absorption into the portal venous system of a variety of macromolecules, such as inflammatory cytokines and intestinal toxins arising as a result of changes in the intestinal bacterial flora. After delivery to the liver, such macromolecules may exacerbate hepatic injury.

A decrease in the intake and absorption of nutritional supplements also may have a negative impact on liver function.

The intestinal bacterial overgrowth in segments of the small intestine bypassed by surgery may result in increased frequency of bowel movements, thereby intensifying nutritional disequilibrium and exacerbating impaired hepatocellular function. The syndrome is associated with susceptibility to thrombogenesis and poor activity of the natural anticoagulant or fibrinolytic system, which predisposes to perisinusoidal microthromboses that lead to hepatocellular necrosis. Bariatric surgery is not a cause of PVT. PVT usually has a normal hepatic histology or can present with mild periportal fibrosis. It usually presents with variceal bleeding and significant liver dysfunction is uncommon.

Reference:

- D'Albuquerque LA, Gonzalez AM, Wahle RC, et al. Liver transplantation for subacute hepatocellular failure due to massive steatohepatitis after bariatric surgery. Liver Transpl 2008; 14(6):881–885.

41. **Answer: D.**

Sequential compression devices alone lead to a low incidence of venous thromboembolism and the American Society for Metabolic and Bariatric Surgery (ASMBS) recommends its use in the position statement. It also recommends heparin as an important adjunct to these methods. Increased intra-abdominal pressure and reverse Trendelenberg position have been shown to independently decrease peak femoral systolic velocity. Sequential compression devices normalize the femoral peak systolic velocities in nonobese but not in obese patients. In one study a decrease in femoral peak systolic velocity of 57% noted during laparoscopic bariatric surgery was only partially normalized by sequential compression device.

References:
- Rocha AT, de Vasconcellos AG, da Luz Neto ER, et al. Risk of venous thromboembolism and efficacy of thromboprophylaxis in hospitalized obese medical patients and in obese patients undergoing bariatric surgery. Obes Surg 2006; 16(12):1645–1655.
- Khouli H, Shapiro J, Pham VP, et al. Efficacy of deep venous thrombosis prophylaxis in the medical intensive care unit. J Intensive Care Med 2006; 21 (6):352–358.
- Magner D, Nguyen NT. Physiology of laparoscopy in morbidly obese. In: Sugerman HJ, Nguyen NT, eds. Management of Morbid Obesity. New York: Taylor and Francis, 2006.
- Nowara HA, Samy H. Venous foot pump prevents venous stasis during laparoscopic bariatric surgery. Egypt J Surg 2002; 21(1):866–870.

42. **Answer: A.**

The patient has endogenous protein loss due to bacterial overgrowth that was resolved with metronidazole. It has an incidence of 27% and if chronic requires a revision surgery with lengthening of the alimentary limb using a part of the biliopancreatic limb in order to increase absorption of carbohydrates.

Reference:
- Scopinaro N. Chapter 13: Malabsorptive procedures: biliopancreatic diversion–scopinaro procedure. In: Pitombo C, Jones K, Higa K, et al., eds. Obesity Surgery: Principles and Practice. Available at: http://www.accesssurgery.com/content.aspx?aID=140666.

43. **Answer: A.**

The most common presenting symptoms of meralgia paresthetica are burning pain and paresthesias in the anterior and lateral portions of the thigh. Mild cases may be interpreted as itching by the patient, and scratching may cause factitious dermatitis. Physical examination may reveal the sensory changes noted above, though the area involved is usually smaller according to objective examination than is described by the patient. Pressure applied just medial and inferior to the anterior superior iliac spine aggravates the pain.

The variable effects of position and movement on the severity of symptoms include worsening with extension of the hip, with flexion of the hip, and even on holding the hip immobile in the neutral position. Some patients are unaffected by walking, but walking and coughing have been reported as aggravating factors.

There are four predisposing variants for the course of lateral femoral cutaneous nerve:

1. passage of the lateral femoral cutaneous nerve through rather than deep to the inguinal ligament,
2. "bowing" of the nerve as it crosses the iliac fascia,
3. passage of the nerve through the sartorius muscle, and
4. passage of the nerve lateral and posterior to the anterior superior iliac spine.

References:

- Macgregor AM, Thoburn EK. Meralgia paresthetica following bariatric surgery. Obes Surg 1999; 9(4):364–368.
- Thoma A, Levis C. Compression neuropathies of the lower extremity. Clin Plast Surg 2003; 30(2):189–201, vi.

44. **Answer: B.**

The management of the condition is initially conservative. In the 277 cases accumulated by Williams conservative treatment was successful in 91%. Removal of inciting agents and the use of anti-inflammatory medication, ice packs, and local injections of local anesthetic and steroids provide relief in the vast majority of cases. Occasionally, surgery is required for intractable pain and disability. While release and transposition may be effective in the presence of a single nerve trunk without neuroma, neurectomy with excision of a portion of the lateral femoral cutaneous nerve appears to produce excellent results with good 15-year follow-up.

Grace et al. reported three cases following RYGB or vertical banded gastroplasty. He utilized a Gomez abdominal retractor, a device that is attached to the operating table by four vertical metal posts, the lower two of which are positioned near the patient's hips. He postulated that compression may occur when the patient's hips are wider than the table. Proper positioning of the patient during surgery can also prevent this condition.

References:

- Macgregor AM, Thoburn EK. Meralgia paresthetica following bariatric surgery. Obes Surg 1999; 9(4):364–368.
- Thoma A, Levis C. Compression neuropathies of the lower extremity. Clin Plast Surg 2003; 30(2):189–201, vi.

45. **Answer: B.**
46. **Answer: C.**

The patient needs a diagnostic laparoscopy as internal hernia is suspected based on her CT scan. The most common site of an internal hernia in a retrocolic gastric bypass is the mesocolic window (through which the Roux limb herniates), not the Petersen's defect.

References:

- Section 6: Complications. In: Inabnet WB, DeMaria EJ, Ikramuddin S, eds. Laparoscopic Bariatric Surgery. Vol. Philadelphia: Lippincott Williams & Wilkins, 2004:230
- Sunnapwar A, Sandrasegaran K, Menias CO, et al. Taxonomy and imaging spectrum of small bowel obstruction after Roux-en-Y gastric bypass surgery. AJR Am J Roentgenol 2010; 194(1):120–128.

47. **Answer: B.**

Though vomiting is less commonly seen with DS, the incidence of heartburn is more after BPD-DS. BPD has a higher revision rate when compared to BPD-DS. BPD and BPD-DS have not been found to be different in their rates of insufficient weight loss.

References:

- Marceau P, Biron S, Hould FS et al. Duodenal switch improved standard biliopancreatic diversion: a retrospective study. Surg Obes Relat Dis 2009; 5 (1):43–47.
- Bruce S, Philip RS. Chapter 27: The surgical management of obesity. In: Brunicardi FC, Andersen DK, Billiar TR, et al., eds. Schwartz's Principles of Surgery. 9th edn. Available at: http://www.accesssurgery.com/content.aspx?aID=5032782.
- Scopinaro N, Adami GF, Marinari GM, et al. Biliopancreatic diversion. World J Surg 1998; 22:936–946.

48. **Answer: D.**

BPD-DS has several advantages over Scopinaro's BPD, which include lower incidence of stomal ulcers and dumping syndrome. It was developed by Hess and

Hess in 1998. BPD-DS also results in better weight loss. The need for revision is decreased after BPD-DS and so is the need for revision due to malnutrition when compared to BPD. After BPD-DS, the levels of calcium, iron, and hemoglobin are significantly greater and the parathyroid hormone level lower than after BPD. There is no difference in mortality between the two procedures at 10 years.

References:
- Marceau P, Biron S, Hould FS, et al. Duodenal switch improved standard biliopancreatic diversion: a retrospective study. Surg Obes Relat Dis 2009; 5 (1):43–47.
- Marceau P, Hould FS, Simard S, et al. Biliopancreatic diversion with duodenal switch. World J Surg 1998; 22(9):947–954.

9 | Revisional bariatric surgery

CHAPTER SUMMARY
- Revisional bariatric surgery should be attempted by surgeons with extensive experience in primary bariatric surgery.
- All revisional surgeries are associated with higher morbidity (complication rate) and mortality.
- Up to 40% of patients with jejunoileal bypass (JIB) may need reversal of JIB for metabolic complications. Another bariatric procedure [usually Roux-en-Y gastric bypass (RYGB)] should always be performed after taking down the JIB. The Roux limb is constructed with the bypassed jejunoileum.
- Vertical banded gastroplasty (VBG) is usually revised to RYGB. The reasons for revision of VBG include inadequate weight loss, vertical staple line dehiscence, stomal stenosis, erosion of the Lap-Band, and reflux. A preoperative upper gastrointestinal contrast study (UGI) is a must to define the anatomy. The RYGB pouch is fashioned such that it lies proximal to the vertical staple line as well as the stoma. No part of the stomach should be left undrained. Weight loss is good after conversion to RYGB.
- Revision of RYGB:
  - Enlarged pouch – in addition to reducing the pouch volume, increasing the Roux limb length and thus decreasing the length of the common limb may be considered.
  - Refractory stricture: When strictures cannot be treated by endoscopic dilation, the gastrojejunostomy (GJ) has to be revised. This is complicated by the high degree of inflammation surrounding the GJ. Sometimes, an esophagojejunostomy may be required.
  - Staple line dehiscence: The pouch is revised and a disconnected RYGB performed.
  - Gastrogastric fistula: Closure of the fistula with limited proximal gastrectomy is done.
  - Unsatisfactory weight loss – if not responsive to nutritional counseling a very very long RYGB can be performed.
  - Revision of RYGB to laparoscopic adjustable gastric banding (LAGB) has been shown to be feasible and has resulted in good weight loss in some studies. Duodenal switch (DS) has also been shown to be a feasible option as a revisional procedure.
- Revision of Lap-Band:
  - Reasons for revision of a Lap-Band include slippage, erosion, rubbing disconnection, and inadequate weight loss.
  - Replacement of Lap-Band is usually not done during the same procedure when the cause of removal of the Lap-Band is erosion. Some surgeons, however, have found good results with replacement of the Lap-Band during the same procedure.
  - Revision of LAGB to RYGB is better than revision of LAGB to another Lap-Band. In the former case weight loss is superior, whereas complication rates are similar to the latter.
  - RYGB is a more reasonable revisional procedure in the presence of esophageal dysmotility.
  - Laparoscopic revision to RYGB takes longer time when compared to open surgery.
  - Bandinaro procedure – it is the conversion of LAGB to biliopancreatic diversion–duodenal switch (BPD-DS) with leaving the Lap-Band in place.

- Revisional surgery for BPD-DS:
  - Reversal
    - May be needed for excess weight loss or for protein energy malnutrition.
    - This is done by side-to-side jejunojejunostomy at the ligament of Treitz between the Roux limb and the biliopancreatic limb.
    - Most common reasons for revisions are also excess weight loss and protein energy malnutrition. This is done by advancing the alimentary limb proximally over the biliopancreatic limb, thus increasing the length of both the common channel and the alimentary limb.
    - For patients with inadequate weight loss, shortening of the common channel and revision of the sleeve gastrectomy are options.
    - Other surgeries are converted into BPD-DS. Some key points are mentioned for such conversions:
      - VBG – the staple line of the sleeve is constructed medial to the vertical staple line.
      - RYGB – the stomach is put back together by joining the pouch to the remnant by interrupted sutures. Continuous sutures should not be used as they will be cut when stapling of the stomach is done during a sleeve gastrectomy. The original anatomy of the intestine is restored before a usual DS is done.

QUESTIONS

1. **A post-bariatric surgical patient may seek a revision for inadequate weight loss or for complications of the bariatric procedure. Identify the <u>CORRECT</u> statement about revisional bariatric surgery.**
   A. The morbidity and mortality after revisional procedures are higher than the primary procedure.
   B. A revision of a revisional procedure is also commonly performed.
   C. A revision of restrictive operation to another restrictive operation is usually not done.
   D. It is better to revise an LAGB to another LAGB than to a gastric bypass when there is inadequate weight loss.

2. **A bariatric surgeon is performing a revisional surgery in a patient with a gastric Lap-Band as he did not attain satisfactory weight loss. The planned procedure is replacement of the Lap-Band. He does the procedure laparoscopically and cuts the Lap-Band and removes it. He notes possible erosion near the gastroesophageal junction where the Lap-Band was initially placed and is unsure about the integrity of the stomach wall. What is the <u>NEXT</u> best step during the surgery?**
   A. Abandon the surgery and do not perform a revisional procedure.
   B. Ask the anesthetist to inject methylene blue dye.
   C. Convert to a laparotomy.
   D. Close the area with an omental patch and then stop the procedure.

3. **A patient who had an adjustable gastric Lap-Band placed 36 months ago, feels over restricted. An UGI contrast study demonstrates a symmetrically dilated pouch. All the saline is removed from the Lap-Band and 6 weeks later, a repeat UGI study showed that the pouch is no longer dilated. After a few adjustments the patient feels overrestricted again, and a repeat UGI contrast study shows a symmetrically dilated pouch. During this period, she follows up a few times with the nutritionist and follows her advice. Which is the <u>BEST</u> management option?**
   A. Remove the adjustable gastric Lap-Band.
   B. Remove the adjustable gastric Lap-Band, and do LRYGB during the same operation.
   C. Remove the adjustable gastric Lap-Band and place another Lap-Band.
   D. Advise her that she will need frequent readjustments of the adjustable gastric Lap-Band for the rest of her life.

4. **VBG is a procedure that has been proven to be inferior to LRYGB and only of historical interest. Identify the TRUE statement about revision of such a procedure.**
   A. The most common reason for revision of a gastroplasty has been Lap-Band erosion.
   B. Revision of gastroplasty to a gastroplasty has a similar outcome as conversion of gastroplasty to RYGB.
   C. Laparoscopic approach and open approach have a similar operating time.
   D. VBG is most commonly revised to RYGB.

5. **Inadequate weight loss, weight regain, diarrhea, and malnutrition after BPD-DS may all lead to the need for a revisional procedure. Identify the FALSE statement about revisional surgery for BPD-DS.**
   A. Inadequate weight loss may be corrected by shortening the common channel.
   B. Inadequate weight loss may be corrected by reducing the volume of stomach.
   C. Malnutrition may be corrected by lengthening the common channel and the alimentary limb.
   D. Adding an LAGB to the sleeve gastrectomy is being investigated as an option for failed BPD-DS.

6. **VBG is a bariatric procedure that is not commonly performed anymore due to its poor long-term efficacy and high incidence of complications. Which of the following is NOT an indication for revision of VBG?**
   A. Barrett's esophagus
   B. Vertical staple line dehiscence
   C. Lap-Band erosion
   D. Stomal stenosis
   E. VBG done in the distant past

7. **A bariatric surgeon is performing a laparoscopic conversion of VBG to RYGB. The preoperative UGI study shows a vertical staple line dehiscence (near the stomal region) as well as complete stomal stenosis. He creates a gastric pouch 4 cm from the gastroesophageal junction and above the Marlex Lap-Band, with thick tissue staples (4.8 mm) fired medial to the vertical staple line. What is the NEXT best course of action during the surgery?**
   A. Do a gastrogastrostomy to drain the distal pouch.
   B. No additional step needed
   C. Remove the Marlex Lap-Band.
   D. Do a partial gastrectomy.

8. **BPD decreases absorption of different nutrients in the intestine, thus predisposing to nutritional deficiencies. Identify the FALSE statement about revisional surgery after BPD and the physiological rationale behind such revision.**
   A. Protein malnutrition is the most common cause of revision of BPD.
   B. The absorption of carbohydrate per unit length of the intestine in the common limb is the same as absorption per unit length in the alimentary limb.
   C. To correct protein malabsorption, the common channel should be elongated by moving the enteroenterostomy further up the alimentary limb.
   D. The absorption of fat per unit length of the intestine is much greater in the common limb compared to the alimentary limb.

9. **Reversal of a BPD with restoration of intestinal continuity is rarely needed. Identify the TRUE statement about restoration of intestinal continuity after BPD.**
   A. This is done most commonly by connecting the disconnected alimentary limb to the proximal end of duodenum.

   B. This is usually done if the patient develops a chronic disease causing inadequate calorie intake or protein loss.

   C. Intractable bone demineralization can be corrected by increasing the length of common limb, and a restoration of continuity is not needed for this purpose.

   D. This is usually done by connecting the gastric pouch to the proximal end of the duodenum.

10. **A patient 1 year after an LRYGB has developed a nonhealing marginal ulcer, and a revisional surgery is planned. Which of the following is a <u>FALSE</u> statement about a revision of the GJ for nonhealing marginal ulcers?**

   A. Laparoscopic approach is contraindicated.

   B. Vagotomy can be performed during revision of a GJ.

   C. One centimeter of gastric pouch is excised above the original GJ.

   D. Patients need to be on postoperative acid suppressive therapy.

ANSWER KEY

1. A	5. B	9. B
2. B	6. E	10. A
3. B	7. B	
4. D	8. C	

ANSWER KEY WITH EXPLANATION

1. **Answer: A.**

   The complication rate of a revisional procedure has been reported to be higher when compared to the primary operation.

   A second revisional procedure is usually considered with skepticism. This is the experience of most bariatric surgeons though there are no published data. A restrictive operation may be changed to another restrictive operation if the reason for revision is a complication arising due to the first surgery. Conversion of LAGB to sleeve gastrectomy has also been found to be successful, with an acceptable complication rate.

   Revision of LAGB to RYGB has been shown to be superior when compared to placement of another Lap-Band.

   References:
   - Patel S, Eckstein J, Acholonu E, et al. Reasons and outcomes of laparoscopic revisional surgery after laparoscopic adjustable gastric banding for morbid obesity. Surg Obes Relat Dis 2010; 6(4):391–398.
   - Gumbs AA, Pomp A, Gagner M. Revisional bariatric surgery for inadequate weight loss. Obes Surg 2007; 17(9):1137–1145.
   - Lim CS, Liew V, Talbot ML, et al. Revisional bariatric surgery. Obes Surg 2009; 19(7):827–832.
   - Cendán JC, Abu-aouf D, Gabrielli A, et al. Utilization of intensive care resources in bariatric surgery. Obes Surg 2005; 15(9):1247–1251.
   - Radtka JF III, Puleo FJ, Wang L, et al. Revisional bariatric surgery: who, what, where, and when? Surg Obes Relat Dis 2010; 6(6):635–642.
   - Gagner M, Gumbs AA. Gastric banding: conversion to sleeve, bypass, or DS. Surg Endosc 2007; 21(11):1931–1935.
   - Jacobs M, Gomez E, Romero R, et al. Failed restrictive surgery: is sleeve gastrectomy a good revisional procedure? Obes Surg 2011; 21:157–160.

2. **Answer: B.**

   Whenever a gastric erosion is suspected during a laparoscopic revisional procedure, it is better to confirm it by injecting methylene blue or testing for leak after insufflating air and placing the stomach under saline. If no leak is found, and if the tissue looks healthy, the revisional procedure can proceed. If an erosion is found, some surgeons do not replace the Lap-Band during the same procedure due to the risk of increased morbidity.

References:

- Cherian PT, Goussous G, Ashori F, et al. Band erosion after laparoscopic gastric banding: a retrospective analysis of 865 patients over 5 years. Surg Endosc 2010; 24(8):2031–2038.
- bu-Abeid S, Bar ZD, Sagie B, et al. Treatment of intra-gastric band migration following laparoscopic banding: safety and feasibility of simultaneous laparoscopic band removal and replacement. Obes Surg 2005; 15(6):849–852.

3. **Answer: B.**

Revision of LAGB to RYGB has been shown to be superior to placing another Lap-Band. Open or laparoscopic revision surgery of LAGB to RYGB produces similar weight loss, although the operative time is higher with a laparoscopic revisional procedure.

Reference:

- Gagner M, Gumbs AA. Gastric banding: conversion to sleeve, bypass, or DS. Surg Endosc 2007; 21(11):1931–1935.

4. **Answer: D.**

The most common reason of revision of gastroplasty is vertical staple line dehiscence. The complication rate of such revisions is very high (approaching 15–20%). Revision of a gastroplasty to an RYGB has a better outcome than revision to gastroplasty again. In one series, one-third of the patients who were revised to VBG required another revisional procedure. Laparoscopic approach has been found to have a longer operating time. VBG is most commonly revised to RYGB.

References:

- Tevis S, Garren MJ, Gould JC. Revisional surgery for failed vertical-banded gastroplasty. Obes Surg 2011; 21(8):1220–1224.
- Hunter R, Watts JM, Dunstan R, et al. Revisional surgery for failed gastric restrictive procedures for morbid obesity. Obes Surg 1992; 2(3):245–252.
- Benotti PN, Forse RA. Safety and long-term efficacy of revisional surgery in severe obesity. Am J Surg 1996; 172(3):232–235.
- Gonzalez R, Gallagher SF, Haines K, et al. Operative technique for converting a failed vertical banded gastroplasty to Roux-en-Y gastric bypass. J Am Coll Surg 2005; 201(3):366–374.
- Behrns KE, Smith CD, Kelly KA, et al. Reoperative bariatric surgery. Lessons learned to improve patient selection and results. Ann Surg 1993; 218(5):646–653.

5. **Answer: B.**

Though reduction of the volume of the stomach was done for the early BPDs done by Hess, these were due to design of an initially large gastric pouch, and further reduction of the pouch does not increase weight loss without complications. Inadequate weight loss can be addressed by shortening the common channel. On the contrary, malnutrition can be addressed by lengthening the common channel as well as the alimentary limb by advancing the alimentary limb proximally over the biliopancreatic limb. Adding an LAGB to sleeve gastrectomy is an option for failed BPD-DS. BPD-DS, done as a revisional procedure for failed Lap-Band patients, with the Lap-Band left in situ during the procedure, has also been shown to be feasible in a small series.

References:

- Slater GH, Fielding GA. Combining laparoscopic adjustable gastric banding and biliopancreatic diversion after failed bariatric surgery. Obes Surg 2004; 14:677–682.
- Hess DS, Hess DW, Oakley RS. The biliopancreatic diversion with the duodenal switch: results beyond 10 years. Obes Surg 2005; 15(3):408–416.

6. **Answer: E.**

Vertical staple line dehiscence is the most common complication after VBG and needs revisional surgery. Gastroesophageal reflux and resulting Barrett's esophagus are an indication for revision. Lap-Band erosion requires removal of the Lap-Band surgically (or sometimes endoscopically) and revision of VBG. Dilation endoscopically is usually not successful for stomal stenosis after VBG. This leads to a dilated pouch and poor emptying of the pouch, and again VBG will need to be revised. VBG done in the distant past is not an indication for revisional surgery. In almost all cases VBG is revised to RYGB.

Reference:
- Gagné D. Chapter 33: Restrictive procedures: laparoscopic revision of vertical banding to gastric bypass. In: Pitombo C, Jones K, Higa K, et al., eds. Obesity Surgery: Principles and Practice. 1st ed. New York: McGraw-Hill, 2007. Available at: http://www.accesssurgery.com/content.aspx?aID=143876.

7. **Answer: B.**

It is important during revisional surgery not to leave any part of the stomach "undrained" to prevent gastric sequestration. Here, though there is stomal stenosis the distal pouch will drain through the vertical staple line dehiscence. Hence no additional step is needed. However, if a silastic ring or a gastric mesh has migrated intragastrically a partial gastrectomy may be necessary.

Reference:
- Gagné D. Chapter 33: Restrictive procedures: laparoscopic revision of vertical banding to gastric bypass. In: Pitombo C, Jones K, Higa K, et al., eds. Obesity Surgery: Principles and Practice. 1st ed. New York: McGraw-Hill, 2007. Available at: http://www.accesssurgery.com/content.aspx?aID=143876.

8. **Answer: C.**

Protein energy malnutrition is the most common cause of revisional surgery after a BPD. Fat is absorbed only in the common limb, whereas the protein and starch digestion/absorption capacity per unit of length of the common limb does not seem to be greater than that of the alimentary limb. Thus, protein absorption after BPD substantially depends on the total intestinal length from the gastroenteroanastomosis to the ileocecal valve. Therefore, elongation of the common limb to correct recurrent protein malnutrition would be ineffective if done along the alimentary limb as this would lengthen the common limb at the cost of the alimentary limb. Moving the alimentary limb along the biliopancreatic limb would lengthen the common limb but keep the alimentary limb constant.

Rarely, diarrhea is due to excessive reduction of ileal bile salt absorption. This condition can be easily diagnosed by cholestyramine administration, and it represents the only indication for the elongation of the common limb along the alimentary limb (two cases in Scopinaro's experience) – 100 cm being sufficient in their experience.

References:
- Scopinaro N, Adami GF, Marinari GM, et al. Biliopancreatic diversion. World J Surg 1998; 22:936–946.
- Biertho L, Biron S, Hould FS, et al. Is biliopancreatic diversion with duodenal switch indicated for patients with body mass index $<50 \, kg/m^2$? Surg Obes Relat Dis 2010; 6(5):508–514.
- Gagner M. Laparoscopic re-operative surgery and biliopancreatic diversion with duodenal switch. In: Inabnet WB, Demaria EJ, Inkramuddin S, eds. Laparoscopic Bariatric Surgery. Philadelphia: Lippincott Williams & Wilkins, 2005:185–193.
- Scopinaro N. Chapter 34: Biliopancreatic diversion: revisional surgery. In: Pitombo C, Jones K, Higa K, et al., eds. Obesity Surgery: Principles and Practice. 1st ed. New York: McGraw-Hill, 2007. Available at: http://www.accesssurgery.com/content.aspx?aID=143988.

9. **Answer: B.**

Restoration of intestinal continuity may be necessary in conditions that can potentially worsen malabsorption like liver cirrhosis, nephrotic syndrome, chronic inflammatory bowel disease, malignancy, or psychosis. It may also be requested by the patient after a long period of recurrent protein energy malnutrition. A full restoration of intestinal continuity can be performed or the alimentary limb can be sectioned distally and anastomosed to the jejunum at the ligament of Treitz. The latter technique, which is more commonly performed, will preserve the effects of the operation on glucose and cholesterol metabolism as the duodenum is still bypassed. If the patient develops intractable bone demineralization and other indications of restoration of intestinal continuity are also present, a full restoration of intestinal continuity can be performed by interposing an ileal segment between the stomach pouch and proximal end of duodenum, thus sacrificing the effects of the operation on glucose and cholesterol metabolism.

Reference:
- Scopinaro N. Chapter 34: Biliopancreatic diversion: revisional surgery. In: Pitombo C, Jones K, Higa K, et al., eds. Obesity Surgery: Principles and Practice. 1st ed. New York: McGraw-Hill, 2007. Available at: http://www.accesssurgery. com/content.aspx?aID=143988.

10. **Answer: A.**

Laparoscopic approach is preferred especially if the surgeon is experienced. The technique involves placement of five trocars, taking adhesions down between the stomach and liver, retracting the liver, dissecting the gastric pouch out from the gastric remnant, completely mobilizing the Roux limb, and, if in the retrocolic position, dividing it 3 to 5 cm distal to the GJ to place it in the antecolic position. Next, the gastric pouch is mobilized and transected 1 cm above the GJ to excise the ulcerated portion, followed by reanastomosis with the use of a linear or circular stapler. An intraoperative endoscopy is performed with the GJ submerged under water to test the anastomosis for air leak. On postoperative day 1 (POD 1), the patient undergoes a UGI gastrografin study to delineate the reconstructed anatomy and rule out leak or obstruction. The patient is started on a bariatric clear liquid diet if the study is normal and discharged on POD 2 with a proton pump inhibitor for 6 to 8 weeks postoperatively. Vagotomy can be performed during the same procedure before performing the revision of the GJ. Some surgeons believe that a truncal vagotomy is unnecessary.

References:
- Datta TS, Steele K, Schweitzer M. Laparoscopic revision of gastrojejunostomy revision with truncal vagotomy for persistent marginal ulcer after Roux-en-Y gastric bypass. Surg Obes Relat Dis 2010; 6(5):561–562.
- Salimath J, Rosenthal RJ, Szomstein S. Laparoscopic remnant gastrectomy as a novel approach for treatment of gastrogastric fistula. Surg Endosc 2009; 23(11):2591–2595.
- Carrodeguas L, Szomstein S, Soto F, et al. Management of gastrogastric fistulas after divided Roux-en-Y gastric bypass surgery for morbid obesity: analysis of 1,292 consecutive patients and review of literature. Surg Obes Relat Dis 2005; 1(5):467–474.

10 | Adolescent obesity

CHAPTER SUMMARY

- At present, adolescent bariatric surgery is recommended to be performed only as a part of an institutional review board (IRB)–approved clinical trial. Some hospitals have established review boards for the purpose of resolving controversial issues regarding selection and management of adolescents undergoing bariatric surgery.
- Though adjustable gastric band is not FDA approved for use in adolescents, data indicate that it is safe. As in adults a high incidence of reoperation is seen.
- Roux-en-Y gastric bypass (RYGB) is considered a safe and effective option in adolescents. Long-term follow-up is necessary.
- Sleeve gastrectomy has been performed in adolescents but data regarding efficacy and safety are limited.
- Biliopancreatic diversion (BPD) and biliopancreatic diversion–duodenal switch (BPD-DS) are not recommended for adolescents due to nutritional concerns.
- There is significant comorbidity improvement in adolescents after bariatric surgery.
  - Resolution of diabetes may be even better than in adults. It should be considered when selecting adolescents for bariatric surgery.
  - Obstructive sleep apnea (OSA), nonalcoholic fatty liver disease, and pseudotumor cerebri also significantly improve after bariatric surgery. They should also be considered during selection of adolescents for surgery.
- Quality of life of adolescents has been shown to improve after RYGB and laparoscopic adjustable gastric band (LAGB).
- Patient selection:
  - Physical maturity is a prerequisite for bariatric surgery. Completion of 95% of adult maturity based on radiographic study should be documented.
  - Patients should be psychologically mature – understand the nature of the operation and should have mature motivations. They should be able to comply with treatment regimens and medical monitoring.
  - Body mass index (BMI) > 99th percentile for any given age/sex is defined as severe obesity, whereas a BMI > 95th percentile is defined as obesity.
  - Even though the mean BMI of adolescents is less than that of adults, BMI cutoffs can be used to identify adolescents at high risk. Surgery is indicated with BMI > 35 with severe comorbidities and BMI > 40 with milder comorbidities.
  - The major risk factors for childhood obesity tracking into adult obesity include parental obesity, increasing age, and increasing BMI. These patients should also be considered for weight loss surgery.
- Bariatric surgery is not effective in producing sustained weight loss in Prader–Willi syndrome. Patients with genetic forms of obesity are chosen on a case-by-case basis.
- Adolescents undergoing RYGB are at an increased risk of calcium, iron, vitamin B_{12}, and vitamin D deficiency. About 50% of total adult bone mass is achieved during adolescence, and hence adequate supplementation of calcium and vitamin D is crucial. Adolescents are at an increased risk for thiamine deficiency.
- Bariatric surgery increases female fertility as was manifested in a twofold increase in teen pregnancies after LRYGB.

- Informed consent:
  - The child must give assent to surgery and the parents should consent to surgery. The adolescent's cognitive, social, and emotional maturity should also be taken into consideration.
  - Informing about risks and benefits of the surgery, medical and surgical alternatives, and need for postoperative follow-up should be a part of obtaining consent from the parents as well as assent from the minor.
- Multicenter studies like Teen-LABS may give more answers regarding risks and benefits of weight loss surgery.

QUESTIONS

1. **The indications and efficacy of adolescent bariatric surgery have not been well established. Identify the <u>FALSE</u> statement about selection of adolescents for bariatric surgery and its overall efficacy.**
   - A. Multidisciplinary review boards for childhood and adolescent bariatric surgery have been developed at some centers.
   - B. RYGB is less effective for diabetes in adolescents when compared to adults.
   - C. RYGB has an acceptable mortality in adolescents.
   - D. Bariatric surgery has been shown to improve quality of life in adolescents.

2. **A 13-year-old boy with a BMI of 40 kg/m^2 and with OSA is brought to the clinic for evaluation for bariatric surgery. Which of the following statements is <u>TRUE</u> about the prerequisites for bariatric surgery in an adolescent?**
   - A. Bariatric surgery is recommended if BMI is $\geq$35 kg/m^2 without comorbidities.
   - B. The sexual maturity should be at least Tanner 4.
   - C. Nutritional evaluation and follow-up are required only till the age of 21 years.
   - D. Physiological immaturity as assessed by a wrist radiograph with bone age films is not a contraindication for this patient to undergo bariatric surgery.

3. **Which of the following statements about bariatric surgery in adolescents is <u>TRUE</u>?**
   - A. Adjustable gastric banding is currently approved by FDA for adolescents.
   - B. Mortality is much higher in adolescents than in adults after bariatric surgery.
   - C. Behavioral therapy for obesity has been shown to be inferior to bariatric surgery for weight loss in pediatric population.
   - D. BPD-DS is currently recommended for weight loss in adolescents.

4. **Identify the <u>FALSE</u> statement about obesity in children/adolescents.**
   - A. The incidence of childhood obesity (age 6–11 years) and adolescent obesity (age 12–19 years) have both increased significantly over the last three decades.
   - B. Adolescent obesity is associated with adverse cardiovascular risk factors.
   - C. Less than 10% of adolescents who are obese remain obese as adults.
   - D. The determinant of obesity in a child is not just the BMI but the percentile into which BMI falls for the child's gender and age.
   - E. Molecular genetic abnormalities contribute to about one-quarter of the prevalence of obesity.

5. **Childhood obesity, like adult obesity, is associated with comorbidities. These comorbidities need to be considered while selecting and working up an adolescent for bariatric surgery. Identify the <u>FALSE</u> statement about the comorbidities of obesity in adolescents.**
   - A. Higher BMI during childhood is associated with increased risk of cardiovascular events in adults.
   - B. Hypertension is more common in obese when compared to nonobese children.
   - C. OSA can present as enuresis and hyperactivity in children.
   - D. Nonalcoholic steatohepatitis (NASH) is very rare (<1%) in childhood obesity.

6. **Obesity in children, like in adults, is also associated with several comorbidities. Identify the <u>FALSE</u> statement about the comorbid problems associated with obesity in children.**
   A. Blount's disease is a disease caused by childhood obesity.
   B. Pseudotumor cerebri is not linked with adolescent obesity.
   C. More than 50% of morbidly obese children have left ventricular hypertrophy.
   D. Slipped capital femoral epiphysis is common in obese adolescents/children.

7. **The father of a morbidly obese boy is researching the Internet regarding the pharmacotherapeutic options for his child. Identify the <u>TRUE</u> statement about pharmacotherapy for childhood obesity.**
   A. Orlistat is a FDA-approved medication for the treatment of obesity in children of 6 to 12 years of age.
   B. Metformin has been FDA approved for treatment of childhood obesity.
   C. Orlistat causes >5% weight loss in one out of four adolescents when used along with behavioral modification.
   D. Sibutramine is FDA approved for children aged >6 years.

ANSWER KEY

1. B	3. C	5. D	7. C
2. B	4. C	6. B	

ANSWER KEY WITH EXPLANATION

1. **Answer: B.**

   Some centers like Cincinnati and Texas Children's Hospital have established review boards, and they have been instrumental in resolving potential controversial patient selection and management decisions.

   Bypass procedures successfully reverse or improve abnormal glucose metabolism in the majority of patients and may be more effective in adolescents than adults. This may be due to short duration of diabetes in adolescents.

   According to one prospective study, RYGB appears to have an acceptable mortality in adolescents.

   Surgical treatment of morbid obesity results in improvement of quality of life in adolescents as shown by improvement in SF-36 and Adolescent Impact of Weight on Quality of Life-Lite scores after gastric bypass.

   References:
   - Inge TH, Zeller M, Garcia VF, et al. Surgical approach to adolescent obesity. Adolesc Med Clin 2004; 15(3):429–453.
   - Leslie DB, Kellogg TA, Ikramuddin S. The surgical approach to management of pediatric obesity: when to refer and what to expect. Rev Endocr Metab Disord 2009; 10(3):215–229.
   - Brandt ML, Harmon CM, Helmrath MA, et al. Morbid obesity in pediatric diabetes mellitus: surgical options and outcomes. Nat Rev Endocrinol 2010; 6(11):637–645 [Epub September 14, 2010].
   - Sugerman HJ, Sugerman EL, DeMaria EJ, et al. Bariatric surgery for severely obese adolescents. J Gastrointest Surg 2003; 7(1):102–107; discussion 107–108.
   - Loux TJ, Haricharan RN, Clements RH, et al. Health-related quality of life before and after bariatric surgery in adolescents. J Pediatr Surg 2008; 43(7):1275–1279.

2. **Answer: B.**

Pediatric bariatric study group (2004) guidelines	Updated pediatric (2009) and standard adult guidelines
BMI $\geq$ 50 kg/m^2	BMI $\geq$ 40 kg/m^2
BMI $\geq$ 40 kg/m^2 with serious comorbidity	BMI $\geq$ 35 kg/m^2 with serious comorbidity
Failure of weight loss after formal program of lifestyle modification	Failure in established weight control program
Family supportive and stable	Not addressed
Patient demonstrates adherence to diet and activity habits	
Tanner 4/5 and final or near-final adult height[a]	Not applicable
Access to experienced surgeon in medical center with team involved in long-term follow-up of patient and family needs	Center of excellence (COE) requires each surgeon to average 50 cases per year and institution to perform 125 cases annually
Patient provides assent to surgery	Patient provides consent to surgery; should be well informed and motivated and have acceptable operative risk
Patient is not pregnant or lactating and agrees to avoid pregnancy for at least 2 years postsurgery	Patient is not pregnant or lactating and agrees to avoid pregnancy during period of rapid weight loss
Eating and psychiatric disorders should be resolved, and patient should not have Prader–Willi syndrome	Psychological evaluation confirming stability of any untreated problems and ability of patient to comply with postoperative regimen
Institution is participating in study of the outcome of bariatric surgery or sharing data	COE requirement: postoperative care, nutritional counseling, and surveillance continue indefinitely
	Monitoring of micro- (vitamin and mineral) and macronutrient indices is lifelong

[a]In case of uncertainty regarding the physiological maturity of patient, the patient should be referred to a specialist in pediatric endocrinology, and radiographs of the hand and wrist should be performed to assess bone age.

References:
- Apovian CM, Baker C, Ludwig DS, et al. Best practice guidelines in pediatric/ adolescent weight loss surgery. Obes Res 2005; 13(2):274–282.
- Inge TH, Krebs NF, Garcia VF, et al. Bariatric surgery for severely adolescents: concerns and recommendations. Pediatrics 2004; 114:217–223.
- Pratt JS, Lenders CM, Dionne EA, et al. Best practice updates pediatric/adolescent weight loss surgery. Obesity 2009; 17:901–910.

3. **Answer: C.**

LAGB is not currently approved by FDA for adolescent patients.

Early postoperative complications or mortality do not seem to be higher in adolescents when compared to adults undergoing bariatric surgery.

Medical/behavioral therapy is inferior to bariatric surgery in causing weight loss in adolescents as compared to surgical treatment.

BPD or the DS procedure is not currently recommended for weight loss in adolescents.

Reference:
- Pratt JS, Lenders CM, Dionne EA, et al. Best practice updates for pediatric/ adolescent weight loss surgery. Obesity (Silver Spring) 2009; 17(5):901–910 [Epub February 19, 2009].

4. **Answer: C.**

About 70% of the obese adolescents were also found to be obese as adults.

About 70% of obese children have at least one cardiovascular risk factor.

The prevalence of obesity among children aged 6 to 11 years increased from 6.5% in 1980 to 19.6% in 2008. The prevalence of obesity among adolescents aged 12 to 19 years increased from 5.0% to 18.1% during the same time. In obesity, adipose tissue increase is combined with an increase in lean body mass (LBM). In children, the height-to-weight ratio changes with growth, and hence BMI growth charts have been developed for children. The definition of adolescent obesity is BMI equal to or above the 95th percentile for gender and age. Children with a BMI between the 85th and 95th percentile are considered overweight. Although numerous genetic markers are linked with obesity and its metabolic consequences, identifiable hormonal, syndromic, or molecular genetic abnormalities are present in less than 5% of obese individuals.

References:
- The NS, Suchindran C, North KE, et al. Association of adolescent obesity with risk of severe obesity in adulthood. JAMA 2010; 304(18):2042–2047.
- http://www.cdc.gov/HealthyYouth/obesity/.

5. **Answer: D.**

Higher BMI during childhood is associated with increased risk of fatal and nonfatal cardiovascular events during adulthood.

Childhood obesity is the leading cause of pediatric hypertension. Systolic blood pressure correlates positively with BMI, skinfold thickness, and waist-to-hip ratio in children and adolescents. Clinical hypertension is three times more common in obese children (BMI > 95th percentile) than children with BMI < 95th percentile, with approximately 50% of the children having hypertension.

There is a strong association between obesity and obstructive sleep apnea syndrome (OSAS), because obese children are four to six times more likely to have OSAS when compared with lean subjects. Symptoms of OSAS may include snoring, poor school performance because of daytime sleepiness, enuresis, and hyperactivity. OSAS is diagnosed by an overnight sleep study to measure the apnea-hypopnea index. Twenty-six percent to 37% of obese children have an abnormal sleep study. Tonsillar enlargement is a differential for OSAS.

NASH is present in about 10% to 40% of obese children.

References:
- Strauss RS, Barlow SE, Dietz WH. Prevalence of abnormal serum aminotransferase values in overweight and obese adolescents. J Pediatr 2000; 136(6):727–733.
- Helmrath MA, Brandt ML, Inge TH. Adolescent obesity and bariatric surgery. Surg Clin North Am 2006; 86(2):441–454.
- Sorof J, Daniels S. Obesity hypertension in children: a problem of epidemic proportions. Hypertension 2002; 40(4):441–447.
- http://www.uptodate.com/contents/comorbidities-and-complications-of-obesity-in-children-and-adolescents#H15. Accessed June 21, 2011.
- http://www.uptodate.com/contents/evaluation-of-suspected-obstructive-sleep-apnea-in-children?source=see_link. Accessed June 21, 2011.
- Weiss R, Dziura J, Burgert TS, et al. Obesity and the metabolic syndrome in children and adolescents. N Engl J Med 2004; 350(23):2362–2374.

6. **Answer: B.**

Blount's disease is due to overgrowth of the medial tibial epiphysis, which then causes bowing of tibia in an overweight child resulting in tibia vara. Slipped capital femoral epiphysis is also common in obese adolescents/children.

Fifty percent of children with pseudotumor cerebri are obese.

Prevalence of left ventricular hypertrophy increases as a function of overweight, with 3% of normal weight, 25% of overweight, 52% of obese, and 86% of morbidly obese youth fulfilling echocardiographic criteria for left ventricular hypertrophy.

References:
- Gettys FK, Jackson JB, Frick SL. Obesity in pediatric orthopaedics. Orthop Clin North Am 2011; 42(1):95–105.
- Helmrath MA, Brandt ML, Inge TH. Adolescent obesity and bariatric surgery. Surg Clin North Am 2006; 86(2):441–454.

7. **Answer: C.**

Orlistat is approved for individuals >12 years of age. About one-quarter of patients taking orlistat (along with diet and exercise modification) have a 5% or higher decrease in BMI.

Metformin is fairly well tolerated and approved by the FDA for the treatment of type 2 diabetes. It is not approved for the treatment of childhood obesity. It has been used primarily in obese adolescents who have polycystic ovarian syndrome to decrease weight and insulin resistance.

Sibutramine was FDA approved for patients >16 years. It has now been withdrawn from the market by the manufacturer.

References:

- Helmrath MA, Brandt ML, Inge TH. Adolescent obesity and bariatric surgery. Surg Clin North Am 2006; 86(2):441–454.
- Chanoine JP, Hampl S, Jensen C, et al. Effect of orlistat on weight and body composition in obese adolescents: a randomized controlled trial. JAMA 2005; 293 (23):2873–2883.

11 | Nutrition

CHAPTER SUMMARY
- Bariatric surgery patients are at an increased risk of malnutrition post surgery. Several nutrient deficiencies are also present before surgery.
- Bariatric surgery patients must be monitored for nutritional deficiencies. The American Society for Metabolic and Bariatric Surgery (ASMBS)/American Association of Clinical Endocrinologists (AACE) guidelines for monitoring are given below:

After a gastric bypass, the following tests are recommended every 3–6 months for the first year and annually thereafter:
- CBC, platelets
- Electrolytes
- Glucose
- Iron studies, ferritin
- Vitamin B_{12}
- Liver function
- Lipid profile
- 25-Hydroxyvitamin D

After a biliopancreatic diversion, the following tests are recommended every 3 months for the first year and every 3–6 months (or as needed) thereafter:
- As above +
- Albumin and prealbumin
- RBC folate
- Fat-soluble vitamins (6–12 mo)
  - Vitamin A
  - 25-Hydroxyvitamin D
  - Vitamin E
  - Vitamin K, INR
- Metabolic bone evaluation
  - Intact PTH (6–12 mo)
  - 24-hr urine calcium (6–12 mo)
  - Urine N-telopeptide (annually)
  - Osteocalcin (as needed)
- Metabolic stone evaluation (annually)
  - 24-hr urine calcium, citrate, uric acid
- oxalate
- Trace elements (annually or as needed)
  - Zinc
  - Selenium
- Routine nutritional supplementation after bariatric surgery:
  - Protein: The recommended intake is 80 to 120 g/day after biliopancreatic diversion (BPD) or biliopancreatic diversion–duodenal switch (BPD-DS). Hospitalization of malabsorptional bariatric surgery patients for protein energy malnutrition is needed in 1% of the patients and parenteral nutrition for 3 to 4 weeks is the treatment for these patients. Lengthening of the common limb + alimentary limb is done if the patient is Total Parenteral Nutrition (TPN) dependent.

- Calcium + vitamin D: Routine supplementation is 1200–2000 mg/day + 400–800 U/day, respectively. Calcium citrate is better than calcium carbonate. Bisphosphonates are an option for osteoporosis but after calcium and vitamin D deficiency have been treated.
- Iron: Routine supplementation is needed – 320 mg twice daily (ferrous sulfate), and iron is more important in menstruating women. Vitamin C increases iron absorption. Iron in multivitamin alone is usually insufficient to prevent deficiency.
- Vitamin B_{12}: Supplementation consists of >350 μg/day orally or 500 μg/wk intranasally or 1000 μg IM monthly.
- Folic acid: Routine supplementation is about 400 μg/day.
- Multivitamin: Supplementation is routinely given.
- Anemia after bariatric surgery is caused mostly by iron and vitamin B_{12} deficiencies, but unexplained anemia could also be due to folate, copper, selenium, and protein deficiencies.
- Treatment of common nutrient deficiencies:
  - Vitamin D: Oral vitamin D in high doses is needed (50,000 IU/wk for 8 weeks). Unresponsive cases may need calcitriol.
  - Iron: Intravenous iron infusion with iron dextran (INFeD), ferric gluconate (Ferrlecit), or ferric sucrose may be needed if oral administration cannot correct deficiency.
  - Vitamin B_{12}: 1000 μg IM monthly or 1000 to 3000 μg every 6 to 12 months.
  - Folate: Treatment of deficiency is by 1000 mg/day of folate. Folate > 1000 mg has the potential to mask vitamin B_{12} deficiency.
  - Thiamine deficiency causing Wernicke's encephalopathy and peripheral neuropathy – aggressive parenteral supplementation with thiamine (100 mg/day) should be administered for 7 to 14 days. Sometimes prolonged treatment may be needed. Glucose should be administered cautiously.
- Protein deficiency – key points:
  - Protein deficiency is not common preoperatively.
  - Postoperative incidence:
    - It is very rare after a standard Roux-en-Y gastric bypass (RYGB).
    - The incidence of protein malnutrition after BPD is not certain with most studies reporting low incidence of the same. The incidence is lower with BPD-DS when compared with BPD.
  - The exact protein requirements after bariatric surgery are not defined but most bariatric programs recommend 1 to 1.5 g/kg of protein daily.
  - Treatment: Liquid protein supplements may be enough for mild deficiency, followed by gradual return to normal diet. Total parenteral nutrition is needed for severe cases. Mechanical and behavioral causes must be ruled out before revisional surgery (lengthening of the common limb) is undertaken.
  - Modular protein supplements should contain all the indispensible amino acids. Protein digestability corrected amino acid (PDCAA) is an excellent method for evaluation of protein quality. It compares the indispensible amino acid content to the estimated average requirement of each amino acid. The PDCAA is 100 for milk, whey, and egg white. Whey is one of the highest-quality proteins. Adequate protein intake with an inadequate content of indispensible amino acids can still cause loss of lean body mass.
- Key points about specific micronutrient deficiencies:
  - Thiamine:
    - Vomiting is an important cause of deficiency.
    - Deficiency presents as Wernicke's encephalopathy or Korsakoff's psychosis or peripheral neuropathy. They may persist even after correction of deficiency.

- Low thiamine levels are common before surgery.
- Thiamine stores in the body are depleted quickly and daily replenishment is necessary. Hence, deficiency can occur in the early postoperative period.
- Vitamin B_{12}:
  - It causes megaloblastic anemia. Others symptoms include paresthesias, polyneuropathy, and psychosis.
  - Gastric acid is necessary for conversion of pepsinogen to pepsin. Pepsin is necessary for release of vitamin B_{12} from protein. Vitamin B_{12} is absorbed in the terminal ileum, and intrinsic factor is essential for the same. Both gastric acid and the intrinsic factor are produced by the parietal cells. These processes are affected more in RYGB compared to laparoscopic adjustable gastric band (LAGB) and BPD (where the parietal cell mass is relatively intact). Hence, vitamin B_{12} is absorbed by passive diffusion, independent of intrinsic factor, in RYGB patients.
  - Some studies have found an increased risk of vitamin B_{12} deficiency in morbidly obese patients.
  - Deficiency usually appears after the first year after surgery. Most studies found that the incidence of postoperative deficiency is around 35%.
  - Methylmalonic acid levels are a more sensitive marker of vitamin B_{12} deficiency as vitamin B_{12} levels may be normal in early deficiency. Patients with symptoms of vitamin B_{12} deficiency may have normal vitamin B_{12} levels. Cutoff for deficiency is around 200 pg/mL.
- Folate:
  - In general, folate deficiency is less common than vitamin B_{12} deficiency after RYGB.
  - One of the greatest concerns of deficiency is the risk of neural tube defects in babies born to deficient women. All enriched grains in the United States are fortified with folate as per FDA guidelines.
  - It also presents with megaloblastic anemia. Other symptoms include psychiatric disturbances.
  - Even though folate absorption mostly occurs in the proximal small bowel, the entire small bowel can absorb folate by postoperative adaptation. Hence, correction of folate deficiency or its prevention is easier than that of vitamin B_{12} deficiency.
  - Homocysteine levels are a sensitive marker for folate deficiency.
- Iron:
  - Absorption of iron mostly occurs in the duodenum and proximal jejunum. Duodenal cytochrome *b* is responsible for conversion of ferric to ferrous iron. Gastric acid also helps in this conversion, which is affected in a RYGB pouch. Etiology of deficiency thus involves bypass of the proximal bowel in malabsorptive procedures. This is further exacerbated by intolerance to red meat, which is a good source of iron. Vitamin C helps in absorption of nonheme iron.
  - Preoperative deficiency is common especially in menstruating women, who comprise a large fraction of the bariatric cases. Preoperative deficiency has also been found to be more common in men. Postoperatively deficiency is found in about 20% to 50% of the patients. Menstruating women who are on oral contraceptives seem to be at a lesser risk for deficiency.
  - Ferritin can be normal in the presence of inflammation. Hence, iron and total iron binding capacity should be used to diagnose iron-deficiency anemia. Decrease in hemoglobin occurs late.
- Vitamin D:
  - It is a fat-soluble vitamin and hence its deficiency can occur due to decreased mixing of bile and resulting fat malabsorption seen in RYGB and BPD.

- It is essential for absorption of calcium by the kidneys. But deficiency does not result in hypocalcemia until skeleton is depleted of calcium stores.
- Preoperative deficiency is very common and higher BMI patients are at a greater risk. This is due to increased clearance by the adipose tissue and decreased exposure to ultraviolet light.
- Decreased vitamin D levels, increased PTH and hypocalcemia are common in post-BPD patients. Decreased bone mineral density (BMD) is also common in post-RYGB patients, and this occurs as early as 3 months postoperatively. Secondary hyperparathyroidism and increased urinary markers for bone turnover are also common in RYGB patients. Secondary hyperparathyroidism seen in postbariatric patients is not easily treated by calcium and vitamin D supplementation. Decreased estradiol after bariatric surgery may play a role in the reduction of BMD.
- Gastric banding patients usually do not have secondary hyperparathyroidism but show negative bone modeling as assessed by urinary markers.
- Vitamin B_6:
  - This is not routinely measured in clinical practice, but postoperative deficiency may be common (around 36% in one study of gastric bypass patients).
  - Erythrocyte aminotransferase levels may be better indicators of deficiency when compared to serum levels of the vitamin.
- Vitamins A, E, and K:
  - Vitamin A: The rate of deficiency after RYGB or BPD varies across studies, with some studies reporting >50%. Ophthalmic symptoms are rare though there are case reports.
  - Vitamin K deficiency has been reported to be more than 50% after BPD, though there have been no reports of bleeding.
  - There is no consensus about prevalence of vitamin E deficiency postoperatively. Preoperatively it was reported in 20% of RYGB patients in one study.
- Zinc:
  - Fat malabsorption contributes to zinc deficiency.
  - Deficiency after BPD is around 50% and that after RYGB is around 35%.
  - Zinc deficiency could also be contributed to by red meat intolerance.
  - Taste changes have been found after bariatric surgery but have not been definitively attributed to zinc deficiency.
- Copper:
  - Copper deficiency causes anemia and myelopathy.
  - Deficiency is very rare with only case reports available.
  - Zinc supplementation over a long period of time can cause copper deficiency.
- Selenium has been found to be deficient in BPD patients both pre- and postoperatively in gastric bypass patients. Selenium deficiency causes cardiomyopathy and heart failure.
- Postoperative diet:
  - Postoperative diet after bariatric surgery is usually progressed in five phases.
    - Clear liquids – they supply electrolytes and a minimal amount of energy. They do not leave any gastrointestinal residue. It is given for 1 to 2 days after surgery.
    - Full liquids – they include milk and milk products. They leave some gastrointestinal residue and provide calories equivalent to a VLCD.
    - Pureed diet – they consist of diet that is blended with adequate fluid resulting in a pudding-like consistency. High-protein food is used. In addition, full liquids are continued. The pureed diet is given till 10 to 14 days after surgery.

- Mechanically altered soft diet – it is a diet that requires minimal chewing, which is obtained by chopping, mashing, grinding, or flaking. It is a transition to the normal diet. It is usually started after 2 weeks.
- Regular diet.
- High-calorie foods like refined sugar are to be avoided. Certain foods like carbonated beverages and caffeine are recommended to be avoided though there is no definitive data to back these recommendations.

QUESTIONS

1. Which of the following is a <u>FALSE</u> statement regarding the biochemistry of thiamine and pathogenesis of Wernicke's encephalopathy?
   A. Thiamine is involved in Kreb's cycle pathway.
   B. Deficiency of thiamine inhibits glucose metabolism in many areas of the brain.
   C. Lactate accumulation is a consequence of thiamine deficiency.
   D. Thiamine is required as a coenzyme in the glycolytic pathway.

2. Both folate and vitamin B_{12} can cause anemia after RYGB. Identify the <u>FALSE</u> statement diagnosis of folate deficiency.
   A. Increased methylmalonic acid levels are specifically seen in folate deficiency.
   B. Increased homocysteine levels are seen in folate deficiency.
   C. RBC folate levels indicate long-term folate stores.
   D. Folate deficiency is rare following RYGB when compared to vitamin B_{12} deficiency.

3. Which of the following is <u>NOT</u> the cause of iron deficiency after RYGB?
   A. Hypoacidity of the gastric pouch
   B. Bypass of the primary site of iron absorption
   C. Intolerance to meat
   D. Gastric restriction

4. Though not proven, it is suspected that vitamin B_{12} is absorbed by an alternate mechanism after RYGB. Identify the <u>TRUE</u> statement for vitamin B_{12} deficiency after RYGB.
   A. In patients receiving multivitamin supplementation, vitamin B_{12} deficiency is less common than folate deficiency.
   B. Patients who do not respond to high dose of oral vitamin B_{12} usually do not respond to IM vitamin B_{12} injections also.
   C. Pancreatic secretions are essential for vitamin B_{12} absorption.
   D. Intranasal vitamin B_{12} is not effective for vitamin B_{12} deficiency.

5. Though obesity is considered an overfed state, nutritional deficiencies do occur in obesity and type 2 DM. Which of the following deficiencies are seen more commonly in obese patients when compared to their lean counterparts?
   A. Vitamin A
   B. Vitamin D
   C. Vitamin E
   D. Thiamine
   E. All of the above

6. Regular follow-up and screening for micronutrient deficiencies is an important part of postoperative care after RYGB. Which of the following nutrient deficiencies is <u>NOT</u> recommended to be screened routinely in an asymptomatic patient after RYGB?
   A. Vitamin B_{12}
   B. Iron

    C. Vitamin D

    D. Vitamin B_6

7. **Iron deficiency is common in obesity as well as after bariatric surgery and the patient needs to be screened for the same both before and after surgery. Which of the following statements is <u>TRUE</u> about iron deficiency and supplementation in obese patients?**
   A. Low serum iron levels are specific for iron-deficiency anemia.
   B. Transferrin levels are decreased iron-deficiency anemia.
   C. Hepcidin is increased in obese patients.
   D. Vitamin C decreases absorption of iron.

8. **A 45-year-old female with a history of a RYGB 4 months ago presents with vomiting, confusion, and lethargy for the past 4 days. She has tolerated small amounts of liquids, but has had increasing difficulty swallowing solids for the past 2 weeks. Her physical examination findings and laboratory studies are as follows:**

   PHYSICAL EXAM AND LABS:

   Vitals: temp: 99.4°F; HR: 110/min; RR: 16/min; BP: 140/90; SpO_2: 95% on room air
   HEENT: pupils – bilaterally equal and reacting to light; lateral nystagmus present; moist oral mucosa; neck supple

   Cardiovascular exam: S_1, S_2 normal; no added sounds or murmurs

   Respiratory system: normal

   Abdominal exam: soft, nondistended, nontender, bowel sounds present

   Neurological exam: retrograde amnesia; deep tendon reflexes 1+ in all extremities; muscle strength 3/5 in all extremities. External Ocular Movements (EOM): bilateral lateral rectus palsy. Gait: ataxic
   Extremities: no cyanosis, clubbing or edema

   Skin: no rash

   Labs: sodium – 136 mmol/L, potassium – 4.1 mmol/L, chloride – 100 mmol/L, bicarbonate – 23 mmol/L, blood urea nitrogen – 10 mg/dL, creatinine – 0.9 mg/dL, and glucose – 86 mg/dL, white blood cell count – 8.6 k/cmm, hemoglobin – 11.2 gm/dL, hematocrit – 41%, and platelet – 300 k/cmm. Urinalysis – negative. Lumbar puncture: protein – 110 mg/dL and glucose – 50 mg/dL, no red blood cells or white blood cells, chest X-ray study was normal. Computed tomography of the brain was normal. In the emergency department, she is given 2 L of normal saline. What is the most important next step in managing this patient?

   A. Give IV dextrose.
   B. CT scan of the abdomen and pelvis.
   C. Prepare the patient for esophagogastroduodenoscopy.
   D. Upper GI swallow study.
   E. Give IV thiamine.

9. **A patient sees you in follow-up 6 weeks after a RYGB, complaining of postprandial epigastric pain and excess gas. After a detailed history, it is clear the patient has not been compliant with all postoperative dietary instructions. You would recommend all of the following <u>EXCEPT</u>.**
   A. Drink fluids through a straw
   B. Avoid drinking carbonated beverages
   C. Avoid combining liquids with solid food during meals
   D. Avoid continuing to eat after feeling full

10. **A patient status post-RYGB has to gradually transition from liquid to solid food after surgery over several weeks to months. Identify the <u>TRUE</u> statement about feeding in a postbariatric patient.**
    A. The most common cause of regurgitation of food and occasional vomiting is improper feeding.
    B. Red meat is recommended as a high source of protein in the first month after RYGB.
    C. Patient should not consume >500 mL of fluids per day to avoid distension of pouch.
    D. The ASMBS recommends post-RYGB diet to be advanced in six stages.

11. **After bariatric surgery, patients need to make a very gradual transition from liquid diet to normal diet over a period of several weeks. All of the following statements about postoperative diet are true <u>EXCEPT</u>.**
    A. Small frequent meals are recommended when the patient can start consuming normal food.
    B. Intake of supplemental proteins is of great importance (60–120 g).
    C. Full liquids taken immediately after discharge may contain up to 50 g of sugar per serving.
    D. Proteins must be taken during the initial part of the meal.

12. **Identify the <u>TRUE</u> statement about protein calorie malnutrition after bariatric surgery.**
    A. Approximately 10% of the patients undergoing BPD-DS are hospitalized for protein energy malnutrition.
    B. Rate of malnutrition after RYGB is about 15% to 20%.
    C. Total parenteral nutrition is the treatment of choice in severe cases.
    D. Surgical management requires reversing the BPD-DS in all cases.

13. **Micronutrient deficiencies need to be screened for before and after bariatric surgery. Restrictive and malabsorptive procedures have different incidences of various micronutrient and macronutrient deficiencies and screening and supplementation should be adapted to the type of procedure. Identify the <u>TRUE</u> statement.**
    A. RYGB has a greater tendency to cause vitamin B_{12} deficiency when compared to sleeve gastrectomy.
    B. Incidence of secondary hyperparathyroidism is equal in RYGB and sleeve gastrectomy patients.
    C. Incidence of vitamins A and E deficiency are equal in RYGB and LAGB.
    D. Protein intolerance seen after RYGB disappears after 3 months of surgery.

14. **There is concern regarding osteoporosis after bariatric surgery. Identify the <u>TRUE</u> statement about vitamin D deficiency and osteoporosis after bariatric surgery.**
    A. Hypocalcemia is seen in less than 10% of patients after BPD.
    B. BMD should be routinely measured before RYGB.
    C. LAGB is associated with decrease in BMD.
    D. Oral bisphosphonate therapy has an increased complication rate in post-RYGB patients.

15. **Nicola Scopinaro has described two types of protein energy malnutrition in his large BPD series. One group has energy and protein deficit and the other has only protein deficit. We would like to call the former group EP and latter P for the purpose of this question. Which of the following statements is <u>FALSE</u> about the two groups?**
    A. EP group is a healthy group that is actually the goal of the operation.
    B. EP group has hyperinsulinemia.
    C. Lipolysis is reduced in P group.
    D. Visceral protein synthesis is reduced in the P group.

16. A 40-year-old male presents with acute onset shortness of breath, leg swelling, and orthopnea 18 months after BPD. The patient has lost a significant amount of weight and now has a BMI of 25. There is no history of recent immobilization and he denies any fever or cough. Patient has a normal mood and has no confabulation. Examination reveals a raised jugular venous pulse, pitting pedal edema, presence of S3 gallop, and crepitation in the bases of both lungs. He has no ataxia or no ophthalmoplegia. The EKG is normal, there is no elevation of cardiac enzymes and a D-dimer assay is normal. A cardiologist is consulted and he makes a diagnosis of acute heart failure. A bolus of furosemide makes the patient more comfortable and sublingual nitroglycerin is administered. What is the most likely diagnosis?
    A. Chromium deficiency
    B. Selenium deficiency
    C. Zinc deficiency
    D. Thiamine deficiency

17. Zinc deficiency is known to occur after bariatric surgery especially after BPD. Identify the symptom which is <u>NOT</u> a manifestation of zinc deficiency.
    A. Acrodermatitis enteropathica
    B. Intercurrent infection
    C. Myelopathy
    D. Hair loss

18. All the following are recommendations to prevent dumping syndrome <u>EXCEPT</u>.
    A. Increasing the frequency of meals to six per day
    B. Decreasing water intake with food
    C. Decreasing dietary fiber
    D. Avoiding excess intake of sweets

19. Recognition of various nutritional deficiencies is crucial in a postbariatric patient. Identify the wrong association between the symptoms and the deficient micronutrient.
    A. Bleeding tendency – vitamin E
    B. Tongue soreness, appetite loss, and constipation – vitamin B_{12}
    C. Bullous-pustular dermatitis – zinc
    D. Posterolateral myelopathy – copper

20. A 45-year-old male 6 months s/p RYGB presents with a 25-hydroxy vitamin D level of 15 (normal > 32 ng/mL) and PTH of 85 (Normal 10 to 55 pg/mL). He seems very compliant and reports that he is currently taking a supplement containing 500-mg calcium citrate and 500 IU of vitamin D twice daily and a multivitamin with iron at least 2 hours apart from the calcium with vitamin D. The patient lives in an area where there is ample sunlight round the year. What would be the <u>BEST</u> recommendation for this patient?
    A. Double his current dosage of calcium citrate.
    B. Prescribe 1000 IU of vitamin D daily.
    C. Sit in the sun for 1 hour daily and drink a few glasses of milk daily.
    D. Prescribe 50,000 IU of vitamin D to be taken once weekly, and recheck labs again in 3 months.
    E. Confirm vitamin D deficiency with measurement of 1,25-dihydroxycholecalciferol (DHCC) levels.

21. When a postbariatric surgery patient with anemia does not respond to iron supplementation, all of the following nutrients may also be deficient <u>EXCEPT</u>.
    A. Folate
    B. Vitamin B_{12}
    C. Selenium

D. Copper

E. Zinc

ANSWER KEY

1. D	7. C	13. A	19. A
2. A	8. E	14. D	20. D
3. D	9. A	15. B	21. E
4. C	10. A	16. B	
5. E	11. C	17. C	
6. D	12. C	18. C	

ANSWER KEY WITH EXPLANATION

1. **Answer: D.**

Thiamine is a water soluble vitamin that is required for the activity of several enzymes including pyruvate dehdrogenase, α-ketoglutarate (of the Kreb's cycle), and transketolase (of the pentose phosphate pathway). Deficiency of thiamine inhibits the activity of these enzymes and inhibits metabolism of pyruvate. Excess pyruvate is converted to lactate, which is toxic to the tissues. The resulting damage to the brain tissues results in Wernicke's encephalopathy. The enzymes in the glycolytic pathway do not require thiamine as a coenzyme.

Reference:
- Bender DA, Mayes PA. Chapter 44: Micronutrients: vitamins & minerals. In: Murray RK, Bender DA, Botham KM, et al., eds. Harper's Illustrated Biochemistry, 28 edn. Available at: http://eresources.library.mssm.edu:2059/content.aspx?aID=5229785.

2. **Answer: A.**

Folate deficiency is rare after RYGB when compared to vitamin B_{12} deficiency because folate absorption occurs throughout the entire small bowel. The first-line tests to diagnose folate deficiency are serum folate and RBC folate levels, the RBC folate levels indicating long-term folate stores. Increased homocysteine levels are observed in folate deficiency. Increased methylmalonic acid levels are specific for vitamin B_{12} deficiency and are seen in only 2% of the patients with folate deficiency without renal failure. Increased homocysteine, however, is also not specific for folate deficiency.

References:
- Wickramasinghe SN. Diagnosis of megaloblastic anaemias. Blood Rev 2006; 20 (6):299–318.
- Koch TR, Finelli FC. Postoperative metabolic and nutritional complications of bariatric surgery. Gastroenterol Clin North Am 2010; 39(1):109–124.

3. **Answer: D.**

The jejunum and duodenum are bypassed in some malabsorptive procedures, which results in loss of the main site of iron absorption. In RYGB, the gastric pouch is hypoacidic, decreasing availability of iron as well as function of iron transport molecules. Heme iron is a form of iron which is easily absorbed but many patients have red meat intolerance, especially after RYGB. Iron deficiency does not usually occur after a purely restrictive procedure unless there is a preoperative deficiency.

References:
- Muñoz M, Botella-Romero F, Gómez-Ramírez S, et al. Iron deficiency and anaemia in bariatric surgical patients: causes, diagnosis and proper management. Nutr Hosp 2009; 24(6):640–654 (review).
- von Drygalski A, Andris DA. Anemia after bariatric surgery: more than just iron deficiency. Nutr Clin Pract 2009; 24(2):217–226 (review).

- Brolin RL, Robertson LB, Kenler HA, et al. Weight loss and dietary intake after vertical banded gastroplasty and Roux-en-Y gastric bypass. Ann Surg 1994; 220:782–790.

4. **Answer: C.**

The prevalance of vitamin B_{12} deficiency is quite high in bariatric surgery patients with some studies reporting a prevalence of up to 30% following RYGB at 1 year. The long-term prevalance varies from 36% to 70%. Comparatively, folate deficiency is rarer after gastric bypass. Multivitamin supplementation seems to reduce the incidence of folate but not vitamin B_{12} deficiency.

Hydrochloric acid releases vitamin B_{12} from proteins. Intrinsic factor produced from the parietal cells of the stomach is essential for absorption of vitamin B_{12} in the ileum. These mechanisms are impaired in gastric resection associated with RYGB. Pancreatic secretions mix with food to release vitamin B_{12} from R protein. Sublingual and oral vitamin B_{12} have been proven to be equally effective in correcting cobalamin deficiency in nonsurgical patients. The usual dose of sublingual vitamin B_{12} is 25,000 U twice weekly or 0.5 mg once daily. Some patients who do not respond to high doses of oral or sublingual vitamin B_{12} may respond to intramuscular vitamin B_{12} injections; 500 µg of intranasally administered vitamin B_{12} has been shown to be effective in reducing the incidence of vitamin B_{12} deficiency.

References:

- von Drygalski A, Andris DA. Anemia after bariatric surgery: more than just iron deficiency. Nutr Clin Pract 2009; 24(2):217–226 (review).
- Mechanick JI, Kushner RF, Sugerman HJ, et al.; American Association of Clinical Endocrinologists; Obesity Society; American Society for Metabolic & Bariatric Surgery. Executive summary of the recommendations of the American Association of Clinical Endocrinologists, the Obesity Society, and American Society for Metabolic & Bariatric Surgery medical guidelines for clinical practice for the perioperative nutritional, metabolic, and nonsurgical support of the bariatric surgery patient. Endocr Pract 2008; 14(3):318–336.
- Slot WB, Merkus FW, Van Deventer SJ, et al. Normalization of plasma vitamin B12 concentration by intranasal hydroxocobalamin in vitamin B12-deficient patients. Gastroenterology 1997; 113(2):430–433.
- Yazaki Y, Chow G, Mattie M. A single-center, double-blinded, randomized controlled study to evaluate the relative efficacy of sublingual and oral vitamin B-complex administration in reducing total serum homocysteine levels. J Altern Complement Med 2006; 12(9):881–885.
- Allied Health Sciences Section Ad Hoc Nutrition Committee; Aills L, Blankenship J, Buffington C, et al. ASMBS allied health nutritional guidelines for the surgical weight loss patient. Surg Obes Relat Dis 2008; 4(5 suppl):S73–S108.

5. **Answer: E.**

Decreased ambulation associated with obesity also results in decreased sun exposure causing vitamin D deficiency. Other factors resulting vitamin D deficiency include excess storage of vitamin D in adipose tissue, ethnicity, and skin tone. Vitamin D is the most common vitamin deficiency in obesity and is found in 40% of the patients. Vitamin E and carotenoids (vitamin A) are considered antioxidants and both of them are decreased in obese patients. Thiamine deficiency is also more common in obesity, though deficiency is likely to be subclinical. Iron deficiency and vitamin B_{12} deficiency are also more common in obese patients.

Reference:

- Kaidar-Person O, Person B, Szomstein S, et al. Nutritional deficiencies in morbidly obese patients: a new form of malnutrition? Part A: vitamins. Obes Surg 2008; 18 (7):870–876.

6. **Answer: D.**

Recommendations for screening and supplementation for nutrient deficiencies in bariatric surgery are based on expert opinions and nonrandomized studies.

Screening after any bariatric procedure is recommended to test the deficiencies of the following nutrients at the baseline, at 6 months after surgery, and then annually – vitamin B_1 (optional), vitamin B_{12}, folate (optional), iron, vitamin D. In addition, testing for vitamins A, E, and K are recommended annually after BPD and BPD-DS. Testing for vitamin B_6, copper, and zinc deficiency is recommended only if symptomatic. Evaluation for metabolic bone disease or for urinary stones is recommended after BPD.

Reference:

- Mechanick JI, Kushner RF, Sugerman HJ, et al.; American Association of Clinical Endocrinologists; Obesity Society; American Society for Metabolic & Bariatric Surgery. Executive summary of the recommendations of the American Association of Clinical Endocrinologists, the Obesity Society, and American Society for Metabolic & Bariatric Surgery medical guidelines for clinical practice for the perioperative nutritional, metabolic, and nonsurgical support of the bariatric surgery patient. Endocr Pract 2008; 14(3):318–336.

7. **Answer: C.**

Low ferritin level is specific for iron deficiency anemia (IDA). Transferrin levels are increased, whereas transferrin saturation is reduced in IDA. Low iron levels are seen with both iron deficiency and anemia of chronic inflammation (ACI). Ferritin is an acute phase reactant. Ferritin levels between 40 and 200 ng/mL with low iron levels must be interpreted with caution as it may be due to coexistent ACI that is known to be present in obesity. Only IDA can be corrected with iron supplementation.

The presence of ACI in obesity is attributed to upregulation of hepcidin. This newly discovered protein blocks the release of iron from the reticuloendothelial stores as well as prevents absorption of iron in the intestine. Hepcidin is an acute phase reactant upregulated by IL-6, which is increased in chronic inflammation along with tumor necrosis factor (TNF)-α, von Willebrand factor and C-reactive protein (CRP), and fibrinogen.

Vitamin C increases absorption of iron and should be included along with iron supplementation.

References:

- Tussing-Humphreys LM, Nemeth E, Fantuzzi G, et al. Decreased serum hepcidin and improved functional iron status 6 months after restrictive bariatric surgery. Obesity (Silver Spring) 2010; 18(10):2010–2016.
- von Drygalski A, Andris DA. Anemia after bariatric surgery: more than just iron deficiency. Nutr Clin Pract 2009; 24(2):217–226 (review).

8. **Answer: E.**

Classical Wernicke's encephalopathy is associated with a triad of mental status changes, gait ataxia, and ophthalmoplegia. This triad is seen in only 10% of the patients. Altered mental status is the most common component of Wernicke's encephalopathy. Approximately 80% of patients with Wernicke's encephalopathy also develop the Korsakoff syndrome that consists of memory impairment and confabulation. Most cases after RYGB present before 6 months of surgery and occur especially in those who have severe prolonged vomiting. ER diagnosis of Wernicke's encephalopathy is a clinical one and serum thiamine should be ordered only if the diagnosis is not certain. Parenteral thiamine must be started as soon as the diagnosis is made. The patient is unlikely to have a leak. Hence, a CT scan or an upper GI contrast study is not appropriate. An upper GI endoscopy may be a subsequent step in the management of this patient. Dextrose should not be given before IV thiamine as it may worsen the condition.

References:

- Escalona A, Pérez G, León F, et al. Wernicke's encephalopathy after Roux-en-Y gastric bypass. Obes Surg 2004; 14(8):1135–1137.

- Galvin R, Bråthen G, Ivashynka A, et al.; EFNS. EFNS guidelines for diagnosis, therapy and prevention of Wernicke encephalopathy. Eur J Neurol 2010; 17 (12):1408–1418.

9. **Answer: A.**

Drinking through a straw may overfill the stomach with fluid and air and may cause discomfort to the patient. Carbonated beverages may cause discomfort by filling the stomach pouch with air. Solids and liquids should not be combined during meals — and liquids must be taken at least 30 min before or after meals. In addition, patient should not continue to eat upon feeling full as this can ultimately result in pouch dilation and poor weight loss.

Reference:
- Strohmayer E, Via MA, Yanagisawa R. Metabolic management following bariatric surgery. Mt Sinai J Med 2010; 77(5):431–445.

10. **Answer: A.**

The ASMBS/AACE recommend that post-RYGB and LAGB diet be advanced in five stages. Initially the patient starts with clear liquids followed by full liquids, and then progresses to a pureed diet, a soft diet, followed by a normal solid diet. Patient must also consume 48 to 64 oz ($\sim$1–2 L) of fluid but should do so at least 30 minutes separate from food. Fluid intake can further be increased after 10 to 14 days. Adequate hydration is crucial in a postbariatric patient who is rapidly losing weight. Vomiting and regurgitation after gastric bypass is commonly due to eating too fast; however, progressively more severe vomiting may suggest a stricture of the gastrojejunal anastomosis. Red meat is usually not well tolerated especially in the first month in post-RYGB patients. Protein is derived mostly from fruits and vegetables.

References:
- Mechanick JI, Kushner RF, Sugerman HJ, et al.; American Association of Clinical Endocrinologists; Obesity Society; American Society for Metabolic & Bariatric Surgery. Executive summary of the recommendations of the American Association of Clinical Endocrinologists, the Obesity Society, and American Society for Metabolic & Bariatric Surgery medical guidelines for clinical practice for the perioperative nutritional, metabolic, and nonsurgical support of the bariatric surgery patient. Endocr Pract 2008; 14(3):318–336.
- Strohmayer E, Via MA, Yanagisawa R. Metabolic management following bariatric surgery. Mt Sinai J Med 2010; 77(5):431–445.

11. **Answer: C.**

Full liquids should contain <15-g sugar per serving (as this can minimize the occurrence of dumping symptoms) and less than 5-g fat per serving; 60 to 120 g of protein should be consumed everyday and the protein component of the meal should be taken first during the meal to avoid satiety later during the meal, which might result in inadequate protein intake. Small frequent meals prevent dumping syndrome and vomiting. For this purpose, patients are advised to eat from small plates and use small utensils to help control portions.

References:
- Strohmayer E, Via MA, Yanagisawa R. Metabolic management following bariatric surgery. Mt Sinai J Med 2010; 77(5):431–445.
- Mechanick JI, Kushner RF, Sugerman HJ, et al.; American Association of Clinical Endocrinologists; Obesity Society; American Society for Metabolic & Bariatric Surgery. Executive summary of the recommendations of the American Association of Clinical Endocrinologists, the Obesity Society, and American Society for Metabolic & Bariatric Surgery medical guidelines for clinical practice for the perioperative nutritional, metabolic, and nonsurgical support of the bariatric surgery patient. Endocr Pract 2008; 14(3):318–336.

12. **Answer: C.**

Rates of protein malnutrition after RYGB is very low, and is in the range of 1% to 5%, although it is more with a >150-cm Roux limb gastric bypass; 3% to 18% of the patients undergoing a BPD develop protein malnutrition. Approximately 1% of the patients who have undergone BPD-DS are hospitalized for protein-energy malnutrition (PEM) and they need to receive parenteral nutrition (PN) for 3 to 4 weeks. If the patient is dependent on PN, lengthening of the common channel may be necessary. PN is rarely required for protein malnutrition occurring after RYGB.

References:
- Mechanick JI, Kushner RF, Sugerman HJ, et al.; American Association of Clinical Endocrinologists; Obesity Society; American Society for Metabolic & Bariatric Surgery. Executive summary of the recommendations of the American Association of Clinical Endocrinologists, the Obesity Society, and American Society for Metabolic & Bariatric Surgery medical guidelines for clinical practice for the perioperative nutritional, metabolic, and nonsurgical support of the bariatric surgery patient. Endocr Pract 2008; 14(3):318–336.
- Malinowski SS. Nutritional and metabolic complications of bariatric surgery. Am J Med Sci 2006; 331:219–225.
- Strohmayer E, Via MA, Yanagisawa R. Metabolic management following bariatric surgery. Mt Sinai J Med 2010; 77(5):431–445.
- Marceau P, Hould FS, Lebel S, et al. Malabsorptive obesity surgery. Surg Clin North Am 2001; 81(5):1113–1127.

13. **Answer: A.**

RYGB has a greater tendency to cause vitamin B_{12} deficiency when compared to sleeve gastrectomy or LAGB. Vitamin D deficiency and secondary hyperparathyroidism are also more common in RYGB when compared to sleeve gastrectomy patients. Fat-soluble vitamin deficiencies (vitamins A and E) are more frequent in RYGB when compared to gastric banding. Protein intolerance is seen up to 1 year following RYGB, though it is much less common with restrictive procedures.

References:
- Gehrer S, Kern B, Peters T, et al. Fewer nutrient deficiencies after laparoscopic sleeve gastrectomy (LSG) than after laparoscopic Roux-Y-gastric bypass (LRYGB)-a prospective study. Obes Surg 2010; 20(4):447–453.
- Ledoux S, Msika S, Moussa F, et al. Comparison of nutritional consequences of conventional therapy of obesity, adjustable gastric banding, and gastric bypass. Obes Surg 2006; 16(8):1041–1049.
- Strohmayer E, Via MA, Yanagisawa R. Metabolic management following bariatric surgery. Mt Sinai J Med 2010; 77(5):431–445.
- Moize V, Geliebter A, Gluck ME, et al. Obese patients have inadequate protein intake related to protein intolerance up to 1 year following Roux-en-Y gastric bypass. Obes Surg 2003; 13:23–28.
- Allied Health Sciences Section Ad Hoc Nutrition Committee, Aills L, Blankenship J, Buffington C, et al. ASMBS allied health nutritional guidelines for the surgical weight loss patient. Surg Obes Relat Dis 2008; 4(5 suppl):S73–S108.

14. **Answer: D.**

Frank hypocalcemia is seen in around half of BPD-DS patients.

BMD need not be routinely measured before bariatric surgery as there is no strong evidence supporting this.

At present, there are no conclusive data regarding the association of altered calcium and vitamin D homeostasis with LAGB surgery. In two reports, LAGB was not associated with significant reduction in BMD.

Bisphosphonate therapy is not indicated routinely in postbariatric patients.

If bisphosphonate therapy is indicated due to decreased BMD, intravenous therapy is recommended as oral therapy can result in inadequate absorption and increased rate of gastric pouch ulceration. Nasal calcitonin is an alternative.

Reference:
- Mechanick JI, Kushner RF, Sugerman HJ, et al.; American Association of Clinical Endocrinologists; Obesity Society; American Society for Metabolic & Bariatric Surgery. Executive summary of the recommendations of the American Association of Clinical Endocrinologists, the Obesity Society, and American Society for Metabolic & Bariatric Surgery medical guidelines for clinical practice for the perioperative nutritional, metabolic, and nonsurgical support of the bariatric surgery patient. Endocr Pract 2008; 14(3):318–336.

15. **Answer: B.**

BPD causes a negative balance for both energy and nitrogen. As such patients can develop both protein and energy deficiency (marasmic form – EP group) or only a protein deficiency (kwashiorkor form – P group). EP group represents the ideal metabolic adaptation to starvation as the resulting hypoinsulinemia ensures lipolysis and proteolysis from skeletal muscle, which supplies amino acids for visceral pool preservation and hepatic synthesis of glucose. The near normal energy supply seen in the P group is associated with hyperinsulinemia, which inhibits lipolysis and proteolysis in the skeletal muscle. When the protein stores cannot be utilized, and in the absence of protein sparing, visceral protein synthesis is reduced, with consequent hypoalbuminemia, anemia, and immune depression.

Reference:
- Scopinaro N, Adami GF, Marinari GM, et al. Biliopancreatic diversion. World J Surg 1998; 22:936–946.

16. **Answer: B.**

Selenium deficiency should be ruled out. Selenium (Se) deficiency has been noted in 14% to 22% of postbariatric surgery patients. This is not unexpected as Se is absorbed in the duodenum and proximal jejunum. Cardiomyopathy is a common manifestation of selenium deficiency. Peripheral muscle involvement with myositis, weakness, and muscle cramps are other manifestations of Se deficiency. Se also has an important role in thyroid hormone production.

Other micronutrients deficiencies do not have a similar presentation as this case.

Reference:
- Shankar P, Boylan M, Sriram K. Micronutrient deficiencies after bariatric surgery. Nutrition 2010; 26(11, 12):1031–1037 [Epub April 3, 2010].

17. **Answer: C.**

Zinc is absorbed in the duodenum and proximal jejunum. Zinc deficiency is known to cause diarrhea, hair loss, emotional disorders, weight loss, intercurrent infection, bullous-pustular dermatitis, and hypogonadism in males. Acrodermatitis enteropathica is characterized by periorificial and acral dermatitis, alopecia, and diarrhea. Myelopathy does not occur with zinc deficiency.

References:
- Allied Health Sciences Section Ad Hoc Nutrition Committee; Aills L, Blankenship J, Buffington C, et al. ASMBS allied health nutritional guidelines for the surgical weight loss patient. Surg Obes Relat Dis 2008; 4(5 suppl):S73–S108.
- Shankar P, Boylan M, Sriram K. Micronutrient deficiencies after bariatric surgery. Nutrition 2010; 26(11, 12):1031–1037.
- Sallé A, Demarsy D, Poirier AL, et al. Zinc deficiency: a frequent and underestimated complication after bariatric surgery. Obes Surg 2010; 20 (12):1660–1670.

18. **Answer: C.**

    Dumping syndrome can be prevented by adhering to specific diet and behavioral modifications. Simple carbohydrates and foods containing them like sweets should be avoided. Liquids should be ingested at least 30 minutes after a meal and the amount of intake during a meal decreased. Increased fiber intake may slow gastric emptying. Patients should chew food thoroughly and consume multiple small meals (about 6/day). Lying down after a meal decreases gastric emptying and helps prevent or minimize symptoms of dizziness if they occur. In severe cases that are unresponsive to these changes, medical therapy with somatostatin analogs or surgical revision or reversal may be required.

    Reference:
    - Strohmayer E, Via MA, Yanagisawa R. Metabolic management following bariatric surgery. Mt Sinai J Med 2010; 77(5):431–445.

19. **Answer: A.**

    Though vitamin E deficiency can cause ataxia and vision abnormalities, its deficiency after bariatric surgery is very rare. There are no documented cases of symptomatic vitamin E deficiency after bariatric surgery. Vitamin E deficiency has not been shown to cause bleeding; however, there are reports of vitamin E toxicity causing bleeding tendency by inhibition of platelet aggregation and vitamin K metabolism. Other associations are correct.

    Reference:
    - Shankar P, Boylan M, Sriram K. Micronutrient deficiencies after bariatric surgery. Nutrition 2010; 26(11, 12):1031–1037.

20. **Answer: D.**

    The patient has vitamin D deficiency based on his labs. The standard recommended treatment for someone post-RYGB with vitamin D deficiency is weekly 50,000 IU of vitamin D for 8 weeks in addition to baseline calcium and vitamin D replacement. DHCC levels may be normal or even increased in vitamin D deficiency.

    Reference:
    - Bringhurst FR, Demay MB, Krane SM, et al. Chapter 346: Bone and mineral metabolism in health and disease. In: Fauci AS, Braunwald E, Kasper DL, et al., eds. Harrison's Principles of Internal Medicine. 17th edn. Available at: http://eresources.library.mssm.edu:2059/content.aspx?aID=2882031.

21. **Answer: E.**

    Zinc deficiency has not been shown to cause anemia. Other nutrient deficiencies should be included in the differential diagnosis of anemia in a postbariatric surgery patient.

    Reference:
    - Russell RM, Suter PM. Chapter 71: Vitamin and trace mineral deficiency and excess. In: Fauci AS, Braunwald E, Kasper DL, et al., eds. Harrison's Principles of Internal Medicine. 17th edn.

12 | Critical care

CHAPTER SUMMARY

- The effect of obesity on intensive care unit (ICU) mortality is not certain as there is no consensus among various studies.
- The factors that predict risk of a bariatric surgery patient for ICU admission include the following:
  - Male sex
  - Age > 50 years
  - Body mass index (BMI) > 60 kg/m^2
  - Diabetes
  - Cardiovascular disease
  - Obstructive sleep apnea (OSA)
  - Venous stasis
  - Intraoperative complications
- Ventilation issues in morbidly obese patients:
  - Obese patients have a restrictive lung pattern. Obstructive pattern has also been reported in some studies.
  - Preexisting pulmonary disease (like asthma) leads to increased postoperative pulmonary complications in the obese. Obesity as such predisposes patients to respiratory complications like hypoxemia and hypoventilation. Bariatric patients are prone for prolonged intubation in the ICU. However, respiratory failure is rare in bariatric surgery patients.
  - Ambulation must be encouraged as early as 2 hours after surgery and frequently thereafter.
  - They have increased risk of aspiration due to the following reasons:
    - Presence of hiatal hernia
    - Increased abdominal pressure
    - Increased amount of gastric fluid (>25 mL)
    - Decreased pH of the gastric fluid (<2.5)
  - The delivered tidal volume should be calculated based on ideal body weight (IBW).
  - Positive end-expiratory pressure (PEEP) would be more helpful for obese when compared to nonobese patients in improving partial pressure of oxygen (PaO$_2$) and partial pressure of carbon dioxide (PaCO$_2$).
  - Reverse Trendelenberg position facilitates not only oxygenation but also early extubation.
  - Issues concerning OSA have been dealt with in chapter 5.
- Cardiovascular issues:
  - Obese patients have an increased preload and afterload.
  - Blood pressure monitoring by using a pressure cuff is inaccurate in obese patients. Invasive arterial monitoring may be necessary. Patients are also poorly tolerant to IV fluids due to diastolic dysfunction. Hence pulmonary arterial catheter may be necessary when large-volume resuscitation is required.
  - Pneumoperitoneum has only a transient effect to decrease the cardiac output. The latter recovers after a few hours due to compensatory mechanisms.
- Nutrition of a critically ill obese:
  - Obese patients mobilize more protein when compared to fat. This increases their risk for early deconditioning. Hence, their feeding regimen should

contain, in addition to protein, calories from carbohydrates (to spare protein) with fats to supply the essential fatty acids.

- Parenteral nutrition has not been shown to be superior to enteral nutrition. When prolonged critical illness is anticipated during surgery, a feeding jejunostomy tube must be placed.
- Enteral feeding regimens must contain 30 kcal/kg and 2.0 g/kg protein per day, based on IBW. Hypocaloric feeds (<20 kcal/kg/day) may be more beneficial as they facilitate early recovery.

- Pharmacology of drugs used in critical care:
  - Renal function is not as such decreased in obesity. On the contrary, glomerular filtration rate (GFR) is increased. Renal function, if decreased, is usually secondary to diabetes and hypertension.
  - Lipophilic drugs, in general, are to be dosed based on actual body weight. Hydrophilic drugs, in general, are to be dosed initially based on IBW. There are exceptions (e.g., fentanyl). Moreover, dosing also depends on clearance and elimination half-life of the drug.
  - Commonly used antibiotics:
    - Vancomycin – to be dosed based on actual body weight. Shorter dosage interval may be required to ensure that the steady-state troughs remain in the therapeutic range.
    - Aminoglycosides: a correction factor is used to calculate dosage based on both actual body weight and IBW.
    - Serum levels of both of the above need to be monitored.

- Rhabdomyolysis:
  - Results from prolonged pressure to the muscles during surgery resulting in release of myoglobin and myoglobinuria.
  - Can be prevented by adequate padding.
  - One needs to maintain high index of suspicion to diagnose it postoperatively. Diagnosis is by serum creatinine phosphokinase (CPK) levels and urinalysis (positive dipstick for hemoglobin).
  - Forced alkaline diuresis is indicated when CPK > 5000 IU/L.
  - Complications include compartment syndrome (treated by fasciotomy) and acute renal failure (treated by renal replacement therapy).

QUESTIONS

1. Several studies have reported that obese patients have an increased mortality in the hospital and ICU when compared to nonobese patients. Which of the following is NOT a risk factor for admission of a bariatric surgical patient to the ICU?
   A. Male sex
   B. OSA
   C. Venous stasis
   D. Revisional surgery

2. Postoperatively, bariatric patients have a higher rate of pulmonary complications. Identify the pathophysiologic mechanism that does NOT contribute to such an increased rate of pulmonary complications.
   A. Increased forced expiratory volume in 1 second to forced vital capacity (FEV1/ FVC).
   B. Redundant oropharyngeal tissue contributing to difficult intubation.
   C. Restrictive pattern due to increased pulmonary blood volume.
   D. Decreased CO_2 production thus removing the hypercapnic drive for ventilation.

3. **A 42-year-old woman, who has a BMI of 52 kg/m², who suffers with diabetes, gastroesophageal reflux disease (GERD), and arthritis, undergoes an uneventful Roux-en-Y gastric bypass (RYGB). Postoperatively she is diagnosed with aspiration and requires admission to the ICU for respiratory failure. However, the patient cannot be extubated for 24 hours after surgery. Identify the <u>FALSE</u> statement about mechanical ventilation of a postbariatric patient.**
   A. Delivered tidal volume should be calculated based on IBW.
   B. A PEEP is more useful in an intubated obese patient than a nonobese patient.
   C. Reverse Trendelenberg position of 30° results in better oxygenation when compared to supine position.
   D. Tracheostomy has not been shown to have an increased complication rate in obese patients in any study.

4. **A patient is 2 weeks status post-LRYGB. He presents with epigastric pain and fever. An UGI study demonstrates a leak at the gastrojejunostomy (GJ). The patient undergoes an open laparotomy. Purulent material and adhesions are found near the GJ site. A redo GJ is done, and the peritoneal cavity is irrigated thoroughly. The surgeon suspects the need for the patient to remain nil per os for a long period. Which of the following is the <u>BEST</u> option for postoperative nutrition for the patient?**
   A. Total parenteral nutrition
   B. Enteral nutrition with a gastrostomy tube with low–protein content feeds
   C. Enteral nutrition with a gastrostomy tube with hypocaloric feeds
   D. Just 5% dextrose infusion till the patient can start oral feeds

5. **A patient is recovering in the ICU after a 4-hour-long RYGB. The patient complains to the nurse of pain in her buttocks. The nurse gives another dose of tramadol but this causes only partial relief of pain. On being informed by the nurse the attending surgeon orders a CPK level that comes back as 5500 IU/L. Her urinalysis is significant for a positive dipstick for blood, with no red blood cells (RBCs) on microscopy. Renal function tests are normal. No pressure elevation in the gluteus maximus compartment was noted. Which is the <u>NEXT</u> best step in management?**
   A. Hemodialysis
   B. Alkaline diuresis
   C. Fasciotomy of the buttock region
   D. IV dantrolene

6. **Rhabdomyolysis is a rare postoperative complication of bariatric surgery. Which of the following statements about the condition is <u>TRUE</u>?**
   A. It does not have external/cutaneous manifestations.
   B. Minimizing the operating time does not prevent rhabdomyolysis.
   C. It is not easy to recognize this complication clinically.
   D. Obesity is not a risk factor.

7. **Pressure sores are a common complication in a morbidly obese patient with prolonged ICU stay and more so in those patients who have prolonged intubation. Identify the <u>FALSE</u> statement about prevention and management of pressure sores.**
   A. Use of pressure reduction mattress is recommended.
   B. Frequent change in position recommended.
   C. MRI has a high sensitivity to diagnose associated osteomyelitis.
   D. Antibiotic cream should be used in the treatment of pressure ulcers in all cases.

8. **Laparoscopic surgery has reduced postoperative pain and recovery time after surgery when compared to open surgery. Identify the <u>FALSE</u> statement about postoperative analgesia after bariatric surgery.**
   A. Infiltration of local anesthetic at the trocar sites decreases postoperative pain.

    B. Morphine when used for patient-controlled analgesia (PCA) is to be calculated based on IBW, not actual body weight.

    C. Hydromorphone (Dilaudid) is commonly used for PCA.

    D. PCA has increased the total dose of opioid use.

9. **Continuous epidural analgesia is one of the choices for PCA after bariatric surgery. How is this method different from IV opioid analgesia?**

    A. It has a faster onset of action.

    B. It causes lesser constipation.

    C. It causes more respiratory depression.

    D. It causes profound sensory disturbances in addition to loss of pain sensation.

10. **OSA is a common complication of obesity and its presence needs to be taken into account during postoperative care. Regarding the management of OSA in a bariatric surgery patient, which of the following statements is FALSE?**

    A. Polysomnography before surgery increases the rate of OSA detection.

    B. Patients with OSA are usually placed continuous positive airway pressure (CPAP) postoperatively.

    C. CPAP increases gastric distension in OSA patients.

    D. CPAP does increase GJ anastomotic failure rates.

ANSWER KEY

1. D	4. C	7. D	10. D
2. D	5. B	8. D	
3. D	6. C	9. B	

ANSWER KEY WITH EXPLANATION

1. **Answer: D.**

   Patients requiring revisional bariatric surgery are no more likely to require emergency critical care admission than the primary cases. Revisional surgery patients, however, do have longer hospital stays, higher hospital costs, and higher mortality. The risk factors for ICU admission of a bariatric surgical patient include the following:
   - Male sex
   - Age > 50 years
   - BMI > 60 kg/m^2
   - Diabetes mellitus
   - Cardiovascular disease
   - OSA
   - Venous stasis
   - Intraoperative complications

   References:
   - Pieracci FM, Barie PS, Pomp A. Critical care of the bariatric patient. Crit Care Med 2006; 34(6):1796–1804.
   - Cendán JC, Abu-aouf D, Gabrielli A, et al. Utilization of intensive care resources in bariatric surgery. Obes Surg 2005; 15(9):1247–1251.
   - Livingston EH, Huerta S, Arthur D, et al. Male gender is a predictor for morbidity and age a predictor of mortality for patients undergoing bypass surgery. Ann Surg 2002; 236:576–582.

2. **Answer: D.**

   Obesity results in a restrictive lung pattern due to both increased pulmonary blood volume and increased chest wall mass from adipose tissue. Abnormal diaphragm position, upper airway resistance, and increased daily CO_2 production exacerbate respiratory load and further increase the work of breathing. The consequences of this restrictive pattern are decreased functional residual capacity, vital capacity, total lung capacity, inspiratory capacity, minute ventilatory volume, and expiratory reserve volume. Patients may also exhibit an obesity-related obstructive air flow pathology that manifests itself as an increased ratio of FEV1:FVC. The relatively short, wide necks and redundant oropharyngeal tissue of obese patients make intubation difficult. Effective preoxygenation is not possible, and rapid arterial desaturation is common after induction of anesthesia.

References:
- Pieracci FM, Barie PS, Pomp A. Critical care of the bariatric patient. Crit Care Med 2006; 34(6):1796–1804.
- Pelosi P, Croci M, Ravagnan I, et al. Total respiratory system, lung, and chest wall mechanics in sedated-paralyzed postoperative morbidly obese patients. Chest 1996; 109:144–151.
- Levi D, Goodman ER, Patel M, et al. Critical care of the obese and bariatric surgical patient. Crit Care Clin 2003; 19:11–32.
- Ray C, Sue D, Bray G, et al. Effects of obesity on respiratory function. Am Rev Respir Dis 1983; 128:501–506.
- Suratt P, Wilheit S, Hsiao H. Compliance of the chest wall in obese subjects. J Appl Physiol 1984; 57:403–409.
- Gibson GJ. Obstructive sleep apnoea syndrome: underestimated and under-treated. Br Med Bull 2004; 72:49–64.

3. **Answer: D.**

Post–bariatric surgery patients in the ICU may benefit from early tracheostomy, in spite of reports of increased perioperative complications associated with tracheostomy in the morbidly obese.

Delivered tidal volume should be calculated based on IBW rather than the actual body weight to avoid high airway pressures, alveolar overdistention, and barotrauma. A PEEP of about 10 mm of H_2O improves lung volumes, PaO_2, $PaCO_2$, elasticity, pressure-volume curves, and intra-abdominal pressure in obese patients when compared to nonobese patients. In a population of critically ill obese patients, the reverse Trendelenburg positioning at $30°$ results in increased PaO_2 and tidal volume and decreased respiratory rate as compared with the supine position.

References:
- Blouw EL, Rudolph AD, Narr BJ, et al. The frequency of respiratory failure in patients with morbid obesity undergoing gastric bypass. AANA J 2003; 71(1): 45–50.
- Pieracci FM, Barie PS, Pomp A. Critical care of the bariatric patient. Crit Care Med 2006; 34(6):1796–1804.
- Pelosi P, Ravagnan I, Giurati G, et al. Positive end-expiratory pressure improves respiratory function in obese but not in normal subjects during anesthesia and paralysis. Anesthesiology 1999; 91:1221–1231.
- Burns SM, Egloff MB, Ryan B, et al. Effect of body position on spontaneous respiratory rate and tidal volume in patients with obesity, abdominal distention and ascites. Am J Crit Care 1994; 3:102–106.
- Poulose BK, Griffen MR, Zhu Y, et al. National analysis of adverse patient safety events in bariatric surgery. Am Surg 2005; 71:406–413.

4. **Answer: C.**

Nutrition in critically ill obese patients should supply enough glucose to spare protein. Calories should be supplied primarily as carbohydrates, with fats given to prevent essential fatty acid deficiency. Most recommended enteral feeding regimens supply 30 kcal/kg and 2.0 g/kg protein per day, based on IBW. However, recent data have reported improved outcomes using hypocaloric feedings, although further well-designed studies are warranted.

Total parenteral nutrition is used often in postoperative bariatric patients when enteral feeding is impossible. However, although data specifically addressing the bariatric patient population are not available, total parenteral nutrition has not been shown to decrease major postoperative complication rates or mortality in critically ill postoperative patients. Placement of a feeding gastrostomy tube at the time of surgery should be considered when a prolonged period of critical illness is anticipated.

References:
- Pieracci FM, Barie PS, Pomp A. Critical care of the bariatric patient. Crit Care Med 2006; 34(6):1796–1804.
- Dickerson RN, Boschert KJ, Kudsk KA, et al. Hypocaloric enteral tube feeding in critically ill obese patients. Nutrition 2002; 18:241–246.
- The Veterans Affairs Total Parenteral Nutrition Cooperative Study Group. Perioperative total parenteral nutrition in surgical patients. N Engl J Med 1991; 325:525–532.
- Heyland DK, MacDonald S, Keefe L, et al. Total parenteral nutrition in the critically ill patient. JAMA 1998; 280:2013–2019.

5. **Answer: B.**

Patients suspected of having rhabdomyolysis should be monitored in the ICU. Treatment is instituted once the CPK concentration increases to >5000 IU/L, including aggressive hydration and diuresis with mannitol to a target urine output of 1.5 mL/kg/hr. Mannitol mobilizes muscular interstitial fluid and increases renal tubular flow. Alkalization of urine with sodium bicarbonate increases the solubility of myoglobin in a pH-dependent manner.

Compartment syndrome, acute renal failure, and mortality may complicate rhabdomyolysis. Acute renal failure (prevalence, 50%) results from hypovolemia, tubular obstruction, acidosis, and free radical release. Factors predictive of renal failure in rhabdomyolysis include age of >70 years, serum CPK concentration of >16,000 IU/L, degree of hypoalbuminemia, and sepsis. Fortunately, complete recovery of tubular function is the norm, albeit after a variable period of renal replacement therapy. Hemofiltration has the added advantage of rapid clearance of myoglobin. This patient does not need any form of renal replacement therapy as she is not in renal failure.

Fasciotomy is to be done only if compartment syndrome is suspected. Dantrolene is the drug of choice for malignant hyperthermia that is side effect of inhalational anesthetics.

References:
- Pieracci FM, Barie PS, Pomp A. Critical care of the bariatric patient. Crit Care Med 2006; 34(6):1796–1804.
- Vanholder R, Sever MS, Erek E, et al. Rhabdomyolysis. J Am Soc Nephrol 2000; 11:1553–1561.

6. **Answer: C.**

Pressure-induced rhabdomyolysis is a rare but well-described postoperative complication that results from prolonged, unrelieved pressure to muscle during surgery. Major risk factors include prolonged operative time and obesity. Rhabdomyolysis after bariatric surgery may affect the lower limbs, gluteal, or lumbar regions. Mean operating room time, mean BMI (67 kg/m^2 vs. 56 kg/m^2), and the prevalence of diabetes mellitus are shown to be significantly greater in patients who developed rhabdomyolysis.

Diagnosis of this condition is difficult as postoperatively patients are under anesthesia. Cutaneous manifestations like epidermolysis and purpura have been described.

Prevention of rhabdomyolysis and related complications includes attention to padding and positioning on the operating table, minimization of operative time, and maintenance of a high index of suspicion postoperatively.

References:
- Pieracci FM, Barie PS, Pomp A. Critical care of the bariatric patient. Crit Care Med 2006; 34(6):1796–1804.
- Bostanjian D, Anthone GJ, Hamoui N, et al. Rhabdomyolysis of gluteal muscles leading to renal failure: a potentially fatal complication of surgery in the morbidly obese. Obes Surg 2003; 13:302–305.
- Wiltshire JP, Custer T. Lumbar muscle rhabdomyolysis as a cause of acute renal failure after Roux-en-Y gastric bypass. Obes Surg 2003; 13:306–313.
- Torres-Villalobos G, Kimura E, Mosqueda JL, et al. Pressure-induced rhabdomyolysis after bariatric surgery. Obes Surg 2003; 13:297–301.

7. **Answer: D.**

Pressure ulcers can be prevented by the use of pressure reduction mattress and frequent change of position of the patient every 2 to 3 hours. Pressure ulcers without infection/cellulitis do not need topical or systemic antibiotics. Debridement should be done in the presence of necrotic tissue. MRI has a 98% sensitivity and 89% specificity for osteomyelitis in patients with pressure ulcers.

Reference:
- Bluestein D, Javaheri A. Pressure ulcers: prevention, evaluation, and management. Am Fam Physician 2008; 78(10):1186–1194.

8. **Answer: D.**

PCA reduces the total dose of opioid in a 24-hour period. Continuous background infusion of medication in addition to PCA offers no advantage.

 The dose of opioids is to be adjusted based on IBW, not actual body weight as opioids are lipophilic drugs. Dexmedetomidine does not have the risk of respiratory depression.

References:
- Brodsky JB, Lerner LC. Chapter 10: Anesthetic concerns. In: Pitombo C, Jones K, Higa K, et al., eds. Obesity Surgery: Principles and Practice. 1st edn. New York: McGraw-Hill, 2007. Available at: http://www.accesssurgery.com/content.aspx?aID=140225.
- Doherty GM. Chapter 4: Postoperative care. In: Doherty GM, eds. CURRENT Diagnosis & Treatment: Surgery. 13th edn. New York: McGraw-Hill, 2010. Available at: http://www.accesssurgery.com/content.aspx?aID=5211176.

9. **Answer: B.**

Continuous infusion of opioids with or without bupivacaine can be used for epidural analgesia. It has the following advantages over IV analgesia:
- Prolonged duration of action
- Lesser respiratory depression
- Similar dose required
- Analgesia is superior
- Lesser depression of consciousness
- Better GI function
- Does not cause sensory disturbance (except pain) or motor or autonomic disturbance

It causes side effects like nausea, pruritus, and urinary retention. It has a delayed onset of action.

Reference:
- Brodsky JB, Lerner LC. Chapter 10: Anesthetic concerns. In: Pitombo C, Jones K, Higa K, et al., eds. Obesity Surgery: Principles and Practice. 1st edn. New York: McGraw-Hill, 2007. Available at: http://www.accesssurgery.com/content.aspx?aID=140225.

10. **Answer: D.**

Although CPAP leads to gastric distension, increased anastomotic failure rates at the GJ site after RYGB have not been demonstrated. There is no consensus on the perioperative management of OSA patients related to non–upper airway surgery. However, polysomnography does increase the rate of detection of OSA. It is also not certain whether OSA increases risk of postoperative hypoxemia.

References:

- Jensen C, Tejirian T, Lewis C, et al. Postoperative CPAP and BiPAP use can be safely omitted after laparoscopic Roux-en-Y gastric bypass. Surg Obes Relat Dis 2008; 4(4):512–514.
- Ahmad S, Nagle A, McCarthy RJ, et al. Postoperative hypoxemia in morbidly obese patients with and without obstructive sleep apnea undergoing laparoscopic bariatric surgery. Anesth Analg 2008; 107(1):138–143.
- Ramirez A, Lalor PF, Szomstein S, et al. Continuous positive airway pressure in immediate postoperative period after laparoscopic Roux-en-Y gastric bypass: is it safe? Surg Obes Relat Dis 2009; 5:544–546.
- Gross JB, Bachenberg KL, Benumof JL, et al. Practice guidelines for the perioperative management of patients with obstructive sleep apnea: a report by the American Society of Anesthesiologists Task Force on perioperative management of patients with obstructive sleep apnea. Anesthesiology 2006; 104:1081–1093.
- Meoli AL, Rosen CL, Kristo D, et al. Upper airway management of the adult patient with obstructive sleep apnea in the perioperative period—avoiding complications. Sleep 2003; 26:1060–1065.
- Weingarten TN, Flores AS, McKenzie JA, et al. Obstructive sleep apnoea and perioperative complications in bariatric patients. Br J Anaesth 2011; 106:131–139.

13 | Anesthesiology

CHAPTER SUMMARY

- There are no guidelines for preoperative laboratory testing of bariatric patients. Lab testing is individualized based on the presence of comorbidities.
- All bariatric patients must be evaluated for airway problems, vascular access, and sleep-disordered breathing on the day prior to surgery. Patients should be asked to quit smoking several weeks prior to surgery.
- At present, routine polysomnography to diagnose obstructive sleep apnea (OSA) is not recommended. Testing should be individualized based on clinical suspicion.
- Continuous positive airway pressure (CPAP) has been shown to improve various abnormalities associated with OSA including systemic and pulmonary hypertension and heart failure. CPAP improves cardiovascular risk.
- Preoperative use of CPAP results in decreased postoperative respiratory difficulty. Patients who are on CPAP are encouraged to use CPAP machine for at least 3 weeks preoperatively.
- Mallampati score >3 is an independent risk factor for difficult intubation. Obesity, increased neck circumference, and OSA as such are not independent predictors of difficult intubation.
- Measurement of blood pressure using a cuff may be difficult, and there should be a low threshold for invasive blood pressure monitoring.
- Induction:
    - Use of a "ramped" position is beneficial.
    - Use of reverse Trendelenberg position increases "safe apnea time" – the time from the onset of apnea during induction to a predefined point of desaturation. This position may also reduce gastroesophageal reflux. The use of noninvasive positive pressure ventilation (NIPPV) also increases the safe apnea time.
    - Use of rapid sequence intubation (RSI) is individualized.
    - Use of laryngeal mask airway (LMA) and videolaryngoscopy may also be useful in cases of difficult intubation in the obese.
    - Intraoperative hypoxemia can be treated with 10 to 15 cm H_2O of positive end-expiratory pressure (PEEP) combined with recruitment maneuvers, carefully balancing their hemodynamic effects.
- Inhalational anesthetics:
    - Nitrous oxide is best avoided in bariatric surgery as it enters the bowels and decreases the space for the surgeon in the abdomen during laparoscopy.
    - Sevoflurane and desflurane are less soluble when compared to other fluranes and therefore allow early recovery from the anesthetic.
- Use of preoperative clonidine and intraoperative dexmedetomidine reduces anesthetic and analgesic requirements. This is important as both clonidine and dexmedetomidine do not have respiratory depressant properties. In addition, use of intravenous (IV) ketorolac, local infiltration of local anesthetics, and use of nonopioid analgesics like ketamine, magnesium sulfate, and methylprednisolone may decrease opioid requirements. Continuous infusion of opioids during patient-controlled analgesia (PCA) should not be given in patients with OSA.
- Dosing of anesthetic agents:
    - Nondepolarizing neuromuscular blocking agents are hydrophilic and are to be dosed based on ideal body weight. Succinylcholine is dosed based on total body weight.

- Propofol can be dosed based on total body weight.
- Remifentanyl and fentanyl dosing should be based on ideal body weight.
- The role of routine CPAP during the early postoperative period is not clear. CPAP is begun postoperatively in the postanesthesia care unit (PACU) for patients who use CPAP preoperatively. In addition, a semi-upright position and lateral decubitus position are recommended for these patients in the PACU for better oxygenation.

QUESTIONS

1. Certain steps can be taken to reduce the risk of anesthesia in a bariatric surgical patient. Which of the following is <u>FALSE</u> regarding the same?
   A. Patient should be encouraged to give up smoking at least 8 weeks prior to surgery.
   B. Patients with proven OSA should receive CPAP at least 3 weeks before surgery.
   C. There is a need to decrease the dosage of medications cleared by the kidney.
   D. Routine preoperative polysomnography is not necessary for all bariatric patients.

2. It is recommended that the use of opioid drugs is minimized in morbidly obese patients. Which of the following have been considered as an "opioid-sparing" agent that can reduce perioperative opioid requirements?
   A. Dexmedetomidine
   B. Local anesthetics
   C. Ketorolac
   D. Clonidine
   E. All of the above

3. Proper positioning of the morbidly obese patient during bariatric surgery can help reduce anesthetic complications during induction of anesthesia. Which of the following positions is <u>NOT</u> considered to be as helpful as others in a bariatric surgery patient?
   A. Ramped position
   B. Trendelenburg position
   C. Sniffing position
   D. Near-sitting position

4. The complications due to OSA can be minimized by certain steps taken in the recovery room postoperatively. Which of the following is <u>NOT</u> recommended?
   A. Lateral decubitus position
   B. Reverse Trendelenberg position
   C. Use of PCA with a basal infusion of hydromorphone
   D. Prolonged monitoring

5. The intraoperative surveillance of pulmonary and cardiovascular functions in obese patients varies according to the surgical intervention and the patient's characteristics. Which of the following statements about the challenges of intraoperative monitoring of the morbidly obese is FALSE?
   A. Pulse oximetry may give wrong readings.
   B. An undersized cuff gives false low blood pressure.
   C. Electrocardiographic monitoring may be unreliable in morbidly obese.
   D. Measurement of ET-CO_2 (end-tidal carbon dioxide) does not reflect $PaCO_2$ (partial pressure of carbon dioxide) in obese patients.

6. A bariatric surgeon performing gastric banding on a 40-year-old female patient with a BMI of 50 kg/m^2 encounters increased difficulty in maintaining the

pneumoperitoneum intraoperatively. Laparoscopic instruments were checked for leaks but none was found. What is his next step?
   A. Abandon the surgery.
   B. Convert to open procedure.
   C. Ask anesthesiologist to check "muscle twitch" monitoring.
   D. Increase CO_2 in flow further.

7. Greater care has to be taken when opioids are used in morbidly obese patients. Identify the <u>FALSE</u> statement about postoperative analgesia after bariatric surgery.
   A. Infiltration of local anesthetic at the trocar sites decreases postoperative pain.
   B. Morphine when used for PCA is to be calculated based on ideal body weight.
   C. Dexmedetomidine does not cause respiratory depression when used for PCA.
   D. PCA has increased the total dose of opioid use.

8. Continuous epidural analgesia is one of the choices for PCA. How is this method different from IV opioid analgesia?
   A. An epidural catheter is best placed after surgery.
   B. It causes lesser constipation.
   C. It causes more respiratory depression.
   D. It causes profound sensory disturbances in addition to loss of pain sensation.

9. A patient with a BMI of 70 kg/m^2 is evaluated preoperatively by the anesthesiologist. He suspects difficult intubation upon assessment of the airway. Which of the following would be the <u>BEST</u> course of management?
   A. Perform an adjustable gastric band procedure under sedation and local anesthesia.
   B. Perform a fiber-optic intubation after paralyzing the patient.
   C. Perform a tracheostomy before surgery.
   D. Perform an awake fiber-optic intubation.

10. Which of the following is <u>TRUE</u> regarding applying cricoid pressure during intubation?
   A. Cricoid pressure is a standard technique that is safe and effective in preventing gastric aspiration.
   B. Possible risk from cricoid pressure includes esophageal injury.
   C. Cricoid pressure is often used consistently and applied properly in all airway management settings.
   D. Applying cricoid pressure has been proven to be a mandatory step in the intubation process.

11. Among the following, the factors that would <u>MOST</u> strongly influence a difficult intubation in obese patients would be
   A. Thyromental distance, sternomental distance
   B. Weight, BMI
   C. Mallampati score
   D. OSA, width of mouth opening
   E. Previous history of laryngospasm, laryngeal edema

12. When performing abdominal surgery, the argument against using nitrous oxide would be associated with its
   A. Diffusion into air-containing cavities
   B. High potency
   C. Dose-dependent reduction in mean arterial pressure
   D. Reduction in net ventilation

ANSWER KEY

1. C	4. C	7. D	10. C
2. E	5. B	8. B	11. C
3. B	6. C	9. D	12. A

ANSWER KEY WITH EXPLANATION

1. **Answer: C.**

   Smoking cessation should be advised with an ideal presurgical duration of at least 8 weeks. Patients with a definitive diagnosis of OSA should receive CPAP/NIPPV treatment as early preoperatively as possible because it improves physical status and reduces perioperative risk. There is no evidence that routine preoperative OSA screening by polysomnography is cost-effective or improves outcomes, and hence it is not recommended by the American Society of Anesthesiologists (ASA).

   There is increased renal blood flow and an increased glomerular filtration rate (GFR) associated with obesity. Renal clearance of drugs may be greater compared to the normal-weight patient.

   Reference:
   - Schumann R. Anaesthesia for bariatric surgery. Best Pract Res Clin Anaesthesiol 2011; 25(1):83–93.

2. **Answer: E.**

   Pain management in bariatric surgical patients should be opioid-sparing or free because of a well-documented risk of sedation and serious respiratory depression from neuraxially or intravenously administered opioids, particularly in obese patients with OSA, and opioid-related side effects, including pruritus, nausea, vomiting, and delayed bowel function. Multimodal analgesic strategies employing multiple non-opioid analgesics and local anesthetics, whenever possible, are able to approach this important goal. Successful strategies include use of nonsteroidal anti-inflammatory drugs (NSAIDs) such as ketorolac and local anesthetic port and wound infiltration or infusion. Less studied nonopioid analgesics reducing perioperative opioid consumption in bariatric surgical patients include ketamine, clonidine, dexmedetomidine, magnesium sulfate, methylprednisolone, and IV lidocaine. Pregabalin has also been used in a group of sleeve gastrectomy patients preoperatively and found to be opioid-sparing. This current evidence suggests that at least NSAIDs and local anesthetic port or wound infiltration should be part of a multimodal postoperative pain management regimen in this patient population, unless contraindicated.

   References:
   - Schug SA, Raymann A. Postoperative pain management of the obese patient. Best Pract Res Clin Anaesthesiol 2011; 25(1):73–81.
   - Schumann R. Anaesthesia for bariatric surgery. Best Pract Res Clin Anaesthesiol 2011; 25(1):83–93.

3. **Answer: B.**

   Creating a "ramped" patient position by placing blankets under the patient's upper body improves laryngoscopic view compared with a standard "sniffing" position. At least three studies showed a longer "safe apnea time" or nonhypoxic apnea – the time from the onset of apnea during induction to a predefined point of desaturation – when bariatric surgical patients were induced in the 25° or 30° reversed Trendelenburg, head up, or the near-sitting position, prolonging the time for safe airway management. A similar result was achieved by using either PEEP (10 cm H_2O for 5 minutes) or NIPPV for preoxygenation at induction of morbidly obese patients.

   Reference:
   - Schumann R. Anaesthesia for bariatric surgery. Best Pract Res Clin Anaesthesiol 2011; 25(1):83–93.

4. **Answer: C.**

The lateral decubitus position structurally improves maintenance of the passive pharyngeal airway and increases its diameter compared with the supine position. Most recent evidence suggests improvement of lung function lasting at least into the first postoperative day when 8-hour NIPPV was begun immediately postextubation versus application on arrival to the PACU. Although some authors suggest that CPAP can be safely avoided in patients with OSA following bariatric surgery, the evidence of its safety and benefits postoperatively clearly favors its use. To minimize hypoxemic events due to the restrictive pulmonary physiology, decreased functional residual capacity (FRC) and airway obstruction associated with the horizontal supine position, a semi-upright recovery position in OSA patients is recommended. Prolonged postoperative monitoring and observation of OSA patients in the PACU following bariatric procedures has been recommended by the ASA to prevent potential OSA-related adverse outcomes.

Reference:
- Schumann R. Anaesthesia for bariatric surgery. Best Pract Res Clin Anaesthesiol 2011; 25(1):83–93.

5. **Answer: B.**

Low voltages may be an artifact caused by excessive tissue impedance. This can complicate electrocardiographic monitoring. Similarly, excess soft tissue thickness can make pulse oximetry unreliable. Alternative sites such as the nose, lip, or smallest finger have been advocated to improve the reliability of this monitor.

Undersized cuffs are known to falsely elevate readings, although the configuration of the arm may also affect readings. Obese patients tend to have conically shaped upper arms in comparison with the cylindrical shape of nonobese patients' arms, and an appropriate cuff sometimes does not fit properly. Use of the forearm has been shown to improve reproducibility, although it has also been shown to overestimate arterial pressure.

ET-CO_2 monitoring is not always accurate in morbidly obese patients. Decreases in FRC, ventilation-perfusion mismatch, and the dead space to tidal volume changes with obesity are cited as factors.

Reference:
- Brenn BR. Anesthesia for pediatric obesity. Anesthesiol Clin North America 2005; 23(4):745–764, x (review).

6. **Answer: C.**

Difficulty in maintaining the pneumoperitoneum as well as difficulty in ventilation calls for checking adequacy of neuromuscular blockade.

7. **Answer: D.**

PCA reduces the total dose of opioid in a 24-hour period. Continuous background infusion of medication in addition to PCA offers no advantage. Morphine is considered drug of choice for opioid analgesia.

The dose of opioids is to be adjusted based on ideal body weight, not actual body weight as opioids are lipophilic drugs. Dexmedetomidine does not have the risk of respiratory depression. It is a sedative that acts on α_{2A} receptors. Other measures to reduce opioid usage include infiltration of local anesthetics into the trocar sites.

References:
- Brodsky JB, Lerner LC. Chapter 10: Anesthetic concerns. In: Pitombo C, Jones K, Higa K, et al., eds. Obesity Surgery: Principles and Practice. 1st ed. New York: McGraw-Hill, 2007. Available at: http://www.accesssurgery.com/content.aspx?aID=140225.
- Doherty GM. Chapter 4: Postoperative care. In: Doherty GM. CURRENT Diagnosis & Treatment: Surgery. 13th ed. New York: McGraw-Hill, 2010. Available at: http://www.accesssurgery.com/content.aspx?aID=5211176.

8. **Answer: B.**

Continuous infusion of opioids with or without bupivacaine can be used for epidural analgesia. It has the following advantages over IV analgesia.

- Prolonged duration of action
- Lesser respiratory depression
- Similar dose required
- Analgesia is superior
- Lesser depression of consciousness
- Better gastrointestinal (GI) function
- Does not cause sensory disturbance (except pain), motor or autonomic disturbance

It causes side effects like nausea, pruritus, and urinary retention. It has a delayed onset of action. Epidural catheters are best placed before the patient is placed under anesthesia.

Reference:

- Brodsky JB, Lerner LC. Chapter 10: Anesthetic concerns. In: Pitombo C, Jones K, Higa K, et al., eds. Obesity Surgery: Principles and Practice. 1st edn. New York: McGraw-Hill, 2007. Available at: http://www.accesssurgery.com/content.aspx? aID=140225.

9. **Answer: D.**

Awake fiber-optic intubation is the best course of action when a difficult airway is suspected. Tracheostomy would be the last resort. Performing a Lap-Band under local anesthesia or performing a fiber-optic intubation after paralysis would not be appropriate.

Reference:

- Schumann R. Anaesthesia for bariatric surgery. Best Pract Res Clin Anaesthesiol 2011; 25(1):83–93.

10. **Answer: C.**

Although widely used, there is little evidence to support the widely held belief that the application of cricoid pressure reduces the incidence of aspiration during an RSI. Concern has been expressed that cricoid pressure may interfere with airway management, obscuring the laryngeal view and creating difficulties in passing the endotracheal tube. This may lead to a failure of airway techniques and subsequent morbidity and mortality.

Reference:

- Ellis DY, Harris T, Zideman D. Cricoid pressure in emergency department rapid sequence tracheal intubations: a risk-benefit analysis. Ann Emerg Med 2007; 50 (6):653–665.

11. **Answer: C.**

BMI alone has not been found to be predictor for difficult intubation. In one study, Mallampati score >3 and male gender were found to be the only predictive factors. Sternomental distance is also suggested as a factor for difficult intubation.

Reference:

- Brodsky JB, Lemmens HJM, Brock-Utne JG, et al. Morbid obesity and tracheal intubation. Anesth Analg 2002; 94(3):732–736.

12. **Answer: A.**

Although nitrous oxide is insoluble in comparison with other inhalation agents, it is 35 times more soluble than nitrogen in blood. Thus, it tends to diffuse into air-containing cavities more rapidly than the bloodstream absorbs nitrogen. For instance, if a patient with a 100-mL pneumothorax inhales 50% nitrous oxide, the gas content of the pneumothorax will tend to approach that of the bloodstream. Because nitrous oxide will diffuse into the cavity more rapidly than the air (principally nitrogen) diffuses out, the pneumothorax expands until it contains 100 mL of air and 100 mL of nitrous oxide. If the walls surrounding the cavity are rigid, pressure rises instead of volume. Examples of conditions in which nitrous oxide might be hazardous include air embolism, pneumothorax, acute intestinal obstruction, intracranial air (tension pneumocephalus following dural closure or pneumoencephalography), pulmonary air cysts, intraocular air bubbles, and tympanic membrane grafting. Nitrous oxide will even diffuse into tracheal tube cuffs, increasing the pressure against the tracheal mucosa.

Because of the effect of nitrous oxide on the pulmonary vasculature, it should be avoided in patients with pulmonary hypertension. Obviously, nitrous oxide is of limited value in patients requiring high inspired oxygen concentrations.

References:
- Becker D, Rosenberg M. Nitrous oxide and the inhalation anesthetics. Anesth Prog 2008; 55(4):124–131.
- Morgan GE, Mikhail MS, Murray MJ. Chapter 7: Inhalation anesthetics. Clinical anesthesiology. 4th edn. New York: Lange Medical Books/McGraw-Hill, 2006.

14 | Endoscopy

CHAPTER SUMMARY
- Preoperative endoscopy is recommended for patients with reflux symptoms, dysphagia, or dyspepsia.
- Endoscopic abnormalities are highly common.
- There is no agreement between studies whether routine preoperative endoscopic assessment changes surgical approach or timing.
- Abnormalities found during endoscopy can change surgical outcome. For example, hiatal hernia can cause increased incidence of band slippage.
- In patients who are not undergoing an endoscopy, noninvasive *Helicobacter pylori* testing followed by treatment is recommended.
- Postoperative routine endoscopy is not recommended and is reserved for symptomatic patients.
- Normal endoscopic findings:
  - Roux-en-Y gastric bypass (RYGB): Small pouch with a stoma is around 10 to 12 mm and has a double-barreled appearance. Care should be taken not to perforate the blind end of the jejunum.
  - Biliopancreatic diversion and duodenal switch (BPD and DS): A stomach pouch of about 200 mL is encountered in a BPD with a double-barreled view of the Roux limb. In a BPD-DS, a tubular stomach with an absent fundus and an intact pylorus is encountered, with an end-to-end duodenoileostomy.
  - Laparoscopic adjustable gastric band (LAGB): A pouch may or may not be visible. If a pouch is seen the distance between the cardia and the stoma is less than 3 cm.
  - Vertical banded gastroplasty (VBG): Consists of a gastric channel 6 to 8 cm in length, and this should be clearly in view as the endoscope passes from the esophagus. The stoma is about 1.5 cm in length and 5 cm wide. Retroflexion of the tip of the endoscope in the distal stomach allows inspection of the caudal aspect of the staple line partition and the remainder of the gastric fundus.
- Indications of endoscopy in a bariatric patient include the following:
  - Vomiting: can indicate stomal stenosis or marginal ulcers in RYGB, prolapse in a band patient, etc.
  - Heartburn/Reflux: can indicate pouch dilation in a band, or stomal stenosis in RYGB.
  - Diarrhea: indicates bacterial overgrowth or malabsorption.
  - Abdominal pain: after gastric bypass surgery, the afferent loop syndrome sometimes with pancreatitis, efferent limb obstruction, anastomotic ulcer, peptic ulcer in the bypassed stomach or duodenum, and pouch outlet obstruction. In a gastric band patient, it may indicate band erosion or tube disconnection.
  - Hematemesis and melena.
  - Weight regain or inadequate weight loss: can be due to stomal dilation or gastrogastric fistula after RYGB, pouch dilation or band erosion after LAGB, and pouch dilation after VBG.
- Endoscopic management of complications – RYGB:
  - Leak: The patient needs to be explored for a leak presenting during the early postoperative period. Covered stents are an option for persisting leaks. Closure rate of >60% has been reported. Other options include application of clips and biological fibrin glue.

- Early obstruction of the gastrojejunostomy (GJ) is usually due to postoperative edema and should be treated with IV fluids and insertion of nasogastric (NG) tube. Stomal stenosis usually occurs 2 to 3 months after surgery. Dilation can be achieved by fluoroscopically guided controlled radial expansion balloons. Dilation should not be performed in the presence of marginal ulcers as it can result in perforation. The goal diameter of dilation is about 10 to 12 mm, not exceeding 15 mm. Complications include bleeding and perforation.
- Acute onset of vomiting after bariatric surgery is due to obstruction of the stoma by food material or foreign body like bezoars. These need to be either removed (as in the case of foreign bodies) or pushed down.
- Marginal ulcers: usually occur during the first 2 years after surgery and have an incidence of 1.8%. They are found on the jejunal side of the GJ. A bleeding marginal ulcer can be cauterized. Prevention is by avoiding smoking, preoperative eradication of *H. pylori*, and prophylactic proton pump inhibitor (PPI) and sucralfate. Treatment is by PPI and sucralfate for 3 to 6 months and revision of GJ for refractory cases.
- Gastrogastric fistula: It is usually due to staple line dehiscence when the stomach is stapled in continuity. It is difficult to diagnose endoscopically and may have the appearance of a diverticulum. The endoscope may be passed into the remnant stomach if the fistula is large. Diagnostic test of choice is an upper gastrointestinal (UGI) contrast study. Patient is put on PPI for 6 to 8 weeks followed by repeat endoscopy. Endoscopic management options include injection of fibrin glue, endoscopic suturing, hemoclips, and argon plasma coagulation.
- Stomal dilation: It causes weight regain or failure of weight loss. Injection of the sclerosing agent sodium morrhuate resulted in a stomal diameter of 1.2 cm or smaller in >60% of patients. Other options include plicating device and endoscopic sutured revision. Refractory cases need revision of the GJ.
- The stomach remnant is difficult to evaluate. Use of the pediatric colonoscope has been found to be successful in about two-thirds of the cases. Other options include percutaneous gastrostomy and endoscopy after dilating the track, and virtual CT gastroscopy. The double-balloon technology has been shown to have a slightly higher success rate (>85%).
- The investigation of choice for a patient suspected of having choledocholithiasis after RYGB is a magnetic resonance cholangiopancreatography (MRCP). Endoscopic retrograde cholangiopancreatography (ERCP) using an enteroscope or a pediatric colonoscope has been shown to be successful in over 80% of the patients. Double-balloon ERCP has also been described. Percutaneous transhepatic cholangiography (PTC) and instrumentation of bile duct after dilation of the tract and percutaneous access to the bypassed stomach by means of a gastrostomy are other options.
- VBG: Bezoars can be removed by endoscopy or dissolved by using meat tenderizers. Stomal stenosis is amenable to dilation by Eder–Puestow dilators, Savary–Guilliard bougies, or balloons. An eroded silastic ring cannot be cut but the stay sutures anchoring it to the stomach can be cut and the ring removed endoscopically. Gortex band can be cut with endoscopic scissors. In the case of staple line disruption, two entrances to the stomach are seen on endoscopy. It is more commonly confirmed by a UGI contrast study. Vertical staple line disruption results weight regain. The latter needs conversion to RYGB.
- Gastric band: Pouch dilation is diagnosed endoscopically by increased distance between the cardia and the band, that is, more than 5 cm, and appearance of a symmetric pouch. Functional stomal stenosis is also observed. This corresponds to a pouch volume of 100 to 200 mL. Barium study shows a dilated pouch with overhanging stomach wall relative to the band. Management is by deflation of the

band and modified liquid diet for 1 to 2 months. If symptoms resolve, the band is reinflated and the patient followed up with frequent UGI studies. Persistent symptoms need revision of the band. Band slippage is diagnosed by the appearance of an asymmetric pouch on endoscopy. This usually needs revision. Stomal stenosis presenting early after surgery is usually due to edema, whereas that presenting late is due to band erosion, slippage, or pouch dilation. It is initially managed by deflation of the band and liquid diet. An upper endoscopy in the presence of a narrow stoma can lead to perforation, and UGI is the initial test of choice. Band erosion is diagnosed by the whitish appearance of the band on endoscopy; the band may look black in late cases due to the influence of bile. Various methods to remove the band endoscopically have been described including the use of a gastric band cutter.

QUESTIONS

1. **A patient presents for follow-up examination to a bariatric surgeon 3 months after RYGB with progressive nausea and vomiting, soon after eating, for the past 1 week, and now cannot even tolerate liquids. Which of the following symptoms is <u>TRUE</u> about the further evaluation of this patient?**
   A. Order a CT scan.
   B. Arrange an endoscopy.
   C. Arrange a stat UGI contrast.
   D. The patient needs a nutritional evaluation only.

2. **From the following scenarios, identify the patient who is <u>NOT</u> usually considered for endoscopy.**
   A. A 62-year-old symptomatic patient suspected of staple line leak on the postoperative day 2 after RYGB.
   B. A 35-year-old asymptomatic patient 2 years s/p RYGB and who present with anemia on examination.
   C. A 45-year-old patient with diarrhea 2 years s/p RYGB who does not respond to a course of levofloxacin.
   D. A 35-year-old patient with dumping syndrome s/p RYGB.

3. **The gastric remnant is very difficult to evaluate by endoscopy. Which of the following is <u>NOT</u> accurate about novel methods used to evaluate the gastric remnant?**
   A. Double-balloon endoscopy uses two balloons one at the end of the enteroscope and the other at the end of an overtube.
   B. ShapeLock technology uses a novel laparoscopic camera that can be "locked" at any angle to facilitate viewing.
   C. Passing an endoscope through a gastrostomy during laparoscopy is a feasible option.
   D. Virtual CT gastroscopy, after distending the stomach remnant with saline injected percutaneously has been shown to be a promising method to evaluate bypassed stomach.

4. **The evaluation of the biliary tree is a challenge in post-RYGB and BPD-DS patients. Identify the <u>FALSE</u> statement about the occurrence of gallstones in these patients.**
   A. Percutaneous transgastric ERCP is technically very easy and most commonly employed when cholangitis is suspected.
   B. MRCP is the first line of investigation of a patient who has undergone a gastric bypass for evaluation of the biliary tree.
   C. ERCP has been reported in RYGB patients but is technically challenging.
   D. ERCP is usually not possible in a BPD patient through the normal route.

5. **A 35-year-old male patient presents 4 weeks post-RYGB with a low-grade fever and epigastric pain for the past 24 hours. Vital signs reveal a HR of 110 and blood pressure of 140/85 mmHg, and physical examination reveals localized epigastric tenderness. The rest of the abdomen is soft, nontender with normal bowel sounds. A UGI contrast study reveals a leak at the GJ anastomosis. A CT scan shows no significant collection. If all options are available, which of the following is the next BEST option?**
   A. Perform an emergency laparotomy.
   B. Perform a diagnostic laparoscopy.
   C. Place a percutaneous drain.
   D. Perform an endoscopy and put a stent across the leak.
   E. C and D.

6. **A 60-year-old male patient presents with repeated episodes of vomiting 6 months after RYGB. Patient's history is significant for an MI 2 months ago. Endoscopy shows a GJ stricture. Dilations are attempted but the stricture recurs even after the fourth attempt. Which of the following is the BEST option?**
   A. Book the patient for an elective revision of the GJ in spite of his poor American Society of Anesthesiologists (ASA) status.
   B. Place a removable stent by endoscopy.
   C. Inform the patient that nothing can be done now and he needs to tolerate his vomiting till he becomes fit for general anesthesia.
   D. Try dilating the stricture once more.

7. **45-year-old male patient came with complaints of fullness and repeated vomiting 5 months after RYGB. Stomal stenosis is suspected. Among the following, what is the NEXT BEST step to be done?**
   A. To diagnose a stricture, first do a UGI contrast study.
   B. Perform an endoscopy and dilate the stoma to 5 to 10 mm.
   C. Perform an endoscopy and dilate the stoma to 10 to 15 mm.
   D. Perform an endoscopy and dilate the stoma to 15 to 20 mm.

8. **Identify the TRUE statement about the endoscopic findings in a bariatric surgical candidate.**
   A. About 20% of the patients have some abnormality on UGI endoscopy.
   B. UGI is less sensitive than upper endoscopy in detecting sliding hiatal hernias.
   C. Monitored anesthesia care has been shown to be less effective than endoscopist-administered anesthesia during endoscopy in a morbidly obese patient.
   D. It has been shown that routine preoperative endoscopy may discover findings that may lead to a delay in surgery or change in surgical approach.

ANSWER KEY

1. B	3. B	5. E	7. C
2. A	4. A	6. B	8. D

ANSWER KEY WITH EXPLANATION

1. **Answer: B.**

   The patient has acute and severe symptoms that are probably not related to his/her compliance with the diet. An endoscopy is a must to rule out stomal stenosis. Abnormal findings on endoscopy are found in >30% of patients with abdominal pain and >60% of the patients with nausea and vomiting. UGI will not be tolerated well by a patient who is vomiting, though it has a good correlation with endoscopy. Endoscopy will also provide a chance for simultaneous treatment of stomal stenosis. The patient does not have fever or abdominal pain, and hence a leak lies low on the differential diagnosis. Hence, a CT scan is not warranted at this time.

References:
- Wilson JA, Romagnuolo J, Byrne TK, et al. Predictors of endoscopic findings after Roux-en-Y gastric bypass. Am J Gastroenterol 2006; 101:2194–2199.
- ASGE Standards of Practice Committee; Anderson MA, Gan SI, Fanelli RD, et al. Role of endoscopy in the bariatric surgery patient. Gastrointest Endosc 2008; 68 (1):1–10.

2. **Answer: A.**

Endoscopy is not routinely recommended after bariatric surgery. A patient who has an acute leak needs percutaneous drainage or exploratory laparotomy, not endoscopy. A chronic leak that persists after initial management can be managed by endoscopic methods like stent placement. Indications for endoscopy include nausea, vomiting, dysphagia, pain, reflux, diarrhea, anemia/bleeding, and weight regain. Patient with anemia can have an anastomotic ulcer or a cancer in the pouch or gastric remnant though the latter two are rare. Patients suspected of dumping syndrome may need an evaluation for other causes of its symptoms through an endoscopy. Bacterial overgrowth can cause diarrhea due to a blind loop syndrome of the excluded small bowel. In patients who do not respond to initial management with antibiotics, breath testing for bacterial overgrowth or endoscopic aspiration for quantitative bacterial culture from the excluded segment should be considered. Obstruction of the excluded segment can also be ruled out with an endoscopy.

Reference:
- Obstein KL, Thompson CC. Endoscopy after bariatric surgery (with videos). Gastrointest Endosc 2009; 70(6):1161–1166.

3. **Answer: B.**

The ShapeLock technology uses a novel overtube that is backloaded over the flexible enteroscope and then, unlike other overtubes, can be locked into a rigid but contorted position. This may overcome the looping of the enteroscope that would generally occur while progressing through an acutely angled jejunojejunal anastomosis. The double-balloon technology uses two balloons, one at the tip of the enteroscope and the other at the end of an overtube. After the enteroscope is advanced beyond the overtube, its balloon is inflated and the small bowel is accordioned back to the overtube. After this, the balloon on the overtube is inflated, and the process is repeated to progressively "walk" down the small bowel. Passing an endoscope through a gastrostomy during laparoscopy would also, obviously, be a good option. Virtual CT gastroscopy has been used to image the bypassed stomach and found to show an excellent intraluminal view of the stomach and duodenum.

References:
- Silecchia G, Catalano C, Gentileschi P, et al. Virtual gastroduodenoscopy: a new look at the bypassed stomach and duodenum after laparoscopic Roux-en-Y gastric bypass for morbid obesity. Obes Surg 2002; 12(1):39–48.
- Pai RD, Carr-Locke DL, Thompson CC. Endoscopic evaluation of the defunctionalized stomach by using ShapeLock technology (with video). Gastrointest Endosc 2007; 66(3):578–581.
- Ross AS, Semrad C, Alverdy J, et al. Use of double-balloon enteroscopy to perform PEG in the excluded stomach after Roux-en-Y gastric bypass. Gastrointest Endosc 2006; 64(5):797–800.

4. **Answer: A.**

MRCP is the initial diagnostic test of choice for evaluation of the biliary tree in a post-RYGB or BPD patient. PTC is an option if there is diagnostic uncertainty, a contraindication to MRI, or if an intervention is necessary. ERCP can be attempted in selected cases in a RYGB patient but needs to be carefully planned as it may not always be feasible. ERCP is even more difficult in a post-BPD patient and usually not possible through the normal anatomical route; one needs to do a laparoscopy-assisted ERCP. In percutaneous transgastric ERCP, a pigtail catheter is inserted under ultrasound or CT guidance. It is then dilated gradually every 1 or 2 weeks to the desired size (14 Fr to 20 or 24 Fr) to introduce the endoscope. It is technically difficult as the remnant stomach cannot be distended with air. Furthermore, as it requires serial dilations, it cannot be employed in emergent situations like cholangitis, where laparoscopy provides a quicker access.

References:
- Kini S, Kannan U. Effect of bariatric surgery on future general surgical procedures. J Minim Access Surg 2011; 7(2):126–131.
- Mutignani M, Marchese M, Tringali A, et al. Laparoscopy-assisted ERCP after biliopancreatic diversion. Obes Surg 2007; 17(2):251–254.

5. **Answer: E.**

Diagnostic laparoscopy or an exploratory laparotomy is usually performed when patient develops a leak in the first few days after surgery, especially in a sick patient. Use of covered stents is reasonable in a stable patient. Endoscopic stents allow oral nutrition to be taken while healing is taking place. A CT-guided placement of a percutaneous drain will drain any collections.

References:
- Marshall JS, Srivastava A, Gupta SK, et al. Roux-en-Y gastric bypass leak complications. Arch Surg 2003; 138(5):520–523; discussion 523–524.
- Labrunie E, Marchiori E, Pitombo C. Chapter 42: Radiographic evaluation and treatment: intervention. In: Pitombo C, Jones K, Higa K, et al., eds. Obesity Surgery: Principles and Practice. 1st edn. New York: McGraw-Hill, 2007. Available at: http://www.accesssurgery.com/content.aspx?aID=145669.
- Fukumoto R, Orlina J, McGinty J, et al. Use of Polyflex stents in treatment of acute esophageal and gastric leaks after bariatric surgery. Surg Obes Relat Dis 2007; 3(1):68–71; discussion 71–72 [Epub December 27, 2006].

6. **Answer: B.**

Expandable stents should be tried before doing a revision of GJ. His poor ASA status also precludes any surgery in the immediate future. Dilating the stricture once more would likely lead to recurrence of the stricture.

References:
- Ryskina KL, Miller KM, Aisenberg J, et al. Routine management of stricture after gastric bypass and predictors of subsequent weight loss. Surg Endosc 2010; 24 (3):554–560.
- Levitzky BE, Wassef WY. Endoscopic management in the bariatric surgical patient. Curr Opin Gastroenterol 2010; 26(6):632–639.

7. **Answer: C.**

The endoscopist needs to dilate the stoma to 10 mm and look for marginal ulcers on the jejunal side before dilating to the full 12 to 15 mm. Even though stomal stenosis can be documented by UGI, it may cause severe vomiting (and possible aspiration) in a patient with stomal stenosis. Dilating beyond 15 mm is not usually recommended. If ulcers are found on the jejunal side dilation is stopped and patient is put on PPIs.

Reference:
- Ryskina K, Miller K, Aisenberg J, et al. Routine management of stricture after gastric bypass and predictors of subsequent weight loss. Surg Endosc 2010; 24(3):554–560.

8. **Answer: D.**

Abnormality on upper endoscopy has been found to be very high in patients undergoing the procedure routinely before bariatric surgery (90% in most series).

UGI is more sensitive and endoscopy more specific for diagnosis of sliding hiatal hernia in bariatric surgical patients. One advantage of endoscopy is the concomitant detection of reflux esophagitis or Barrett's esophagus if present.

Endoscopy can discover findings that can lead to a delay in surgery or change in surgical approach in about 60% of patients. It is not certain whether routine UGI contrast study can change or delay surgical approach.

Patients undergoing monitored anesthesia with propofol tend to remember the scope being placed in the mouth less often when compared to surgeon-administered anesthesia with benzodiazepines and narcotics. Though it did not reach statistical significance in a study, it needs to be confirmed whether monitored anesthesia care is better in terms of patient recovery and incidence of gagging.

References:
- Sharaf RN, Weinshel EH, Bini EJ, et al. Endoscopy plays an important preoperative role in bariatric surgery. Obes Surg 2004; 14(10):1367–1372.
- Greenwald D. Preoperative gastrointestinal assessment before bariatric surgery. Gastroenterol Clin North Am 2010; 39(1):81–86.
- Fornari F, Gurski RR, Navarini D, et al. Clinical utility of endoscopy and barium swallow X-ray in the diagnosis of sliding hiatal hernia in morbidly obese patients: a study before and after gastric bypass. Obes Surg 2010; 20(6):702–708 [Epub September 12, 2009].
- Madan AK, Tichansky DS, Isom J, et al. Monitored anesthesia care with propofol versus surgeon-monitored sedation with benzodiazepines and narcotics for preoperative endoscopy in the morbidly obese. Obes Surg 2008; 18(5):545–548.
- Madan AK, Speck KE, Hiler ML. Routine preoperative upper endoscopy for laparoscopic gastric bypass: is it necessary? Am Surg 2004; 70(8):684–686.
- Ghassemian AJ, Donald KGM, Cunningham PG, et al. The workup for bariatric surgery does not require a routine upper gastrointestinal series. Obes Surg 1997; 7:16–18.
- ASGE Standards of Practice Committee; Anderson MA, Gan SI, Fanelli RD, et al. Role of endoscopy in the bariatric surgery patient. Gastrointest Endosc 2008; 68 (1):1–10.

15 | Radiology

CHAPTER SUMMARY

- Roux-en-Y gastric bypass (RYGB):
  - Upper gastrointestinal (UGI) studies are done in the immediate postoperative period to rule out leaks. Normal anatomy consists of a gastric pouch, free flow of contrast from the pouch into the jejunum, and appearance of jejunal plicae indicating flow into the jejunum. One must be aware that the contrast flows into the jejunal blind limb and that gastric fluid and air can be seen in the stomach remnant. The former should not be confused with a gastrogastric fistula and the latter should not be confused with a gastrojejunostomy leak.
  - Leak: Radiological contrast material is seen at the left upper quadrant during fluoroscopy. Before administration of contrast, air may be seen in the left upper quadrant. The nasogastric (NG) tube should be removed before the procedure. Leak can also occur at the jejunojejunostomy though rare.
  - Strictures: Fluoroscopy shows narrowing of the gastrojejunal anastomosis, enlargement of the pouch, and delayed flow of contrast from the pouch to the jejunum. Stricture may also occur (<1% incidence) at the jejunojejunostomy. The Roux limb is distended and oral contrast flows retrograde into the afferent limb.
  - Gastrogastric fistulae and staple line disruption are best assessed with a fluoroscopy as one cannot ascertain whether contrast in the stomach remnant resulted due to a flow through the fistula or due to retrograde flow through the afferent limb on the CT scan.
  - The diagnostic test of choice for bowel obstruction after bariatric surgery is a CT scan with oral contrast.
  - Mesocolic window stenosis: seen only with retrocolic gastric bypass. Distension of the Roux limb is seen above the level of the mesocolic window with variable passage of contrast into the distal Roux limb depending on the degree of obstruction.
  - Herniation through the mesocolic window: usually the Roux limb herniates, sometimes to such an extent that the jejunojejunostomy is pulled through the defect causing an obstruction of the afferent limb. CT shows small-bowel obstruction, clustered small-bowel loops, central displacement of the colon, no overlying omental fat, displacement of the mesenteric trunk and engorgement, and stretching of the mesenteric vessels. It is differentiated from a mesocolic window stenosis by obstruction at a point beyond the level of the mesocolic window and by affection of the afferent limb. A hernia through the jejunojejunostomy defect displaces the transverse colon upwards, whereas that through the mesocolic window displaces the transverse colon downwards.
- Laparoscopic adjustable gastric banding (LAGB):
  - Stomal stenosis: usually due to edema of the stomach wall in the postoperative period. It can also be due to an overtight band. Fluoroscopy reveals delayed emptying of contrast from the pouch with enlargement of the pouch and gastroesophageal reflux in advanced cases. Normally, the size of the pouch is about 3 to 4 cm and that of the stoma is about 3 to 4 mm on contrast study.
  - Prolapse: anterior prolapse results in a medial eccentric gastric pouch with a phi angle less than 4°. Posterior prolapse results in a lateral eccentric gastric pouch with a phi angle greater than 58°. Normal phi angle is between 4° and 58°.

- Band system leakage can be discovered when fluoroscopy is done during adjustment of a band. In equivocal cases, ^{99m}Tc-albumin study can help locate the leak.
- Early band erosions cannot be detected by UGI study. Late erosions can be detected by flow of contrast around the band.
- Vertical banded gastroplasty (VBG):
  - The patient is evaluated during a UGI contrast study in the right posterior oblique position. The vertical staple line is viewed in a tangent. Initial scout film enables identification of the staple line and the band.
  - Stomal stenosis: Delayed emptying of the contrast is seen with pouch dilation and gastroesophageal reflux. Rarely a diverticulum may be observed in the gastric pouch. Stoma may also be blocked because of food particles.
  - Vertical staple line dehiscence: Contrast can be seen flowing from the pouch laterally into the rest of the stomach.
- Sleeve gastrectomy:
  - UGI contrast study can detect a leak from the staple line. This is usually present in the upper part of the sleeve gastrectomy staple line.
- Biliopancreatic diversion–duodenal switch (BPD-DS):
  - Sleeve gastrectomy leak can be detected as above.
  - Obstruction of duodenoileostomy can occur immediately after surgery or in the long term and can be diagnosed by UGI study.

QUESTIONS
1. A 45-year-old patient with a BMI of 45 is seen on the postoperative day 2 after a laparoscopic Roux-en-Y gastric bypass (LRYGB). He complains of fever and abdominal pain. Physical examination shows nondistended abdomen without guarding or rebound. Bowel sounds are positive. A UGI contrast study is performed (see figure below). Identify the <u>TRUE</u> statement.

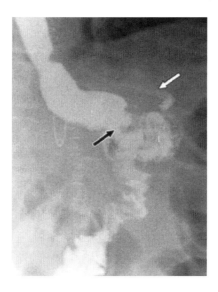

Source: From the *American Journal of Roentgenology*.

    A. The patient has an abscess collection near the gastrojejunostomy.
    B. The patient has a leak at the jejunojejunostomy.
    C. This is a normal fluoroscopic exam.
    D. The fluoroscopic exam is equivocal and CT abdomen is warranted.

2. **A postoperative contrast study after LAGB may be helpful for identification of late complications arising after LAGB. Identify the <u>FALSE</u> statement with respect to a normal fluoroscopic exam after LAGB.**
   A. The gastric pouch should be symmetric and about 3 to 4 cm in size when fully distended with contrast.
   B. The stoma should measure 3 to 4 mm in size.
   C. No delayed emptying of contrast.
   D. The phi angle should measure about 70°.

3. **Identify the <u>TRUE</u> statement about the correct diagnosis in a post-RYGB patient from the fluoroscopic image given below.**

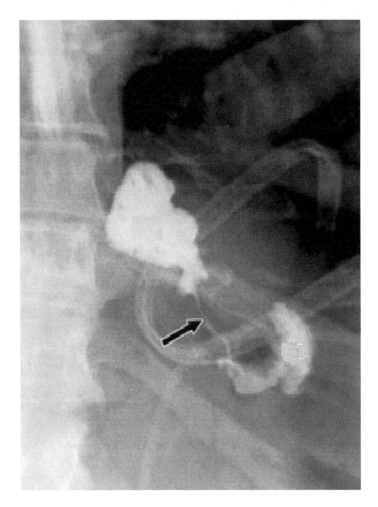

Source: From the *American Journal of Roentgenology*.

   A. The patient has an internal hernia.
   B. The patient has a stricture at the gastrojejunal anastomosis.
   C. The patient has a staple line leak.
   D. The patient has a leak at the jejunojejunostomy.
   E. The patient has mesocolic window stenosis.

4. Identify the <u>CORRECT</u> diagnosis in this patient who presented with abdominal pain, distension, and vomiting 4 months after a laparoscopic retrocolic, antegastric RYGB.

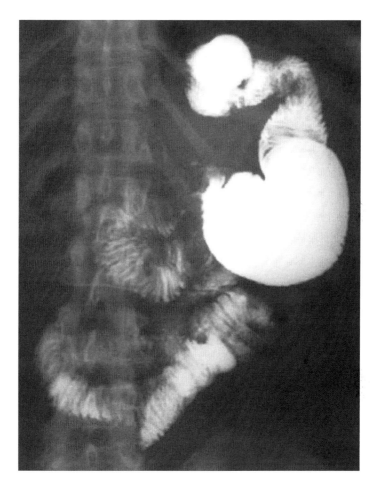

Source: From the *American Journal of Roentgenology*.

    A. Petersen's hernia
    B. Mesocolic window stenosis
    C. Obstruction at jejunojejunostomy
    D. Gastric remnant dilation

5. A 32-year-old woman who had a BMI of 45 and has lost a significant amount of weight after a retrocolic LRYGB and now has a BMI of 34 presents 8 months after surgery with vomiting, abdominal distension, and constipation. Examination reveals borborygmi. Small-bowel obstruction is suspected and a CT is done that shows dilated bowel loops in the right upper quadrant of abdomen. A water-soluble UGI contrast study is shown below. Identify the <u>CORRECT</u> diagnosis.

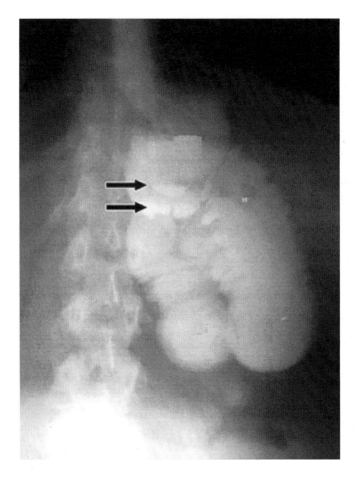

Source: From the *American Journal of Roentgenology*.

    A. Small-bowel herniation through mesocolic defect
    B. Mesocolic window stenosis
    C. Petersen's hernia
    D. Biliopancreatic limb obstruction

6. **Identify the <u>TRUE</u> statement about radiological diagnosis of staple line disruption and gastrogastric fistula.**
    A. A CT scan with oral contrast is the best way to diagnose.
    B. The flow of contrast into the proximal Roux limb during a UGI series can mimic flow into the gastric remnant.
    C. Appearance of jejunal plicae is not useful in the diagnosis of gastrogastric fistula during a fluoroscopy.
    D. One should not suspect gastrogastric fistula when abdominal symptoms appear <3 months after RYGB.

7. **Gastric prolapse is a diagnosis that should never be missed as it requires surgical management in all cases. Identify the <u>TRUE</u> statement about radiological diagnosis of gastric prolapse.**
    A. The phi angle is greater than 58° in anterior gastric prolapse.
    B. The phi angle is less than 4° in posterior gastric prolapse.
    C. A lateral eccentric gastric pouch is found in anterior gastric prolapse.
    D. Stomal obstruction is not a prerequisite for diagnosis of gastric prolapse.

8. Intussusception is a rare complication of gastric bypass. Identify the <u>FALSE</u> statement about this condition.
   A. Patients sometimes present with intermittent abdominal pain.
   B. It is retrograde and occurs at the jejunojejunostomy.
   C. The classic CT scan finding is a target sign.
   D. It is very rare for intussusception to progress to frank obstruction due to the resistance offered by jejunojejunal junction.

9. Gastric dilation is a known complication in the immediate postoperative period after RYGB. Identify the <u>TRUE</u> statement about acute gastric dilation after RYGB.
   A. CT scan shows dilation of the gastric pouch and edema of gastroejejunostomy.
   B. Percutaneous drainage is the definitive treatment for this condition even in sick patients.
   C. The type of gastrojejunostomy (antegastric or retrogastric) has no effect on the outcomes.
   D. It represents a closed loop obstruction.

10. A patient presents with postprandial abdominal pain 3 months after LRYGB (retrocolic). An internal hernia is suspected and a CT scan demonstrates dilated loops anterior to the gastric pouch and a caudally displaced transverse colon. Routine labs demonstrate an increased alkaline phosphatase and transaminases. Which of the following is the most likely site of obstruction?
   A. The biliopancreatic limb at the jejunojejunostomy
   B. The Roux limb at the jejunojejunostomy
   C. The Roux limb at the transmesenteric defect
   D. The biliopancreatic limb at the mesocolic defect

ANSWER KEY

1. C	4. B	7. D	10. D
2. D	5. A	8. D	
3. B	6. B	9. D	

ANSWER KEY WITH EXPLANATION

1. Answer: C.

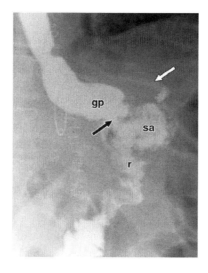

Source: From the *American Journal of Roentgenology*.

A radiologist or a bariatric surgeon should be aware of the appearance of the LRYGB anatomy on a fluoroscopic exam. This is a normal exam with the contrast flowing into the Roux limb (r) from the gastric pouch (gp). The flow of contrast into the blind jejunal limb (sa) should not be mistaken for a leak or gastrogastric fistula. A drain is depicted by the white arrow.

Reference:
- Chandler RC, Srinivas G, Chintapalli KN, et al. Imaging in bariatric surgery: a guide to postsurgical anatomy and common complications. AJR Am J Roentgenol 2008; 190(1):122–135.

2. **Answer: D.**

On postoperative day 1, patients may undergo fluoroscopic evaluation to assess gastric pouch size for possible contrast extravasation from occult iatrogenic gastric injury and for unhindered passage of orally administered contrast material into the remainder of the stomach via the surgically created stoma. The gastric pouch should be relatively symmetric in shape and measure approximately 3 to 4 cm in maximum dimension when distended with contrast material. The stoma should measure approximately 3 to 4 mm in diameter. Another factor assessed on every fluoroscopic examination is the phi angle. The phi angle is created by intersecting a line drawn parallel to the spinal column with a line drawn parallel to the plane of the gastric band, on an anteroposterior projection. Normally, this angle should range from 4° to 58° and lie approximately 4 to 5 cm below the left hemidiaphragm.

Reference:
- Chandler RC, Srinivas G, Chintapalli KN, et al. Imaging in bariatric surgery: a guide to postsurgical anatomy and common complications. AJR Am J Roentgenol 2008; 190(1):122–135.

3. **Answer: B.**

The gastrojejunostomy is severely narrowed as shown by the black arrow. There is also a dilation of the gastric pouch. On fluoroscopy, a delayed passage of contrast into the Roux limb will be observed (gp = gastric pouch; sa = short afferent limb or blind end of the jejunum).

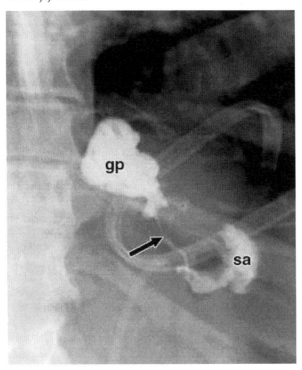

Source: From the *American Journal of Roentgenology*.

Reference:
- Chandler RC, Srinivas G, Chintapalli KN, et al. Imaging in bariatric surgery: a guide to postsurgical anatomy and common complications. AJR Am J Roentgenol 2008; 190(1):122–135.

4. **Answer: B.**

The Roux limb is obstructed at the area where it passes through the transverse mesocolon. The Roux limb is dilated. One of the dreaded complications of any obstructed hernia after RYGB is a gastrojejunostomy leak (gp = gastric pouch; r = Roux limb).

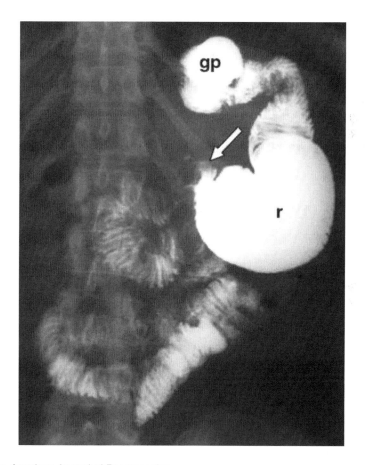

Source: From the *American Journal of Roentgenology.*

Reference:
- Chandler RC, Srinivas G, Chintapalli KN, et al. Imaging in bariatric surgery: a guide to postsurgical anatomy and common complications. AJR Am J Roentgenol 2008; 190(1):122–135.

5. **Answer: A.**

The figure shows distention and herniation of entire Roux limb (r) above expected region of mesocolic window, air-contrast levels (*arrows*), and distended gastric pouch (gp).

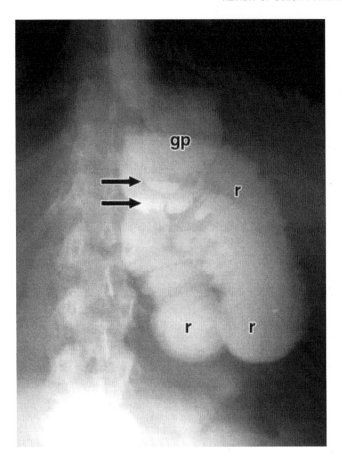

Source: From the *American Journal of Roentgenology*.

Reference:
- Chandler RC, Srinivas G, Chintapalli KN, et al. Imaging in bariatric surgery: a guide to postsurgical anatomy and common complications. AJR Am J Roentgenol 2008; 190(1):122–135.

6. **Answer: B.**

The incidence of gastric staple line disruption varies from 0.7% to 8.3%. Early disruption is due to suboptimal surgical technique or gastric ischemia. Disruption can also occur due to dietary noncompliance resulting in distension that leads to increased tension on the staple line. With a CT it is difficult to discern whether contrast material in the remnant stomach resulted from a gastrogastric fistula or retrograde flow through the biliopancreatic limb. Fluoroscopy allows progression of contrast to be visualized and may demonstrate either extravasation into the peritoneal cavity or a communication with the remnant stomach, if a gastrogastric fistula has formed. A potential pitfall is filling of the short stump of jejunum at the gastrojejunal anastomosis. Sometimes, contrast material will opacify this segment of jejunum and mimic leakage into the gastric remnant. Distinguishing features include lack of contrast progression into the gastric antrum and afferent loop and visualization of jejunal plicae. Gastrogastric fistula is known to be diagnosed as early as 1 month after RYGB.

References:

- Cho M, Kaidar-Person O, Szomstein S, et al. Laparoscopic remnant gastrectomy: a novel approach to gastrogastric fistula after Roux-en-Y gastric bypass for morbid obesity. J Am Coll Surg 2007; 204(4):617–624.
- Chandler RC, Srinivas G, Chintapalli KN, et al. Imaging in bariatric surgery: a guide to postsurgical anatomy and common complications. AJR Am J Roentgenol 2008; 190(1):122–135.

7. **Answer: D.**

Gastric prolapse can be anterior or posterior.

The phi angle is created by intersecting a line drawn parallel to the spinal column with a line drawn parallel to the plane of the gastric band, on an anteroposterior projection. Anterior gastric prolapse shows a medial eccentric dilated pouch and a phi angle less than 4°. Posterior gastric prolapse shows a lateral eccentric dilated pouch and a phi angle greater than 58°. Mild to moderate prolapse does not present with stomal obstruction.

Reference:

- Chandler RC, Srinivas G, Chintapalli KN, et al. Imaging in bariatric surgery: a guide to postsurgical anatomy and common complications. AJR Am J Roentgenol 2008 Jan; 190(1):122–135.

8. **Answer: D.**

The exact cause of an intussusception is unknown; however, various theories propose the possibility of lead points from suture lines, adhesions, lymphoid hyperplasia, and submucosal edema. Electrolyte imbalance, ectopic gut pacemaker foci, chronic bowel dilatation, and altered bowel motility have also been suggested. Regardless of cause, intussusception is usually retrograde and located at or just distal to the jejunojejunostomy. CT shows the classic target sign consisting of the invaginating bowel segment (intussusceptum) and its mesentery telescoping into the lumen of the receiving bowel segment (intussuscipiens). With obstruction, varying degrees of proximal dilatation of the Roux limb, afferent limb, gastric remnant, and gastric pouch will be seen.

Reference:

- Chandler RC, Srinivas G, Chintapalli KN, et al. Imaging in bariatric surgery: a guide to postsurgical anatomy and common complications. AJR Am J Roentgenol 2008; 190(1):122–135.

9. **Answer: D.**

Acute gastric dilation occurs due to edema at the jejunojejunostomy site and resulting dilation of the biliopancreatic limb and the gastric remnant. It is thus a closed loop obstruction. In an antegastric anastomosis, this dilation may cause leak at the gastrojejunostomy site by putting tension on the Roux limb. A CT scan is the diagnostic test of choice. A sick patient needs to be reoperated, whereas percutaneous drainage may provide temporary relief in nontoxic patients.

Reference:

- Merkle EM, Hallowell PT, Crouse C, et al. Roux-en-Y gastric bypass for clinically severe obesity: normal appearance and spectrum of complications at imaging. Radiology 2005; 234(3):674–683.

10. **Answer: D.**

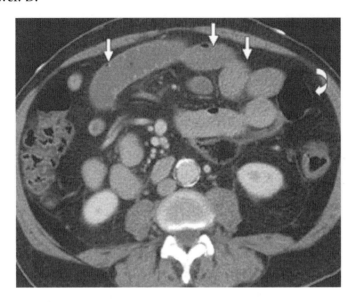

Source: From the *American Journal of Roentgenology.*

In a transmesocolic herniation, dilated bowel loop displaces the transverse colon caudally. Sometimes the biliopancreatic limb can be pulled through the mesocolic defect and be obstructed. Obstruction of the biliopancreatic limb can cause elevation of liver and pancreatic enzymes.

A transmesenteric herniation shows superiorly displaced transverse colon with absent overlying omental fat, displacement of the mesenteric trunk, and stretched and engorged mesenteric vessels on CT scan.

Reference:
- Sunnapwar A, Sandrasegaran K, Menias CO, et al. Taxonomy and imaging spectrum of small bowel obstruction after Roux-en-Y gastric bypass surgery. AJR Am J Roentgenol 2010; 194(1):120–128.

16 | Cancer

CHAPTER SUMMARY

- Cancer, in general, is not a contraindication for bariatric surgery.
- The incidence of several cancers is increased by obesity. Examples include endometrial cancer, renal cancer, liver cancer, and pancreatic cancer.
- Bariatric surgery decreases cancer incidence. This benefit has been demonstrated in women only.
- Barrett's esophagus has been related to obesity in a meta-analysis. Definitive diagnosis requires a four-quadrant biopsy. Length of Barrett's esophagus has been shown to be decreased after Roux-en-Y gastric bypass (RYGB) in 80% of the patients.
- Esophageal adenocarcinoma is, however, a contraindication for bariatric surgery. Esophagectomy should be performed and the stomach remnant can be used as conduit in a post-RYGB patient presenting with esophageal cancer.
- Gastrointestinal stromal tumors (GISTs): They are exophytic and may not be discovered during an endoscopy. They can be resected with adequate margins during bariatric surgery. Frozen section is performed during surgery to rule out cancer. Negative margin is the most important prognostic indicator. Follow-up of the patient is 3 to 6 months for the first 5 years and then yearly thereafter. Imatinib is indicated for positive tumor margins and for recurrent tumors.
- Gastric carcinoids are very rarely detected during upper GI endoscopy. Small carcinoids may be managed by endoscopic polypectomy. Large gastric carcinoids, >5 carcinoids, and type 3 carcinoids can be managed by subtotal gastrectomy during an RYGB.
- Gastric polyps are commonly encountered during preoperative endoscopy in a bariatric surgery patient, and their management is the same as in the general population. Remnant gastrectomy is opted if follow-up endoscopic surveillance after polypectomy is necessary due to technical difficulties in reaching the bypassed stomach during an endoscopy.
- Other tumors that are commonly encountered by bariatric surgeons include lymphoma, hepatic tumors, adrenal tumors, renal tumors, and gynecological tumors.

QUESTIONS

1. A 50-year-old Caucasian woman with a BMI of 50 kg/m^2 undergoes preoperative tests and is scheduled for a laparoscopic Roux-en-Y gastric bypass (LRYGB). During the initial diagnostic laparoscopy, a smooth 1-cm nodular lesion is visible on the distal greater curvature of the stomach, 10 cm proximal to pylorus. Which of the following is the next **BEST** step in management?
   A. Do a distal resection of stomach.
   B. Do a sleeve gastrectomy.
   C. Excise the lesion and wait for the frozen section.
   D. Do an RYGB after taking biopsy of the mass and investigate postoperatively.

2. A patient with gastroesophageal reflux disease (GERD) and BMI 65 kg/m^2 is scheduled to undergo an LRYGB and undergoes a preoperative endoscopy. Columnar-lined esophagus is found 3 cm above the squamocolumnar junction. Biopsy reveals Barrett's esophagus without dysplasia. Which of the following is the **BEST** course of action to manage this condition?

   A. Perform a Nissen's fundoplication instead.
   B. Perform endoscopic surveillance every year.
   C. Perform the RYGB.
   D. Repeat endoscopy after 3 months.

3. **Obesity is a risk factor for cancer, and bariatric surgery is hence thought to decrease cancer risk. Identify the <u>TRUE</u> statement about the beneficial effect of bariatric surgery on cancer.**
   A. Epidemiologically, obesity is not an important cause of cancer.
   B. The mortality risk reduction for cancer in various studies has been <5% after bariatric surgery.
   C. Bariatric surgery reduces cancer risk more in women than in men.
   D. Bariatric surgery reduces cancer incidence by <5%.

4. **Obesity causes increased risk of cancer and cancer mortality. Identify the <u>TRUE</u> statement from the following regarding cancer mortality in obese patients.**
   A. The strongest relation between cancer death and obesity in women is with endometrial cancer.
   B. In men the strongest relation of obesity with cancer death is with that of the prostate.
   C. Risk of renal cancer is not increased in obese patients.
   D. Increasing BMI has no correlation with increasing cancer risk.

ANSWER KEY

1. C	2. C	3. C	4. A

ANSWER KEY WITH EXPLANATION

1. **Answer: C.**

This is probably a GIST. All GISTs are currently considered to have some malignant potential. The patient cannot undergo an RYGB as one needs to wait for permanent section. If not cancer, one can proceed with the RYGB. If it turns out to be cancer, the patient needs to undergo a thorough workup.

References:
- Sanchez BR, Morton JM, Curet MJ, et al. Incidental finding of gastrointestinal stromal tumors (GISTs) during laparoscopic gastric bypass. Obes Surg 2010; 20 (3):393–396.
- Beltran MA, Pujado B, Méndez PE, et al. Gastric gastrointestinal stromal tumor (GIST) incidentally found and resected during laparoscopic sleeve gastrectomy. Obes Surg 2005; 15(10):1384–1388.

2. **Answer: C.**

RYGB is an excellent antireflux procedure due to decreased acid content of the pouch as well as absence of bile reflux owing to the Roux-en-Y anatomy. RYGB has been shown to cause regression of Barrett's esophagus in a few patients. Moreover, endoscopic surveillance is possible even after surgery. Nissen's fundoplication will not address the patient's morbid obesity.

References:
- Csendes A, Burgos AM, Smok G, et al. Effect of gastric bypass on Barrett's esophagus and intestinal metaplasia of the cardia in patients with morbid obesity. J Gastrointest Surg 2006; 10(2):259–264.
- Sharaf RN, Weinshel EH, Bini EJ, et al. Endoscopy plays an important preoperative role in bariatric surgery. Obes Surg 2004; 14(10):1367–1372.

3. **Answer: C.**

Obesity is the second largest preventable cause of cancer next only to smoking.

Bariatric surgery has been shown to decrease the incidence of various cancers and shown to be more effective in decreasing cancer risk as well as mortality in women, and such a benefit has not been found for men (as was seen in the Swedish obese subject (SOS) study and the Adams et al. study). The decrease in mortality for cancer has been found to be 42% to 60% after bariatric surgery. Bariatric surgery has been show to decrease cancer incidence by 30% to 38%.

References:

- http://www.cbsnews.com/stories/2007/10/31/earlyshow/health/main3434821. shtml. Accessed June 20, 2011.
- Ashrafian H, Ahmed K, Rowland SP, et al. Metabolic surgery and cancer: protective effects of bariatric procedures. Cancer 2011; 117(9):1788–1799.

4. **Answer: A.**

Obesity increases the rate of death due to cancer of the esophagus, colon and rectum, liver, gallbladder, pancreas, kidney, non-Hodgkin lymphoma, and multiple myeloma. In men, there is also a significant increased rate of death due to cancer of the stomach and prostate, while in women, this increased risk was found for cancer of the breast, uterus, cervix, and ovary.

The highest relative risk of death in men with obesity was seen with liver cancer. The second highest was with pancreatic cancer. The highest relative risk of death in obese women was seen with endometrial cancer and the second highest with kidney cancer. Increasing risk of cancer is found in both sexes with increasing BMI.

Reference:

- Calle EE, Rodriguez C, Walker-Thurmond K, et al. Overweight, obesity, and mortality from cancer in a prospectively studied cohort of U.S. adults. N Engl J Med 2003; 348(17):1625–1638.

17 | Pregnancy

CHAPTER SUMMARY

- Women represent >80% of the patients undergoing bariatric surgery.
- The prevalence of obesity in pregnant patients ranges from 10% to 35%.
- Maternal complications during pregnancy include miscarriage, hypertension, gestational diabetes (GDM), cesarian delivery, postpartum hemorrhage, and thromboembolic events.
- Fetal complications due to obesity include macrosomia, birth defects, stillbirth, premature birth, and childhood obesity.
- Fertility increases postoperatively after bariatric surgery. This risk of pregnancy seems to be even higher in adolescents after bariatric surgery.
- It is recommended by most bariatric surgeons that pregnancy should be delayed till 18 to 24 months after bariatric surgery.
- The risk of iron deficiency anemia is increased in pregnant patients after bariatric surgery.
- One study reported a relatively higher rate of band slippage in pregnant patients. It is not certain whether pregnancy predisposes to increased rate of intestinal obstruction.
- Maternal complications like hypertension and diabetes are decreased after bariatric surgery. Cesarian rates have not been shown to be definitively decreased.
- Bariatric surgery decreases the rate of macrosomia and increases the rate of appropriately grown neonates and small-for-gestational-age neonates.
- Weight gain during pregnancy is decreased after Roux-en-Y gastric bypass (RYGB), laparoscopic adjustable gastric banding (LAGB), and biliopancreatic diversion (BPD).
- Maternal obesity in a pregnant woman can cause obesity in the child.
- The rate of obesity in children born to mothers after BPD and biliopancreatic diversion/duodenal switch (BPD-DS) has been shown to be reduced when compared to obese women before surgery. The former also have a better metabolic profile.
- High rate of protein energy malnutrition (14%) was seen after pregnancy in one study in mothers after BPD.
- In a comparative study, LAGB has been shown to produce greater weight gain during pregnancy when compared to RYGB. There was no difference in the incidence of low birth weight (LBW) or macrosomia or in the maternal complications.
- There is no fixed protocol for management of LAGB during pregnancy. "Active management of the band" with removal of all the fluid causes increased weight gain during pregnancy.
- The oral glucose tolerance test can precipitate dumping symptoms in pregnant women with an RYGB. Hence, daily fasting and postprandial blood glucose for 1 week during 24- to 28-week period are recommended to diagnose GDM.

QUESTIONS

1. A bariatric surgeon needs to be aware of changes in weight that occur in obese pregnant women in order to manage weight loss in his/her patient effectively. Identify which of the following is <u>TRUE</u> regarding the weight changes of obese women during pregnancy.
   A. Obese women gain more weight during pregnancy when compared to nonobese women.
   B. Obese women do not differ in weight gain during pregnancy when compared to nonobese women.

    C. Obese women are recommended to gain the same amount of weight as nonobese women during pregnancy.

    D. Obese women are recommended to gain less weight than nonobese women during pregnancy.

2. **A 35-year-old lady who is 18 months s/p adjustable gastric band placement is referred by her Ob/Gyn practitioner. She is 30 weeks pregnant and has gained 10 kg during the course of her pregnancy. She is asymptomatic other than occasional nausea. Her counseling should include which of the following?**

    A. She should have her band loosened during the course of her pregnancy.

    B. She is at increased risk for revision of band.

    C. She is at increased risk for preeclampsia when compared to her obese counterparts.

    D. She should have her band tightened.

3. **A 35-year-old woman who is pregnant (30 weeks of gestation) has presented to her bariatric surgeon for a routine postoperative visit 2 years after a laparoscopic RYGB. She has lost a significant amount of weight. She complains of intermittent postprandial epigastric abdominal pain (about 6/10 in severity and radiating to the back) and vomiting episodes for the past 3 days. This episode has lasted 2 hours. She has had a recent upper GI endoscopy that revealed no stomal stenosis or marginal ulcers. Which of the following is the next BEST step in management?**

    A. Upper GI contrast study

    B. Diagnostic laparoscopy

    C. Repeat upper GI endoscopy

    D. CT scan with oral contrast

4. **A woman who has a BMI of 40 kg/m² would like to know what complications she is likely to suffer during her pregnancy and childbirth. All of the following are reproductive complications of obesity EXCEPT.**

    A. Increased likelihood of a cesarian section

    B. Low birth weight

    C. Preeclampsia

    D. GDM

5. **Obese mothers have an increased incidence of congenital anomalies in their offspring. Which of the following congenital anomalies is NOT associated with obesity and pregnancy?**

    A. Neural tube defects

    B. Congenital heart disease

    C. Gastroschisis

    D. Cleft palate

6. **There is a concern that BPD/DS may cause nutritional deficiencies during pregnancy. Identify the FALSE statement regarding outcomes of pregnancy in a woman conceiving after BPD/DS.**

    A. Most patients gain weight normally during pregnancy.

    B. There is a decrease in rate of fetal macrosomia.

    C. The rate of miscarriage is unchanged.

    D. Women who become euglycemic after BPD have a high chance of reappearance of diabetes during pregnancy.

7. **Obesity surgery increases fertility of a female after surgery. Identify the FALSE statement about the use of contraceptives after bariatric surgery.**

    A. Intrauterine devices (IUDs) are safe in adolescents.

    B. Oral contraceptives (OCPs) in female patients after BPD have been shown to be as effective as in the general population.

C. It is recommended that closer follow-up of the maternal and fetal health status may be beneficial if failure of contraception occurs within the first year after bariatric surgery.

D. Most bariatric surgeons recommend that women wait for at least 12 to 24 months after bariatric surgery before they conceive.

8. **Nutritional supplementation during pregnancy needs to be modified in the post–bariatric surgery patient. Which of the following statements is <u>TRUE</u>?**
   A. Bariatric surgery in the mother is not responsible for nutritional deficiencies in the breastfeeding baby.
   B. Patients who are overweight after bariatric surgery need to be on calorie restriction to prevent pregnancy complications.
   C. Supplemental doses of vitamin A should be at least 10,000 IU/day during pregnancy.
   D. Pregnant patients who have had bariatric surgery should take prenatal vitamins along with a multivitamin.

9. **Oral glucose tolerance test is used to screen for GDM. This test, however, is not well tolerated by pregnant post–bariatric surgery patients who have dumping syndrome. Which one of the following is considered to be a suitable alternative in a post-RYGB pregnant patient with dumping syndrome?**
   A. One reading of fasting blood glucose at 28 weeks of gestation
   B. One reading of postprandial blood glucose at 28 weeks of gestation
   C. Hemoglobin A_1c (HbA_1c) measurement at 28 weeks of gestation
   D. Fasting and postprandial blood sugar daily for approximately 1 week during 24 to 28 weeks of gestation

ANSWER KEY

1. D	4. B	7. B	9. D
2. B	5. C	8. D	
3. D	6. D		

ANSWER KEY WITH EXPLANATION

1. **Answer: D.**

   Obese women tend to gain less weight when compared to nonobese women during pregnancy, while they gain more weight in between pregnancies. Current recommended gestational weight gain is 11.2 to 15.9 kg for women with a normal BMI, 6.8 to 11.2 kg for overweight women, and no more than 6.8 kg for obese women.

   References:
   - Dixon JB, Dixon ME, O'Brien PE. Pregnancy after Lap-Band surgery: management of the band to achieve healthy weight outcomes. Obes Surg 2001; 11(1):59–65.
   - Edwards LE, Hellerstedt WL, Alton IR, et al. Pregnancy complications and birth outcomes in obese and normal-weight women: effects of gestational weight change. Obstet Gynecol 1996; 87(3):389–394.
   - Institute of Medicine. Nutritional status and weight gain. In: Nutrition during pregnancy. Washington, DC: National Academies Press, 1990:27–233.

2. **Answer: B.**

   Routine loosening of the band in early pregnancy may lead to increased weight gain during pregnancy. Routine tightening and associated malnutrition may lead to fetal complications. Adjustment of the band during pregnancy should be based on the amount of weight gained or lost.

Pregnancy after gastric banding has not been shown to increase the rate of revisional surgery. However, decreased time interval between surgery and pregnancy is associated with increased primary revisions.

Many studies have shown that LAGB decreases the complications associated with pregnancy like preeclampsia.

References:

- Carelli AM, Ren CJ, Youn HA, et al. Impact of laparoscopic adjustable gastric banding on pregnancy, maternal weight, and neonatal health. Obes Surg 2011; 21(10):1552–1558.
- Haward RN, Brown WA, O'Brien PE. Does pregnancy increase the need for revisional surgery after laparoscopic adjustable gastric banding? Obes Surg 2011; 21(9):1362–1369.
- Karmon A, Sheiner E. Pregnancy after bariatric surgery: a comprehensive review. Arch Gynecol Obstet 2008; 277(5):381–388.
- Lapolla A, Marangon M, Dalfrà MG, et al. Pregnancy outcome in morbidly obese women before and after laparoscopic gastric banding. Obes Surg 2010; 20(9):1251–1257.

3. **Answer: D.**

The patient is suspected of having an intestinal obstruction that may be due to an internal hernia. She needs to undergo a CT scan with oral contrast to diagnose the same. Laparoscopy is an invasive procedure, and surgery is to be avoided in the first and the third trimester if possible. If internal hernia is diagnosed or very strongly suspected, a laparoscopy should be performed. Given that her recent upper GI endoscopy was normal, a repeat endoscopy or upper GI study is unlikely to reveal any pathology. The maximal limit of ionizing radiation to which the fetus should be exposed during pregnancy is a cumulative dose of 5 rad. CT scan has a radiation exposure of 2.6 rad. CT scan can therefore be used during pregnancy when no safer alternative for adequate diagnosis is available. The greatest risk for central nervous system teratogenesis is between 10 and 17 weeks of gestation.

References:

- Toppenberg KS, Hill DA, Miller DP. Safety of radiographic imaging during pregnancy. Am Fam Physician 1999; 59(7):1813–1818, 1820.
- Gagné DJ, DeVoogd K, Rutkoski JD, et al. Laparoscopic repair of internal hernia during pregnancy after Roux-en-Y gastric bypass. Surg Obes Relat Dis 2010; 6 (1):88–92.
- Torres-Villalobos GM, Kellogg TA, Leslie DB, et al. Small bowel obstruction and internal hernias during pregnancy after gastric bypass surgery. Obes Surg 2009; 19(7):944–50.

4. **Answer: B.**

Obese patients have an increased rate primary and repeat cesarian delivery. They also have an increased rate of preeclampsia and GDM. A recent meta-analysis shows an increased risk of preterm deliveries has no significant effect on low birth weight (after accounting for publication bias). Without including imputed studies, obesity was protective against low birth weight. However, outcomes regarding postpartum hemorrhage, urinary tract infections, wound infections, fetal macrosomia, intrauterine growth restriction (IUGR), intrauterine fetal demise (IUFD), placental abruption, and operative vaginal delivery have been conflicting.

References:

- McDonald SD, Han Z, Mulla S, et al.; Knowledge Synthesis Group. Overweight and obesity in mothers and risk of preterm birth and low birth weight infants: systematic review and meta-analyses. BMJ 2010; 341:c3428.
- Weiss JL, Malone FD, Emig D, et al.; FASTER Research Consortium. Obesity, obstetric complications and cesarean delivery rate—a population-based screening study. Am J Obstet Gynecol 2004; 190(4):1091–1097.

5. **Answer: C.**

Maternal overweight or obesity is associated with a greater risk of developing a neural tube defect in the offspring. One study found that multivitamins were not as effective in reducing this risk compared to normal weight controls.

The offspring of obese women have higher risks for congenital heart diseases like atrial septal defect, hypoplastic left heart syndrome, aortic stenosis, pulmonic stenosis, and tetralogy of Fallot.

The incidence of cleft lip and palate is also increased in offsprings of obese women. The incidence of gastroschisis is reduced in offsprings of obese women.

In one of the larger series of obese women who have undergone bariatric surgery, no cases of congenital anomalies were reported in the offsprings.

References:
- Scialli AR; Public Affairs Committee of the Teratology Society. Teratology Public Affairs Committee position paper: maternal obesity and pregnancy. Birth Defects Res A Clin Mol Teratol 2006; 76(2):73–77.
- Abodeely A, Roye GD, Harrington DT, et al. Pregnancy outcomes after bariatric surgery: maternal, fetal, and infant implications. Surg Obes Relat Dis 2008; 4 (3):464–4671.
- Kral J, Biron S, Simard S, et al. Large maternal weight loss from obesity surgery prevents transmission of obesity to children who were followed for 2 to 18 years. Pediatrics 2006; 118:e1644–e1649.
- Stothard KJ, Tennant PW, Bell R, et al. Maternal overweight and obesity and the risk of congenital anomalies: a systematic review and meta-analysis. JAMA 2009; 301(6):636–650.

6. **Answer D.**

The data on outcomes of pregnancy after BPD are very limited. BPD does not change the rate of miscarriage. It does decrease the incidence of fetal macrosomia. Most BPD patients tend to gain normal weight during their pregnancy. Obese women who had diabetes before BPD and had resolution of the same were found to maintain normal blood glucose levels during pregnancy.

References:
- Marceau P, Kaufman D, Biron S, et al. Outcome of pregnancies after biliopancreatic diversion. Obes Surg 2004; 14(3):318–324.
- Adami GF, Murelli F, Briatore L, et al. Pregnancy in formerly type 2 diabetes obese women following biliopancreatic diversion for obesity. Obes Surg 2008; 18 (9):1109–1111.

7. **Answer: B.**

Pregnancy must be avoided during the first 12 to 24 months after bariatric surgery, especially in adolescents, as this is the period of rapid weight loss and mother is prone to nutrient deficiencies. However, there is no evidence to indicate that conception during this period increases bariatric surgery complications or has adverse pregnancy outcomes for all types of bariatric procedures. Early conception does increase the revision rate of gastric bands. No adverse effects on maternal or perinatal outcomes have been found when conception occurs early after RYGB. Should pregnancy occur during this time period, closer surveillance of maternal weight and nutritional status may be beneficial. Use of ultrasound for serial monitoring of fetal growth may also be beneficial. About 22% of patients taking OCPs developed unforeseen pregnancy after BPD in one series, and larger studies are required to confirm the decreased efficacy of OCPs in post-BPD patients. IUDs are a safe and effective long-term contraceptive method with no increase in risk of pelvic inflammatory disease, tubal infertility, or ectopic pregnancies. Because adolescents contribute disproportionately to the epidemic of unintended pregnancy, IUDs should be considered as a first-line contraceptive choice regardless of parity.

References:

- Wax JR, Cartin A, Wolff R, et al. Pregnancy following gastric bypass for morbid obesity: effect of surgery-to-conception interval on maternal and neonatal outcomes. Obes Surg 2008; 18(12):1517–1521.
- Gerrits EG, Ceulemans R, van Hee R, et al. Contraceptive treatment after biliopancreatic diversion needs consensus. Obes Surg 2003; 13(3):378–382.
- Division of Reproductive Health, National Center for Chronic Disease Prevention and Health Promotion; Centers for Disease Control and Prevention (CDC); Farr S, Folger SG, Paulen M, et al. U. S. Medical Eligibility Criteria for Contraceptive Use, 2010: adapted from the World Health Organization Medical Eligibility Criteria for Contraceptive Use. 4th ed. 2010; 59(RR-4):1–86.
- Merhi ZO. Challenging oral contraception after weight loss by bariatric surgery. Gynecol Obstet Invest 2007; 64(2):100–102.
- Gold MA, Johnson LM. Intrauterine devices and adolescents. Curr Opin Obstet Gynecol 2008; 20(5):464–469.

8. **Answer: D.**

Vitamin A is teratogenic and should be limited to 5000 IU/day during pregnancy. Patients who become pregnant after bariatric surgery should take a prenatal vitamin along with the multivitamin. Patients who are overweight after bariatric surgery should not attempt further calorie restriction as this has been shown to impair fetal growth and has no benefit in reducing pregnancy comorbidities. There are several case reports of nutritional deficiencies in infants who have been breast-fed by women who had undergone bariatric surgery.

References:

- Eerdekens A, Debeer A, Van Hoey G, et al. Maternal bariatric surgery: adverse outcomes in neonates. Eur J Pediatr 2010; 169(2):191–196.
- American College of Obstetricians and Gynecologists. ACOG practice bulletin no. 105: bariatric surgery and pregnancy. Obstet Gynecol 2009; 113(6):1405–1413.

9. **Answer: D.**

HbA_1c is not used for diagnosis of GDM at 28 weeks. American Diabetes Association (ADA) recommends the use of HbA_1c for the detection of diabetes in the nonpregnant population as it does not require a fasting state, thus encouraging more number of people to get tested and leads to higher detection rates. HbA_1c can also be used to screen for diabetes at the first prenatal visit in patients who are at high risk for diabetes like the following:

- Severe obesity
- Prior history of GDM or delivery of large-for-gestational-age infant
- Presence of glycosuria
- Diagnosis of polycystic ovary syndrome (PCOS)
- Strong family history of type 2 diabetes

All women of greater than low risk of GDM, including those above not found to have diabetes early in pregnancy, should undergo GDM testing at 24 to 28 weeks of gestation. The 50-g oral glucose tolerance test to screen for GDM is not well tolerated by post–malabsorptional surgery patients with dumping syndrome. Hence, daily measurement of fasting and postprandial blood glucose for 1 week is recommended during 24 to 28 weeks of gestation.

References:

- American Diabetes Association. Standards of medical care in diabetes—2010. Diabetes Care 2010; 33(suppl 1):S11–S61.
- American College of Obstetricians and Gynecologists. ACOG practice bulletin no. 105: bariatric surgery and pregnancy. Obstet Gynecol 2009; 113(6):1405–1413.

18 | Plastic surgery

CHAPTER SUMMARY
- Plastic surgery/body contouring procedures are to be performed only when the patient's weight has been stable for 1 year or more.
- Most plastic surgical procedures are deferred until a BMI < 35 is attained.
- Preoperatively, a thorough history including the type of bariatric procedure, comorbidities, and nutritional intake should be obtained. Documentation of functional problems is also essential.
- Excision of skin and soft tissue for the purpose of body contouring must be weighed against the need for an incision that will produce a scar.
- A post–bariatric surgery patient may have excess skin in multiple areas of the body. Plastic surgery in such patients aims to remove such excess skin, unwanted fatty deposits and restore fullness to areas such as breast and buttocks.
- Contouring procedures for the torso include the following:
  - Panniculectomy – removal of abdominal tissue without umbilical transposition.
  - Abdominoplasty – removal of abdominal tissue, undermining of the superior abdominal flap, plication of the rectus muscles, and umbilical transposition.
  - Belt lipectomy – abdominoplasty along with lateral thigh and buttock lift.
  - Medial thigh lift – excision of medial thigh tissue.
- Mastopexy: excision of mostly breast skin for the purpose of repositioning the nipple-areolar complex and restoring fullness. It may require placement of a silicone implant if more volume is required.
- Brachioplasty – excision of medial arm tissue to treat skin laxity. The incision for this is placed on the inner arm where it may be concealed.
- Multiple body contouring procedures can be performed in a single setting but often it is more prudent to stage several procedures.
- Proper protein and micronutrient intake should be ensured during the perioperative period to allow for proper wound healing.

QUESTIONS
1. Weight loss after bariatric surgery results in skin laxity, and body contouring procedures are hence performed to provide the patients better cosmesis. Which of the following statements about selection of bariatric surgery patients for plastic surgery/body contouring is **FALSE**?
   A. Body contouring needs to be performed even before weight is stabilized, as greater weight loss usually means greater incidence of nutritional deficiencies.
   B. Most body contouring procedures are performed only on patients with BMI < 35.
   C. Nutritional deficiencies should be corrected before proceeding to plastic surgery.
   D. Documentation of functional disturbances like sexual dysfunction and intertriginous skin rash will help the patient to get insurance coverage for the procedure.

2. Known in lay terms as the "tummy tuck" the abdominoplasty is useful to provide a firm-looking abdomen to the bariatric patients after their weight loss surgery. This involves a combination of surgical procedures. Identify the procedure that is usually **NOT** done as a part of abdominoplasty.
   A. Undermining of the upper abdominal flap
   B. Diastasis recti correction if present
   C. Umbilical transposition

D. Panniculectomy
E. Suction lipectomy

3. **Bariatric surgery usually leaves women with a flat breast that is not cosmetically pleasing. Three types of plastic surgery procedures may be done on breasts to improve their appearance in women – augmentation, breast lift, and breast reduction. Identify the <u>INCORRECT</u> statement regarding breast contouring procedures done for post–bariatric surgery patients.**
   A. Breast volume decreases after bariatric surgery.
   B. Breast reduction is never required in a post–bariatric surgery patient.
   C. Breast augmentation can be done using patient's own tissue.
   D. The breast lift procedure consists of centralizing the nipple on the breast mound.

4. **It is common for post–bariatric surgery patients to undergo a combination of plastic surgery procedures on various parts of their body. This woman has no midline abdominal incision but has a low suprapubic skin crease incision and incisions on both breasts. Identify which combination of procedures has been performed in the lady in the figure shown below.**

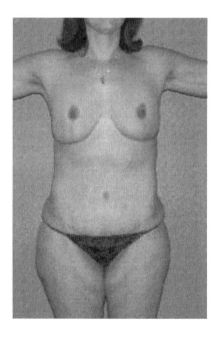

   A. Breast reduction and abdominoplasty
   B. Mastopexy and abdominoplasty
   C. Breast reduction and fleur-de-lys abdominoplasty
   D. Breast augmentation and fleur-de-lys abdominoplasty

5. **Wound-related complications in bariatric patients after body contouring are very high. Identify the <u>FALSE</u> statement about management of patients undergoing body contouring procedures.**
   A. All body contouring procedures are performed as staged procedures and never done in a single setting.
   B. Patients should be educated about nutrition and given vitamin supplementation.
   C. All patients usually require 4 to 6 weeks off from work.
   D. Use of anti–deep vein thrombosis (anti-DVT) measures is crucial in a post–bariatric surgery patient.

6. **A lax abdomen leads to a great demand for "tummy tuck" or abdominoplasty procedures after bariatric surgery. Investigators have also looked into how this procedure could be refined to produce better outcomes. Identify the <u>FALSE</u> statement regarding abdominoplasty.**
   A. More superficial flap elevation can decrease the duration for which a drain is placed in the postoperative period.
   B. Abdominoplasty has been shown to positively affect self-esteem and mental health.
   C. Nearly half the number of patients can develop wound-related complications.
   D. Abdominoplasty with liposuction has greater complication rate when compared to traditional abdominoplasty.

7. **Though all body contouring procedures improve cosmesis, they may result in complications. This is also true of the brachioplasty procedure. Identify the <u>FALSE</u> statement relating to brachioplasty.**
   A. Sensory loss is common after brachioplasty.
   B. The brachioplasty incision is on the lateral side of the arm.
   C. Complication rates increase when arm liposuction is combined with brachioplasty.
   D. Seromas not responding to repeated aspiration can be injected with sclerosing agent.

ANSWER KEY

1. A	3. B	5. A	7. B
2. E	4. B	6. D	

ANSWER KEY WITH EXPLANATION

1. **Answer: A.**

   Body contouring procedures should be performed once the patient's weight has stabilized as future skin laxity will compromise an otherwise adequate result. Most insurance companies require 6 to 12 months of stable weight to be documented. Other than panniculectomy, most body contouring procedures are performed when the BMI is less than or equal to 35. At the initial visit, a history is taken regarding the initial and the current BMI, dietary intake, and functional disturbances. Psychiatric evaluation is also required. The presence of functional disturbances, like sexual dysfunction, intertriginous skin rashes, and difficulty with exercise, are important to document. The latter will also help the patient to get medical insurance for the procedure.

   References:
   - Borud LJ, Warren AG. Body contouring in the postbariatric surgery patient. J Am Coll Surg 2006; 203(1):82–93 [Epub May 2, 2006].
   - Collwell AS. Current concepts in post-bariatric body contouring. Obes Surg 2010; 20(8):1178–1182.

2. **Answer: E.**

   Traditional abdominoplasty is performed via a horizontal incision at the level of the pubis and extended bilaterally to the anterior superior iliac crests. It typically involves dissection of the abdominal wall in a suprafascial plane around the umbilicus and up to the level of the xiphoid process. As such the umbilicus is transposed with excision of the excess skin and subcutaneous tissue (panniculectomy) and closure. Any laxity of the fascia is addressed with plication of the rectus muscles. Suction lipectomy is not always part of the procedure.

   References:
   - Borud LJ, Warren AG. Body contouring in the postbariatric surgery patient. J Am Coll Surg 2006; 203(1):82–93 [Epub May 2, 2006].

- Collwell AS. Current concepts in post-bariatric body contouring. Obes Surg 2010; 20(8):1178–1182.

3. **Answer: B.**

Breast reduction is occasionally done in a post–bariatric surgery patient when the patient retains enough volume. After bariatric surgery the breast volume decreased, requiring breast augmentation. This can be done using implants or using adjacent tissue flaps from either the back and/or axilla. More obese patients have an inferior displacement of the nipple-areola complex requiring repositioning through a breast lift procedure.

References:
- Borud LJ, Warren AG. Body contouring in the postbariatric surgery patient. J Am Coll Surg 2006; 203(1):82–93.
- Collwell AS. Current concepts in post-bariatric body contouring. Obes Surg 2010; 20(8):1178–1182.

4. **Answer: B.**

Patients with breast ptosis following massive weight loss often have volume loss without contraction of the skin. Most of these patients require excision of the skin and redraping of the skin and remaining breast tissue (mastopexy). Some even require the addition of an implant. Few retain sufficient breast volume to consider improvement in the shape of the breast – a true reduction. The incisions noted in the abdomen indicate that the patient underwent a standard abdominoplasty as evidenced by the lower horizontal incision. If she had horizontal skin excess, an additional midline incision would be required (fleur-de-lys).

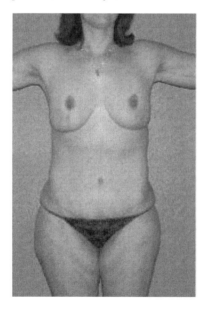

Reference:
- Collwell AS. Current concepts in post-bariatric body contouring. Obes Surg 2010; 20(8):1178–1182.

5. **Answer: A.**

All procedures can be performed in a single sitting by experienced surgeons and if the patient's health permits. Otherwise it is safer to do staged procedures that are separated by 3 to 6 months. Patients should be educated to get adequate proteins in their diet and take vitamin supplements to allow proper healing of wounds. Most patients remain in the hospital for 1 to 2 days and require 4 to 6 weeks off from work.

The use of pneumatic compression devices and blood thinners is crucial in these patients to minimize the risk of venous thromboembolism.

References:

*   Borud LJ, Warren AG. Body contouring in the postbariatric surgery patient. J Am Coll Surg 2006; 203(1):82–93.
*   Collwell AS. Current concepts in post-bariatric body contouring. Obes Surg 2010; 20(8):1178–1182.

6. **Answer: D.**

Flap elevation in a plane superficial to the standard suprafascial approach during abdominoplasty may decrease the length of time required for drains in the postoperative period in the abdominoplasty patient. A significant positive impact on body image, self-esteem, and mental health was found 1 to 6 months postoperatively in one study. In a study by Zuelzer et al., it was found that more than 50% of the patients developed one or more wound-related complications. Abdominoplasty with liposuction is not associated with a statistically significant increase in perfusion-related complication rates as compared with traditional abdominoplasty, despite the fact that it involves potential trauma to the vascularity of the elevated abdominoplasty flap. This holds true even in patients who are at increased risk for perfusion-related complications secondary to a history of active smoking or a previous supraumbilical scar.

References:

*   Fang RC, Lin SJ, Mustoe TA. Abdominoplasty flap elevation in a more superficial plane: decreasing the need for drains. Plast Reconstr Surg 2010; 125(2):677–682.
*   de Brito MJ, Nahas FX, Barbosa MV, et al. Abdominoplasty and its effect on body image, self-esteem, and mental health. Ann Plast Surg 2010; 65(1):5–10.
*   Zuelzer HB, Ratliff CR, Drake DB. Complications of abdominal contouring surgery in obese patients: current status. Ann Plast Surg 2010; 64(5):598–604.
*   Samra S, Sawh-Martinez R, Barry O, et al. Complication rates of lipoabdomino-plasty versus traditional abdominoplasty in high-risk patients. Plast Reconstr Surg 2010; 125(2):683–690.

7. **Answer: B.**

Any brachioplasty technique is associated with a certain degree of sensory loss. Incisions to remove skin and subcutaneous tissue from the arms by brachioplasty are designed to be as inconspicuous as possible. In general, they are designed to run in the brachial groove of the arm so that they lie on the medial aspect making them difficult to visualize from either an anterior or posterior viewpoint. The medial cutaneous nerve of arm runs in the medial aspect of the arm and is at risk with resection of skin and subcutaneous tissue. Injury to the nerve and any associated comorbidity may be avoided by placing the incision in a more posterior position. Liposuction when done along with a brachioplasty increases the rate of wound complications. Seromas are common after brachioplasty and initially managed with repeated aspiration. If this is not successful, injection of a sclerosing agent can be done many times. The last resort for management of a seroma would be exteriorization of the cavity by making a small opening through the scar into the cavity, inserting a Penrose drain, and leaving the drain in place until the cavity fills itself in and stops draining.

References:

*   Aly A, Soliman S, Cram A. Brachioplasty in the massive weight loss patient. Clin Plast Surg 2008; 35(1):141–147; discussion 149.
*   Symbas JD, Losken A. An outcome analysis of brachioplasty techniques following massive weight loss. Ann Plast Surg 2010; 64(5):588–591.
*   Chowdhry S, Elston JB, Lefkowitz T, et al. Avoiding the medial brachial cutaneous nerve in brachioplasty: an anatomical study. Eplasty 2010; 10:e16.

- Gusenoff JA, Coon D, Rubin JP. Brachioplasty and concomitant procedures after massive weight loss: a statistical analysis from a prospective registry. Plast Reconstr Surg 2008; 122(2):595–603.
- Knoetgen J III, Moran SL. Long-term outcomes and complications associated with brachioplasty: a retrospective review and cadaveric study. Plast Reconstr Surg 2006; 117(7):2219–2223.

19 | Miscellaneous

CHAPTER SUMMARY
- Management of ventral hernias in bariatric surgery:
  - Ventral hernias are more common in bariatric surgery patients – 8% of patients who presented for Roux-en-Y gastric bypass (RYGB) had ventral hernias.
  - Open bariatric surgery has a high incidence of incisional hernias, and prophylactic mesh can be used in preventing them. Laparoscopic bariatric surgery has decreased to a large extent the incidence of ventral hernias, but port site hernias still occur. Meshes are also available that can be prophylactically used to prevent port site hernias.
  - All obese patients need to be examined for hernias as operative management may need to be modified in their presence.
  - During an RYGB, if a ventral hernia is detected intraoperatively and reduced, it is best to repair it primarily as the use of meshes has a high rate of infection. Hernias with small neck need to be repaired as they are more likely to cause obstruction postoperatively.
  - Meshes of any type can be used for repair of hernias during Lap-Band surgery as enterotomies are not done in this bariatric procedure. Biological meshes (absorbable meshes) have a relatively low risk of infection and are preferred for bariatric procedures where enterotomies are created.
  - If the hernia is not reduced or repaired during the bariatric procedure, the patient needs to be followed up closely postoperatively to detect bowel obstruction.
  - Plastic surgery procedures can be done along with open hernia repair postoperatively.
  - Component separation technique is an excellent option for repair of large ventral hernias in morbidly obese patients. This consists of medial advancement of the rectus muscles after separation of the external oblique aponeurosis from the anterior rectus fascia and the underlying internal oblique muscle along with relaxing incisions over the posterior rectus sheath. The downside is weakening of the abdominal wall and recurrence of the hernia.
  - Port site hernias are very difficult to detect by physical examination. One needs to maintain a high index of suspicion and order a CT scan when bowel obstruction is suspected in a post–bariatric surgery patient.
- Renal transplantation:
  - Data are very sparse.
  - Obese patients who undergo renal transplantation have a high rate of wound infection, delayed graft function, and worse graft survival.
  - Renal failure patients who undergo bariatric surgery have a higher mortality.

QUESTIONS
1. **It is not uncommon for a bariatric surgeon to encounter an obese patient who has undergone a renal transplant. Renal transplantation influences outcomes of bariatric surgery and bariatric surgery can impact graft survival. Which of the following is <u>FALSE</u> regarding the same issue?**
   A. Weight loss in morbidly obese patients who have had renal transplantation or have end-stage renal disease (ESRD) is very poor after bariatric surgery.
   B. RYGB does not change dose of the immunosuppressants in renal transplant patients.

    C. Protein need not be restricted in a post-RYGB post–renal transplant patient.

    D. Magnesium supplementation should be given to post-RYGB post–renal transplant patient.

2. **The management of ventral hernias in morbidly obese patients can be challenging. Identify the <u>FALSE</u> statement about the problem of ventral hernias in morbidly obese.**

    A. Obesity is a risk factor for recurrence of incisional hernia after repair.

    B. Five to ten percent of patients who undergo gastric bypass have ventral hernias.

    C. Increased BMI is associated with an increased incidence of incisional hernias after open surgery.

    D. Incisions that avoid the umbilicus can decrease the incidence of incisional hernia.

3. **Port site hernias are notorious for the difficulty they present in their diagnosis. Identify the <u>TRUE</u> statement about the problem of port site hernias.**

    A. Post site hernias occur at a rate of about 10% in abdominal surgeries in general.

    B. Port sites caused by radially dilating trocars need routine closure.

    C. Hernias that present within 2 weeks have a lower incidence of obstruction.

    D. Hernias that occur ≤2 weeks do not have a peritoneal sac.

4. **During an LRYGB, a ventral hernia with a small neck with incarcerated omentum is encountered just above the umbilicus. The surgeon has to reduce the contents of the hernia to be able to proceed with the surgery. He then completes a standard LRYGB. What is the <u>NEXT</u> ideal step?**

    A. Do not repair the hernia.

    B. Repair the hernia primarily with sutures.

    C. Place a polypropylene mesh.

    D. Place a Gore-Tex mesh.

5. **The nurse is measuring the vitals of a morbidly obese patient who has just arrived at the ambulatory clinic to consult her bariatric surgeon. What advice would you give her about measuring the blood pressure?**

    A. The width of the cuff should be about 80% of the circumference of the arm.

    B. The length of the cuff has to be about 50% of the circumference of the arm.

    C. The length/width of the cuff does not matter – she could use any cuff as long as it can be wrapped around the arm.

    D. The width of the cuff should be about 50% of the circumference of arm.

6. **Nurses often have problems in administering medications to morbidly obese patients. Identify the step that does <u>NOT</u> overcome such difficulties.**

    A. Use longer needles to administer IM injections.

    B. Use transillumination to help identify veins.

    C. Pierce the skin at a greater angle and use longer cannulas.

    D. Take measures to preserve IV lines that are in situ for a long time.

7. **Medicaid and Medicare are two governmental programs that provide medical and health-related services to specific groups of people in the United States. Although the two programs are very different, they are both managed by the Centers for Medicare and Medicaid Services, a division of the U.S. Department of Health and Human Services. Identify the <u>FALSE</u> statement about Medicaid and Medicare coverage for bariatric surgery.**

    A. Laparoscopic sleeve gastrectomy is not covered by Medicare.

    B. Open adjustable gastric banding procedure is covered by Medicare.

    C. Medicaid covers bariatric surgery in most states.

    D. The surgery must be performed in American Society for Metabolic and Bariatric Surgery (ASMBS)-accredited Center of Excellence or American College of Surgeons (ACS)-certified Level 1 Bariatric Surgery Center in order to be covered by Medicare.

8. **Identify the <u>TRUE</u> statement about the characteristics of the "defense" in litigations involving bariatric surgery.**
   A. About 90% of the surgeons sued have less than 1 year of experience.
   B. Only one in four of the surgeons involved in the litigation had performed <100 cases.
   C. Less than 1% of the surgeons with training in laparoscopic or bariatric surgery were involved.
   D. About 1% of all litigations also target the hospital in general in addition to the primary surgeon.

9. **Identify the <u>TRUE</u> statement about the incidents that provoke litigations.**
   A. Most litigations are for complications that occur after discharge.
   B. The most common complication resulting in litigation is a gastrointestinal leak.
   C. The most common cause of alleged negligence is a wrong diagnosis.
   D. Major disability is the outcome in patients involved in most litigations.

10. **Which of the following statement <u>TRULY</u> reflects the meaning of the term "dropped baton phenomenon" that is used in medicolegal language?**
    A. Complications occur during a surgery due to an incompetent assistant.
    B. The patient does not follow the physician's advice thus resulting in a complication.
    C. A physician performs a management error due to a misprint in a textbook.
    D. The primary surgeon had left town or stopped practice, and his/her practice is taken over by a junior surgeon who is less experienced.

11. **Proper patient selection is an important aspect of bariatric surgery practice, which if done in a proper manner can minimize malpractice claims. Identify which of the following does <u>NOT</u> help a bariatric surgeon decrease chances of malpractice claims.**
    A. Adhering to the National Institutes of Health (NIH) guidelines.
    B. Documentation of conservative methods of weight loss before surgery.
    C. Documentation of significant impairment of lifestyle of the patient.
    D. Minimizing the number of specialists involved in selection of the patient.

12. **A patient looks at an advertisement in a local newspaper. It is about a bariatric surgery program that proclaims being the best bariatric program in the country that performs a large number of gastric bypass procedures that is "routine in the hands of our experienced team." The patient visits the center and views an hour long tape that describes the operation, its preoperative workup, and expected weight loss. After that she signs a consent form. She undergoes a psychological evaluation and nutritional evaluation the same day, has blood tests, and undergoes a gastric bypass 2 days later. Two years after surgery she develops severe malnutrition and sues the hospital and the surgeon. She claims that she was never informed about such a complication. The lack of which of the following could have potentially contributed to such a lawsuit?**
    A. Lack of a detailed informed consent
    B. Careless marketing
    C. Rushing with the process of informed consent
    D. All of the above

13. **A bariatric surgeon needs to follow his/her patients for clinical reasons and also to avoid medicolegal problems. Identify which of the following is NOT a step toward decreasing such medicolegal problems.**
    A. Training of nurses in bariatric surgery–specific problems
    B. Good physician–patient relationship
    C. Good physician relationship with nurses
    D. Decreasing the involvement of primary care physicians

14. **A 55-year-old female patient presents to her bariatric surgeon for a routine checkup 1 week after an LRYGB. She has been taking over-the-counter (OTC) phenylephrine and chlorpheniramine for her cold. Her vitals include HR, 121/min; RR, 16/min; BP, 110/70 mmHg; and temperature, 98.4°F. Her abdomen is soft, nontender, and nondistended with normal bowel sounds. The surgeon notes that the OTC medication that she is taking can cause tachycardia but orders an upper gastrointestinal (UGI) contrast study, which is reported as normal. The patient is discharged home. Two weeks later, the surgeon's office gets a phone call from a lawyer saying that the same patient had died and that he was being sued for negligence. The forensic pathologist reports the cause of death as peritonitis due to staple line leak. Which of the following statements is MOST ACCURATE regarding the same issue?**
    A. Give a β-blocker to counter the effect of the OTC medication.
    B. The surgeon should not have ordered a UGI contrast study as it was not indicated.
    C. The surgeon should have performed a laparotomy in spite of a normal UGI.
    D. The surgeon is not at any fault as his management was in accordance with best practice guidelines.

15. **Which one of the following has been identified as the LEAST common cause of lawsuits?**
    A. Lack of detailed bariatric surgery–specific informed consent
    B. Inappropriate documentation by the attending surgeon
    C. "Dropped baton phenomenon"
    D. Fraudulent billing

16. **The Surgical Review Committee and ACS grant "Center of Excellence" status to hospitals and practices. Which of the following is NOT a consideration for granting such status?**
    A. Long-term patient follow-up
    B. Critical care support
    C. Presence of a panel of administrative directors consisting of people who are not doctors
    D. Patient support groups
    E. Surgical experience and volumes

ANSWER KEY

1. A	5. D	9. B	13. D
2. D	6. D	10. D	14. C
3. D	7. B	11. D	15. D
4. B	8. B	12. D	16. C

ANSWER KEY WITH EXPLANATION

1. **Answer: A.**

   Data concerning renal transplantation in bariatric surgery patients or bariatric surgery in renal transplant patients are very sparse. Weight loss after surgery appears to be good in patients who have had a renal transplant or have ESRD (and are hence listed for transplant). However, mortality in such patients after bariatric surgery is higher. RYGB has no effect on the dosage of immunosuppressants. There is no need to restrict protein after renal transplant in a bariatric surgery patient. Magnesium supplementation should be given to all renal transplant patients who also have a bariatric procedure as some of the immunosuppressants like cyclosporine cause decreased magnesium absorption.

References:
- Lightner AL, Lau J, Obayashi P, et al. Potential nutritional conflicts in bariatric and renal transplant patients. Obes Surg 2011; 21(12):1965–1970.
- Szomstein S, Rojas R, Rosenthal RJ. Outcomes of laparoscopic bariatric surgery after renal transplant. Obes Surg 2010; 20(3):383–385.
- Modanlau K, Muthyala U, Xiao H, et al. Bariatric surgery among kidney transplant candidates and recipients: analysis of the United States renal data system and literature review. Transplantation 2009; 87(8):1167–1173.

2. **Answer: D.**

Ventral hernias are more common in the morbidly obese population. Morbidly obese patients have an increased intra-abdominal pressure that has been shown to correlate with increased incidence of hernias. Datta et al. reported that 8% of the patients who underwent gastric bypass procedure had ventral hernias. All patients chosen to undergo bariatric surgery need to be examined for ventral hernias as operative approach and follow-up may have to be modified in their presence.

Open bariatric operations are associated with a high incidence of incisional hernia. The risk of incisional hernias after open bariatric surgery increases with increasing BMI. Sugerman et al. reported in their series that incisional hernias occurred in 20% of the open gastric bypass patients with an even higher rate of occurrence in those with previous incisional hernia. Similar incidence has been reported in other studies. Strzelczyk et al. reported that characteristics of patients undergoing bariatric surgery could not be correlated with occurrence of ventral hernia (other than their BMI), which has also been the finding of another study. Capella et al. reported that small incisions that were located in the upper abdomen and that avoided the umbilicus decreased the incidence of incisional hernias.

References:
- Rao RS, Gentileschi P, Kini SU. Management of ventral hernias in bariatric surgery. Surg Obes Relat Dis 2011; 7(1):110–116.
- Graziano A, Santangelo M, Umana D, et al. Risk factors for hernia after gastroplasty. Acta Chirurgica Mediterranea 2008; 24:5.
- Sauerland S, Korenkov M, Kleinen T, et al. Obesity is a risk factor for recurrence after incisional hernia repair. Hernia 2004; 8(1):42–46.

3. **Answer: D.**

The true incidence of port site hernias after bariatric surgery is not known. In a series by Susmallian et al. access port site hernia after laparoscopic adjustable gastric banding (LAGB) was reported in 0.65% of the patients. In abdominal surgeries their incidence is reported between 0.8% and 2.8%. In a prospective study by Hussain et al. they occurred after a mean postoperative period of 43 months.

Port sites where radially dilating trocars are used generally do not require closure, thus saving valuable time during the procedure. Early port site hernias (<2 weeks) usually do not have a hernia sac and are more likely to be obstructed.

References:
- Rubenstein JN, Blunt LW Jr., Lin WW, et al. Safety and efficacy of 12-mm radial dilating ports for laparoscopic access. BJU Int 2003; 92(3):327–329.
- Rao RS, Gentileschi P, Kini SU. Management of ventral hernias in bariatric surgery. Surg Obes Relat Dis 2011; 7(1):110–116.

4. **Answer: B.**

Placing a mesh increases the chance of infection. If the surgeon desires to place a mesh, however, an absorbable mesh like Surgisis would be the best choice. Both Prolene and Gore-Tex are nonabsorbable meshes and should not be used. Repairing primarily does not carry the risk of mesh infection and its associated morbidity but has a higher chance of recurrence. Mesh infection will necessitate further trips to the OR, one for removal of the mesh and the second for repair of the hernia once infection has resolved. Not repairing the hernia carries the risk of postoperative bowel incarceration and blowout of anastomosis.

Reference:
- Rao RS, Gentileschi P, Kini SU. Management of ventral hernias in bariatric surgery. Surg Obes Relat Dis 2011; 7(1):110–116.

5. **Answer: D.**

The width of the cuff bladder must be 40% to 50% of the arm's circumference, and the length of the bladder must be 80% of the circumference to obtain an accurate reading.

Reference:
- Palatini P, Parati G. Blood pressure measurement in very obese patients: a challenging problem. J Hypertens 2011; 29(3):425–429.

6. **Answer: D.**

This is to be done only if other veins cannot be found and there are no local signs of inflammation. The Centers for Disease Control and Prevention's Guidelines for the Prevention of Intravascular Catheter-Related Infections recommend routinely restarting peripheral IV sites every 72 to 96 hours in adults to prevent phlebitis. Use of longer cannulas and piercing the skin more vertically are also recommended to overcome the difficulty offered by thick subcutaneous tissue during establishment of a peripheral IV line. Use of transillumination can help identify veins better in the obese and in infants. Use of longer needles is recommended for IM injections to avoid injecting into subcutaneous tissue in obese patients.

Reference:
- http://www.cdc.gov/mmwr/preview/mmwrhtml/rr5110a1.htm.

7. **Answer: B.**

The bariatric surgeries covered by Medicare include open RYGB and LRYGB, open and laparoscopic biliopancreatic diversion–duodenal switch (BPD-DS), and LAGB. Sleeve gastrectomy through any approach is not covered by Medicare. The surgery must be performed at an ASMBS-accredited Center of Excellence or ACS-certified Level 1 Bariatric Surgery Center in order to be covered by Medicare. Medicaid covers bariatric surgery in most states.

Reference:
- http://www.cms.gov/(https://www.cms.gov/manuals/downloads/ncd103c1_Part2.pdf).

8. **Answer: B.**

In a study by Cottam et al. of 100 consecutive medicolegal cases, the mean age of patients who were involved in litigation was 40 years (range 18–65); 75% of patients were women, 81% had a BMI of <60, 31% were diabetic, and 38% had sleep apnea. Of the primary surgeons, 42% had <1 year of experience in performing bariatric operations, 26% had performed <100 cases, and 38% of surgeons had performed <300 cases. For 69% of the surgeons, a general surgery residency was their only formal training; 29 surgeons had completed fellowships (laparoscopic and/or bariatric surgery), and two had completed a focused 4- to 6-week training experience in laparoscopic bariatric surgery.

About 45% of the litigations involve the hospital in addition to the surgeon.

Reference:
- Cottam D, Lord J, Dallal RM, et al. Medicolegal analysis of 100 malpractice claims against bariatric surgeons. Surg Obes Relat Dis 2007; 3(1):60–66; discussion 66–67.

9. **Answer: B.**

In the study by Cottam et al., the most common adverse patient events initiating litigation were intestinal leak (53%), intra-abdominal abscess (33%), bowel obstruction (18%), major airway events (18%), organ injury (10%), and pulmonary embolism (8%). Of the events that initiated litigation, 69% had occurred on the day of operation, 32% had occurred intraoperatively, 8% had occurred on postoperative day 1 to 3, and 23% had occurred within a wide range (postoperative days 4–192). The overall outcomes in this series of 100 legal cases were death (53%), major disability (7%), minor disability (12%), and near full recovery (28%). Evidence of potential negligence was found in 28% of cases. Of these cases, 82% resulted from a delay in diagnosis and 64% from misinterpreted vital signs.

Reference:
- Cottam D, Lord J, Dallal RM, et al. Medicolegal analysis of 100 malpractice claims against bariatric surgeons. Surg Obes Relat Dis 2007; 3(1):60–66; discussion 66–67.

10. **Answer: D.**

In 15% of the cases in the case series by Cottam et al., it was noted that the primary surgeon had left town or transferred coverage immediately before the occurrence of a complication. In each case, it was noted that a delay in diagnosis and treatment occurred and was thought to be related to either poor communication between surgeons and/or inadequate training or familiarity on the part of the covering surgeon. This phenomenon has been likened to runners at relay race who fumble the transfer of the baton, resulting in a dropped baton, which almost always brings defeat – hence the term "dropped baton."

Reference:
- Cottam D, Lord J, Dallal RM, et al. Medicolegal analysis of 100 malpractice claims against bariatric surgeons. Surg Obes Relat Dis 2007; 3(1):60–66; discussion 66–67.

11. **Answer: D.**

Patient selection and indications for surgery are often issues in any medical malpractice case involving bariatric surgery. Careful selection is crucial. Appropriate documentation outlining the thought process of the surgeon is vital. Often, questions arise whether the patient was appropriately screened. Does the patient fit the surgical candidacy guidelines as recommended by the NIH? Does the patient fit other guidelines for optimal candidates for bariatric surgery? Does the medical record accurately document the events leading up to surgery? Has the physician considered factors beyond BMI? Is there significant impairment on the lifestyle of the patient? Has the patient undergone conservative measures that have not worked? Are these documented? Are there other contraindications to the procedure, and have they been considered and documented? It is important to consult with a number of appropriate specialists to clear the patient for surgery and to document their agreement in the medical chart. It is difficult for a plaintiff lawyer to prove that several well-qualified health care providers all committed malpractice at the same time.

Reference:
- Eagan MC. Bariatric surgery: malpractice risks and risk management guidelines. Am Surg 2005; 71(5):369–375.

12. **Answer: D.**

The process of giving informed consent should not be rushed. It should be a drawn-out process so that the patient has ample time and opportunity to review the information and reflect upon it. The documentation must be accurate and complete. In the area of informed consent, fraud and misrepresentation allegations have stemmed from careless marketing documents fraught with superlatives. These documents, including Web site information, must be carefully worded and reviewed with counsel so not to warrant the procedure as "safe and successful" or "routine in the hands of our experienced team."

Reference:
- Eagan MC. Bariatric surgery: malpractice risks and risk management guidelines. Am Surg 2005; 71(5):369–375.

13. **Answer: D.**

Nurses should be trained in bariatric surgery–specific problems and complications. The bariatric surgeon should maintain a good relationship with both the nurses and the primary care physicians. In addition, good doctor–patient relationship is vital.

Reference:
- Eagan MC. Bariatric surgery: malpractice risks and risk management guidelines. Am Surg 2005; 71(5):369–375.

14. **Answer: C.**

Evidence of potential negligence was found in 28% of the 100 legal cases reviewed by Cottam et al. In the same series, the most common cause of negligence was considered to be a delay in diagnosis of an intestinal leak or abscess (82%). In the vast majority of cases involving a delay in diagnosis, misinterpretation of vital signs (64%) was the most common surgeon error. Most notable was the error in failing to recognize sustained tachycardia as an early sign of peritonitis. The misinterpretation of other studies, including UGI contrast studies, abdominal CT, and chest radiography, accounted for the remainder. A technical error in the performance of the operation was noted in only 8% of the cases.

Reference:
- Cottam D, Lord J, Dallal RM, et al. Medicolegal analysis of 100 malpractice claims against bariatric surgeons. Surg Obes Relat Dis 2007; 3(1):60–66; discussion 66–67.

15. **Answer: D.**

In a series of medicolegal cases by Cottam et al., although in none of the cases was the lack of informed consent a primary allegation, only 22% of the cases had detailed, bariatric surgery–specific consent forms. Patients were noncompliant with perioperative management recommendations in 23% of cases, but in only 19% of these cases did the noncompliance have a perceived effect on the patient outcome. The patients' dietary habits potentially contributed to complications in 7% of the cases. Twelve percent of the patients were noncompliant in adhering to return visits for follow-up. In two cases, unconfirmed fraudulent billing was alleged and may have been a factor precipitating the lawsuit. Finally, 15% of the charts reviewed had inappropriate documentation by the staff or attending surgeon.

The "dropped baton phenomenon" has been described in a previous question, and this contributed to 15% of the litigations.

Reference:
- Cottam D, Lord J, Dallal RM, et al. Medicolegal analysis of 100 malpractice claims against bariatric surgeons. Surg Obes Relat Dis 2007; 3(1):60–66; discussion 66–67.

16. **Answer: C.**

Centers are fully approved for the Bariatric Surgery Center of Excellence (BSCOE) designation when they comply with the hospital requirements that are in effect when they submit their applications for designation. A comprehensive site inspection is conducted to verify compliance. The following are taken into consideration while granting BSCOE status:
1. Institutional commitment to excellence
2. Surgical experience and volumes
3. Responsive critical care support
4. Appropriate equipment and instruments

5. Surgeon dedication and qualified call coverage
6. Clinical pathways and standardized operating procedures
7. Bariatric nurses, physician extenders, and program coordinator
8. Patient support groups
9. Long-term patient follow-up

Reference:
• http://www.surgicalreview.org/asmbs/requirements/hospitals/.

GASTROINTESTINAL HORMONES AND ADIPOKINES

Section Summary

- Central regulation of energy homeostasis:
  - The arcuate nucleus of the hypothalamus (ARH) is an important center for long-term regulation of energy balance.
  - The ARH contains neuropeptide Y (NPY), pro-opiomelanocortin (POMC), and Agouti-related peptide (AgRP) neurons and is responsive to leptin.
  - Alpha–melanocyte-stimulating hormone (α-MSH) is derived from POMC. It is an agonist of the MC4R (melanocortin 4 receptor). MC4R mutation is the most common cause of monogenic obesity in humans.
  - NPY and AgRP are orexigenic (hunger causing) and POMC is anorexigenic (satiety inducing).
  - NPY receptors NPY5 and NPY1 are strongly implicated in regulation of feeding.
  - Cocaine and amphetamine-regulated transcript is another neurotransmitter that is thought to have mostly anorexigenic properties.
  - Endocannabinoids are orexigenic neurotransmitters. There are two endogenous cannabiniods – 2-arachnidoglycerol and anandamide. There are various types of cannabinoid receptors of which CB1 is located in the human brain. Rimonabant is a CB1 receptor antagonist, which is not approved for weight loss by the FDA.
- Leptin:
  - It is derived from *ob* gene, located on chromosome 7. The leptin receptor is located on chromosome 1.
  - It is an anorexigenic hormone.
  - It is a product of the adipose tissue, and is released in a greater amount from the subcutaneous adipose tissue.
  - Leptin levels are an indicator of the body's energy stores and correlates with body fat content.
  - Leptin crosses the blood–brain barrier and CSF leptin has been correlated with the body mass index (BMI).
  - Though considered an indicator of energy stores, leptin levels are increased by short as well as long-term overfeeding. Fasting for only 3 days has been shown to decrease leptin levels. Leptin has been suggested to be involved in short-term regulation of food intake.
  - Leptin has an effect on the orexigenic and anorexigenic peptides of the hypothalamus. It inhibits release of NPY and AgRP.
  - In addition to regulation of food intake, leptin also regulates resting energy expenditure.
  - Leptin decreases after all types of bariatric surgery.
  - Leptin resistance is present in obese humans and this is attributed to various causes like deceased leptin transport into the CSF, defects in downstream mediators of leptin like AgRP, and presence of negative regulators of leptin signaling like suppressor of cytokine signaling 3 (SOCS3).
- Adiponectin:
  - Adiponectin is a 244–amino acid protein that shares a high degree of structural homology with molecules like collagen 7, complement C1q, and tumor necrosis factor (TNF)-α.

- It is secreted from white adipose tissue and is the most abundant adipokine secreted from the adipose tissue.
- Basal adiponectin is reduced in obese patients, whereas adiponectin response to meal is increased in the same patients.
- Adiponectin is correlated inversely with waist-hip ratio, fasting insulin, and fasting glucose levels. It has been correlated with insulin resistance.
- Adiponectin levels increase after all types of bariatric surgery.
- Ghrelin:
  - Ghrelin acts through growth hormone secretagogue receptor 1a present in the hypothalamus.
  - Ghrelin acts at the level of the hypothalamus to stimulate release of NPY and AgRP. It inhibits the POMC neurons.
  - In addition to acting on the hypothalamus, ghrelin may also act via the vagus nerve.
  - The levels of ghrelin are highest preprandially, and decrease to basal levels after intake of food. There is also intermeal diurnal variation in ghrelin levels. The above variations are absent in obesity.
  - Obese patients have low circulating ghrelin levels and the levels of ghrelin increase with weight loss. The exception to this is the Prader–Willi syndrome; a monogenic cause of obesity is associated with high ghrelin levels when compared to healthy subjects.
  - Ghrelin is a meal initiating signal, and infusion of ghrelin has been shown to cause hunger and food intake in healthy and obese humans.
  - Ghrelin increases gastric emptying, and ghrelin infusion has been shown to be useful in patients with gastroparesis.
  - Change in ghrelin levels after all types of bariatric surgery is controversial; the exception is sleeve gastrectomy, which has been able to consistently decrease ghrelin levels.
  - Animal studies have shown that ghrelin is not critical for growth, appetite, and fat deposition.
- Peptide YY (PYY):
  - It is a 36–amino acid peptide, the letter Y standing for tyrosine residues.
  - PYY (1-36) is activated by DPP-4 (dipeptidyl peptidase 4) to PYY (3-36).
  - It is secreted by the L cells of the small intestine, which are present throughout the gut but are found in highest concentration in the distal part of the intestine.
  - It is a satiety hormone. Its levels are low in obesity.
  - Postprandial PYY is increased after Roux-En-Y gastric bypass (RYGB) and this has been shown to contribute to weight loss. Increase in PYY occurs within a few days even before significant weight loss. Laparoscopic adjustable gastric banding (LAGB) patients have a lower PYY response when compared to RYGB patients. Sleeve gastrectomy increases PYY to the same extent as RYGB.
  - It slows gastric emptying and has been implicated in the ileal brake mechanism.
- Glucagon-like peptide 1 (GLP-1):
  - It is released from the intestinal L cells in two forms: GLP-1 (1-36)amide and GLP-1 (1-37). Further cleavage of the N terminus produces GLP-1 (7-36)amide and GLP-1 (7-37), which are biologically active.
  - It has a short half-life.
  - GLP-1 is inactivated by DPP-4.
  - It is an incretin – induces glucose-dependent insulin secretion. Other actions include inhibition of gastric motility, lipolysis, and inhibition of glucagon secretion.
  - The levels of fasting or postprandial GLP-1 levels in obese patients are not clear. RYGB has been shown to increase postprandial GLP-1 response.

- Glucose-dependent insulinotropic polypeptide (GIP):
  - It is a 42–amino acid peptide, which is degraded by DPP-4.
  - Actions of GIP include the following:
    - Incretin effect – secretion of insulin from the β cells in a glucose-dependent manner.
    - Stimulation of production of glucagon from pancreatic islets.
    - No appreciable effect on stomach emptying.
    - Proliferation of the β cells.
    - Increased deposition of fat in the adipose tissue.
  - Resistance to action of GIP has been suspected to be present in obese patients.
  - GIP levels (both basal and meal stimulated) are increased in obese patients.
  - RYGB and biliopancreatic diversion with duodenal switch (BPD-DS) decrease GIP levels.
- Cholecystokinin (CCK):
  - In addition to its well-known effect to inhibit gall bladder and gastric motility, it is also a satiety hormone.
  - It is secreted by the I cells of the duodenum, jejunum, and proximal ileum.
  - The change in the levels of this hormone after bariatric surgery is controversial, with most studies reporting no change.

Questions

1. There are various types of melanocortin receptors, with different types being expressed in different tissues in the human body. The type 4 receptors are mainly responsible for regulation of food intake. Identify the <u>TRUE</u> statement about melanocortin (MC4R) receptors.
   A. MC4R stimulation causes decreased feeding.
   B. α-MSH inhibits MC4R.
   C. AgRP stimulates MC4R.
   D. Melanocortin receptor mutation has not been described as a genetic cause of obesity.

2. The arcuate nucleus plays a pivotal role in regulating appetite and food intake. It contains various orexigenic and anorexigenic neurons and is influenced by hormones like ghrelin and leptin. Which letter in the picture represents the arcuate nucleus?

Coronal section of hypothalamus

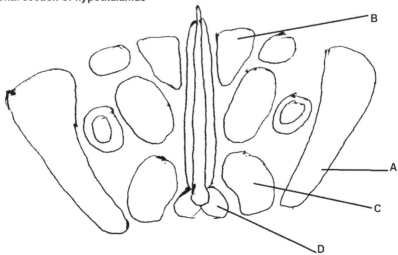

A. A
B. B
C. C
D. D

3. **NPY, POMC, and AgRP neurons are affected by leptin signaling and have an important role in energy homeostasis. Which of the following statements regarding the effects of these neurotransmitters is <u>TRUE</u>?**
   A. Both AgRP and POMC are anorexigenic.
   B. NPY is anorexigenic, POMC is orexigenic.
   C. Both NPY and POMC are orexigenic.
   D. POMC is anorexigenic and AgRP is orexigenic.

4. **A 4-month-old male baby is brought to the endocrinologist by his mother with the concern that the baby looked too "fat and big" and had red-colored hair. She is surprised because both she and her husband have black hair. Baby looks very lethargic. Vitals are significant for hypotension. Laboratory studies reveal decreased adrenocorticotropic hormone (ACTH). Which of the following is the <u>MOST LIKELY</u> diagnosis?**
   A. POMC null mutation
   B. MC4R haploinsufficiency
   C. AgRP null mutation
   D. NPY gene mutation

5. **Leptin deficiency is responsible for prolonged activation of the "pleasure center" in the brain even after sufficient feeding has occurred. Identify the location of this center from the following coronal slice in MRI.**

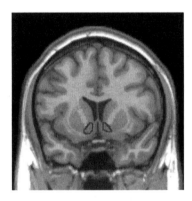

Source: http://en.wikipedia.org/wiki/File:Nucleus_accumbens_MRI.PNG

   A. Amygdala
   B. Nucleus accumbens
   C. Caudate nucleus
   D. Putamen

6. **Ghrelin has many actions in addition to being an orexigenic hormone. Identify the <u>FALSE</u> statement about ghrelin.**
   A. Ghrelin acts by inhibiting the NPY pathway.
   B. Ghrelin acts on a type of growth hormone receptor.
   C. Ghrelin crosses the blood–brain barrier.
   D. Ghrelin decreases gastric emptying.

7. Ghrelin-producing cells are mainly present in the body of the stomach. Ghrelin-producing cells are removed in a sleeve gastrectomy and they lose contact with the food in an RYGB. Changes in serum ghrelin levels after bariatric surgery is a matter of debate and controversy. Identify the <u>TRUE</u> statement regarding changes in ghrelin levels that have been *consistently* shown in *most* studies.
   A. RYGB – decreased
   B. BPD-DS – no change
   C. Sleeve gastrectomy – decreased
   D. LAGB – no change

8. Ghrelin circulates in blood in two forms that have differing actions. The role of ghrelin in resolution of diabetes after bariatric surgery is controversial. The main receptor for ghrelin action is the growth hormone receptor 1a (GHR1a). Identify the <u>TRUE</u> statement about the action of the different forms of ghrelin on pancreas and on glucose homeostasis.
   A. Ghrelin has no influence on the β-cell mass.
   B. Acylated ghrelin binds to GHR1a.
   C. Desacylated ghrelin binds to GHR1a.
   D. The most commonly used assays of ghrelin measure acylated ghrelin only.

9. Ghrelin levels are found to be meal-related as well as to be changed in certain disease states. What are the expected changes in ghrelin levels in the following situations?

	Obesity (fasting levels)	2 hr postprandial	Immediately before a meal
A	Increased	Decreased	Increased
B	Decreased	Baseline	Baseline
C	Decreased	Decreased	Baseline
D	Decreased	Baseline	Increased

10. GLP-1 is secreted by the L cells of the intestine, and is an insulin secretagogue. Its effect may partially explain the effect of bariatric and metabolic surgery on the resolution of diabetes mellitus. Identify the <u>FALSE</u> statement about metabolism of GLP-1.
    A. GLP-1 is activated by DPP-4.
    B. GLP-1 and PYY are cosecreted by the same cells.
    C. GLP-1 has a short half-life of a few minutes.
    D. The insulinotropic activity of GLP-1 is preserved to a large extent in patients with well-controlled diabetes.

11. GIP was found to have an incretin effect in 1973 and GLP-1 was found to have an incretin effect in 1987. Identify the <u>CORRECT</u> statement about the "incretin effect."
    A. It is the effect of a substance to inhibit insulin release.
    B. It is the effect of a substance to cause increase in glycemia.
    C. It is the greater amount of insulinemia after oral than intravenous glucose.
    D. It is the increase in insulin secretion that occurs when the glucose is given intravenously when compared to when it is given orally.

12. Though both GIP and GLP-1 are incretins, there are certain differences between the two. Identify the <u>FALSE</u> statement.
    A. There is "GIP resistance" in type 2 diabetes.
    B. GLP-1 contributes more to the incretin effect in healthy subjects after a meal.

C. GIP and GLP-1 have opposing effects on glucagon secretion.

D. GLP-1 causes delayed gastric emptying whereas GIP does not affect gastric emptying.

13. **An investigator wants to test the effect of food intake on GLP-1 levels in a group of RYGB patients. He uses obese patients who are age, sex, and BMI matched as controls. He also uses a group of lean patients as controls. Identify the <u>TRUE</u> statement about GLP-1.**

A. Fasting GLP-1 has been definitively shown to be reduced in obesity.

B. Postprandial GLP-1 response is typically reduced in obese when compared to lean subjects.

C. Fasting GLP-1 has consistently been shown to increase after RYGB.

D. Patients after RYGB have an impaired GLP-1 response to a meal.

14. **PYY has been identified as a satiety factor that may contribute to decreased food intake after bariatric surgery. Identify the <u>CORRECT</u> statement about the postsurgical change of PYY levels after bariatric surgery.**

A. BPD causes same degree of increase in postprandial PYY compared to RYGB.

B. The postprandial PYY response after RYGB is more than that of sleeve gastrectomy.

C. PYY has been shown to be increased after ileal transposition in humans.

D. Postprandial PYY response is normal in obesity.

15. **An investigator working on rats wants to find out the change of PYY and GLP-1 that can occur after an experimental bariatric procedure. He uses a particular enzyme inhibitor to prevent alteration of the hormone levels he wants to assay. Which of the following facts that the investigator needs to know about PYY is <u>TRUE</u>?**

A. PYY is inactivated by DPP-4.

B. PYY (1-36) is the predominant form of circulating hormone.

C. PYY acts on the arcuate nuclues.

D. PYY is a promising obesity pharmacotherapy.

16. **The delivery of food into the distal small intestine decreases gastric emptying that has been termed the "ileal brake." This mechanism may have an important role in weight loss and improvement of metabolic parameters after bariatric surgery. Identify the <u>FALSE</u> statement about the ileal brake mechanism.**

A. It contributes to decreased food intake.

B. One of the mediators is neurotensin.

C. Presence of food in stomach leads to "braking" of ileal motility.

D. This is a humoral as well as a neural mechanism.

17. **Amylin is a peptide hormone that is cosecreted with insulin by β cells at roughly 1 amylin:100 insulin ratio, and analogues of amylin have been used as pharmacotherapy for the treatment of diabetes. Which of the following statements about amylin is <u>FALSE</u>?**

A. Amylin increases insulin secretion.

B. The combination of amylin and metreleptin has been found to be more effective in the treatment of obesity than either of them alone.

C. Low amylin levels are found in diabetes.

D. Low meal-stimulated amylin levels are found in obesity.

18. **Leptin is regarded as an indicator of long-term energy stores. Identify the <u>TRUE</u> statement about leptin levels in humans.**

A. Subcutaneous fat is the main source of leptin.

B. Leptin is higher in obese type 2 diabetes patients compared to patients with obesity without diabetes.

C. Leptin levels are inversely correlated with insulin in obese patients with insulin resistance.

D. Low leptin levels induce negative energy balance.

19. **Obese people have leptin resistance due to which they do not respond to leptin when it is administered as pharmacotherapy. Which of the following factors has been definitively implicated as a cause of leptin resistance in humans?**
    A. Mutated leptin receptor
    B. Decreased levels of adiponectin
    C. Defect in leptin signaling
    D. Mutated leptin gene

20. **Adiponectin is the most abundant adipokine secreted from the adipose tissue. Despite being produced in the adipose tissue, adiponectin was found to be decreased in obesity. Identify the <u>FALSE</u> statement about adiponectin.**
    A. Adiponectin is produced more from the subcutaneous fat when compared to visceral fat.
    B. Adiponectin has been implicated in NASH, independent of insulin resistance.
    C. Unlike leptin resistance, adiponectin resistance has not been shown to exist in obesity.
    D. Adiponectin causes lipolysis and increased glucose uptake.

21. **Studies have reported changes in adiponectin after bariatric surgery, which could possibly be the reason behind resolution of metabolic abnormalities in obesity after bariatric surgery. Identify the <u>TRUE</u> statement about adiponectin.**
    A. Adiponectin stimulated by meal is decreased in obesity.
    B. Most studies have not been able to show a significant increase of adiponectin after RYGB.
    C. Adiponectin is negatively correlated with insulin resistance.
    D. Gastric banding does not increase adiponectin.

22. **The adipose tissue is an important contributor to the metabolic syndrome and the fat mass has been positively correlated with insulin resistance in many studies. Which of the following does <u>NOT</u> describe the mechanism by which adipose tissue contributes to insulin resistance?**
    A. Increased production of TNF-α by the adipose tissue.
    B. Increased release of free fatty acids (FFAs) by the omental adipose tissue.
    C. Increased production of interleukin-6 (IL-6) by the adipose tissue.
    D. Visceral adipose tissue only causes peripheral insulin resistance but no hepatic insulin resistance.

23. **The existence of an intestinal hormone that had a choleretic action was first proposed by Bayliss and Starling in 1902. CCK has long been suspected to be involved in metabolic changes after bariatric surgery. Identify the <u>FALSE</u> statement about CCK.**
    A. CCK and leptin have a synergistic action.
    B. Fats and proteins are potent stimulators for its release.
    C. CCK agonists are promising weight loss drugs.
    D. CCK has an action on the CNS.

24. **Two novel adipokines, resistin and visfatin, have been postulated to be involved in type 2 diabetes mellitus (T2DM). Resistin was observed to be the cause of insulin resistance in obese rodents and hence the name. Visfatin is nicotinamide phosphoribosyltransferase, whose levels have been reported to be altered by bariatric surgery. However, it has not been linked to human insulin resistance.**

Which of the following is definitely known to be <u>TRUE</u> about resistin and visfatin?
A. Resistin levels have been found to be increased in obesity and T2DM in all studies.
B. Resistin has been found to be decreased after bariatric surgery in all studies.
C. There is no consensus on the levels of visfatin in obese when compared to lean patients.
D. Visfatin is consistently decreased after bariatric surgery.

GENETICS

Section Summary
- Prader–Willi syndrome (PWS) is a monogenic form of obesity and is attributed to a deletion in chromosome 15q13. It is a classic example for genomic imprinting. The patient presents with PWS or Angelman syndrome depending on whether the defect is paternally inherited or maternally inherited.
- At birth, the infant has hypotonia, feeding difficulties, and *poor* weight gain. During childhood, these patients develop hyperphagia and morbid obesity.
- Unique problems of these patients include osteoporosis, growth hormone deficiency, hypogonadism, altered pain threshold, and inability to vomit.
- Medical management includes growth hormone administration and limiting access to food.
- Bariatric surgery does not produce good weight loss in these patients.

Questions
25. PWS is one of the rare genetic obesity syndromes occurring in 1 in 15,000 children, which is also associated with hypogonadism. Identify the <u>FALSE</u> statement about the diagnosis of PWS in which most bariatric surgeons do not perform weight loss surgery.
    A. DNA methylation test is very sensitive for diagnosis of PWS.
    B. Obesity is not present at birth.
    C. This syndrome is often due to deletion of the paternally derived autosomal chromosome.
    D. Holm's criteria can help in the diagnosis of this syndrome.

26. Treatment of PWS is challenging due to hyperphagia in these children. Identify the <u>TRUE</u> statement about PWS and bariatric surgery.
    A. Growth hormone (GH) has no role in the treatment of PWS.
    B. Ghrelin is decreased in PWS.
    C. Current opinion is that conservative methods of weight control be tried in patients with PWS instead of bariatric surgery.
    D. Bariatric surgery produces sustained weight loss in PWS.

27. The thrifty gene hypothesis is one of the hypotheses put forward to explain as to how "natural selection" has paradoxically favored obesity. Identify the <u>FALSE</u> statement about the thrifty gene hypothesis.
    A. It was initially proposed as an explanation for obesity and then later expanded to diabetes.
    B. It hypothesizes that "thrifty genes" exist to allow people who have them to accumulate fat stores during abundant periods so that they can better survive during famines.

    C. It hypothesizes that these "thrifty genes" were advantageous in hunter-gatherer populations but not in today's world, resulting in diabetes and obesity.

    D. No single convincing candidate for this "gene" has been discovered.

28. **The thrifty gene hypothesis is not accepted by many authorities. James Neel, the founder of this theory, himself found many contradictions to this theory upon more careful examination. Identify which of the following statements have <u>NOT</u> been proposed as arguments against the thrifty gene hypothesis.**

    A. People who die during famines have had a high rate of obesity.

    B. The prevalence of obesity between famines is too low.

    C. Frequency of famines is insufficient to account for intensity of selection.

    D. Many of the populations that later developed high rates of obesity and diabetes appeared to have no discernible history of famine or starvation.

BODY COMPOSITION

Section Summary

- Bioelectrical impedance analysis (BIA):
  - It is based on two-compartment body composition model.
  - It measures resistance to electrical current as it travels through the total body water pool, and body composition is derived using formulae.
  - Single-frequency BIA is most commonly used. It cannot distinguish intracellular from extracellular water.
  - Multifrequency devices can distinguish between intracellular and extracellular water.
  - They are not recommended in the presence of a pacemaker.
  - Its validitiy is influenced by age, sex, and ethnicity.
- Dual-energy X-ray absorptiometry (DEXA):
  - It is considered accurate, reproducible, and produces accurate results in the presence of disease states.
  - It is based on certain assumptions: minimal effects of hydration on lean tissue estimates; lack of an effect of variations in regional (e.g., chest, leg, and arm) thickness on soft-tissue estimates; and that the fat content of the area being analyzed (nonbone-containing area or pixels) is comparable with the fat content of the unanalyzed area. This can lead to inaccuracies.
  - Though radiation is used, radiation exposure is very low.
- Dilution techniques:
  - Isotopes like deuterated, tritated, or oxygen-labeled water is used to determine total body water, from which other measures of body composition are derived.
- Air displacement plethysmography:
  - It is similar to the underwater weighing technique but is obviously more comfortable to the participant requiring no sedation, is quick, and requires no radiation exposure.
- MRI:
  - Imaging methods like MRI and CT are the most accurate methods for measurement of body composition.
  - Their primary application has been in quantifying the distribution of adipose tissue into visceral, subcutaneous, and more recently intermuscular depots.
  - Patients with very large BMI cannot fit into MRI or CT scanners. The technique is also relatively costly.
  - MRI has been used to quantify resting energy expenditure of organs in vivo.
  - Proton MRI has been used to quantify intramyocellular lipid.
- Other methods include three-dimensional body scanner, quantitative magnetic resonance, and positron emission tomography (PET).

Questions

29. **DEXA is the most commonly used technique to measure body composition in clinical practice. Identify the <u>TRUE</u> statement about the measurement of body composition by DEXA scan.**
    A. DEXA is an acronym for double-emission X-ray absorbance.
    B. It depends on absorption of photons of different energy levels by different tissues.
    C. Hydrodensitometry is a simpler method than DEXA for the measurement of body composition.
    D. One of the disadvantages of DEXA is the exposure of the patient to a relatively high radiation dose.

30. **BIA devices are in widespread use as they are quick, nonexpensive, and easily performed by the patients themselves. Identify the <u>TRUE</u> statement about bioelectrical impedance for measurement of body fat.**
    A. Bioelectrical impedance is measured by the passage of an electrical current through the body; equations are then used to convert impedance into an estimate of fat.
    B. Single-frequency devices are advantages over multifrequency devices in the presence of electrolyte abnormalities.
    C. Single-frequency devices are advantageous over multifrequency devices in the presence of edema due to cardiac failure.
    D. In general, BIA devices tend to overestimate percent body fat.

31. **MRI though highly accurate for measuring body fat is very expensive. Identify the <u>FALSE</u> statement about the use of MRI as a tool to assess body composition.**
    A. It can measure regional fat distribution.
    B. T1-weighted images are useful for differentiating adipose from nonadipose tissue.
    C. Weight of super-super-obese patients is not an issue unlike the CT scan.
    D. The MRI can quantify the lipid content of muscle.

32. **In 1988, Gerald Reaven proposed that central obesity is associated with insulin resistance and hypertension. This was initially termed syndrome X, and is now known as the metabolic syndrome. Which of the following is <u>NOT</u> considered in the diagnosis of metabolic syndrome.**
    A. Waist circumference
    B. HDL cholesterol
    C. Fasting glucose
    D. Plasma triglyceride levels
    E. LDL cholesterol

33. **Which of the following statements about measurement of body fat is <u>FALSE</u>?**
    A. Hydrodensitometry and DEXA are recognized to be the best methods for body fat measurement.
    B. A single CT slice at L4 level is used to measure abdominal fat.
    C. Dilution techniques use radioactive substances.
    D. Air displacement plethysmography requires radiation exposure.

34. **Waist circumference is a criterion for diagnosis of the metabolic syndrome. Which of the following statements about waist circumference is <u>TRUE</u>?**
    A. BMI > 25 is assumed to correspond to increased waist circumference.
    B. The site for measurement of waist circumference is not standardized.
    C. BMI is a better predictor of diabetes risk than waist circumference.
    D. Waist circumference does not account for subcutaneous abdominal adipose tissue (SAAT).

ANIMAL MODELS OF BARIATRIC SURGERY

Section Summary

- Both small and large animals are used as models for bariatric surgical procedures and a researcher needs to be aware of the anatomy and physiology of these models.
- Pigs are the most commonly used large animals – anatomy of the stomach consists of a diverticulum ventriculi and thick perigastric membranes. Duodenum is intraperitoneal. Colon is of the same caliber as the small bowel. It has a spiral colon and lacks a proper transverse colon. The staple line of the stomach needs to be reinforced due to the thick perigastric membranes. The thin intestinal wall also leads to frequent leakage from the anastomosis.
- Other than in the classic experiment by Dr Scopinaro using BPD, dogs have rarely been used as models of bariatric surgery. The anatomy of their stomach is similar to humans. The duodenum is composed of a cranial and a caudal flexure, which is interposed by the descending duodenum. The caudal flexure continues as the ascending duodenum and then as jejunum. The ileum is very short and does not open into the cecum.
- In rats, the esophagus opens into the lesser curvature. The stomach consists of a forestomach separated from the glandular stomach by the margo plicatus. The jejunum is the longest segment. The ileum is characterized by bumps on the surface due to the presence of lymph nodes.
- The various rat models used are
  - Wistar and Sprague-Dawley – which are nonobese and nondiabetic.
  - Zucker fatty – which are obese and nondiabetic.
  - Zucker diabetic fatty – which are obese and diabetic.
  - Goto-Kakizaki – which are nonobese and diabetic rat models.
- The physiologic changes associated with bariatric surgery including the hormonal, metabolic, and neurobiologic changes are best studied using small animals like rats and mice.

Questions

35. The study of animal models of obesity has given insight to the developments in obesity treatment and is important for future advances in the bariatric field. *ob/ob*, *db/db* mice, and *fa/fa* rats have all served as models of obesity. Identify the <u>TRUE</u> statement about these animals.
    A. *ob/ob* mice have a full length but truncated leptin receptor.
    B. *db/db* mice have an absence of circulating leptin.
    C. *fa/fa* rats have an absence of leptin receptors.
    D. *ob/ob* mice have an absence of circulating leptin.

36. Pigs are one of the most widely used models of bariatric surgery due to their large nature and resemblance to the human anatomy. Knowing the basic anatomy of these animals is crucial for a surgeon engaged in bariatric surgery research. Identify the <u>FALSE</u> statement about the gastrointestinal anatomy of this animal.
    A. Pig intestine has variable length.
    B. Duodenum is intraperitoneal.
    C. Colon is of the same caliber as the small bowel.
    D. Pig stomach has thin perigastric membranes which facilitates transection with staplers.

37. Rats are widely used small animal models for bariatric surgery and are more useful to study the metabolic aspects of bariatric surgery. A surgeon involved in bariatric surgery research needs to know the basic facts about the anatomy of a rat in order

to perform bariatric procedures. Identify the <u>FALSE</u> statement about the anatomy of these animals.
A. Jejunum has the greatest length.
B. Ileum has bumps on its surface.
C. Esophagus opens into the fundus.
D. The forestomach and pylorus are separated by the margo plicatus.

38. Identify the <u>FALSE</u> statement about the technical challenges encountered when using pigs as models of bariatric surgery.
A. It is difficult to identify the ligament of Treitz.
B. A retrocolic gastric bypass is not possible in pigs.
C. Intestinal anastomosis in pigs very rarely produces leakage as a complication.
D. Pigs are not a very good survival model.

39. Various types of diabetic and obese rat models are being used in bariatric surgery research. Identify the <u>TRUE</u> statement about various rat models that have been used in bariatric surgery experiments.
A. Wistar rats do not develop obesity even when fed a high-fat diet.
B. Female Zucker diabetic fatty rats can be used as controls for their male counterparts.
C. Goto-Kakizaki rats have only decreased insulin secretion but no peripheral insulin resistance.
D. F-344 is a nondiabetic and obese rat model.

APPLIED ANATOMY AND PHYSIOLOGY

Chapter Summary
- Physiology of laparoscopic bariatric operations:
  - CO_2 is used for pneumoperitoneum and is absorbed into the blood and finally eliminated by the lungs. To prevent hypercapnia, close monitoring of $PaCO_2$ or end-tidal CO_2 is essential. Amount of CO_2 absorbed from the peritoneum ranges from 19 to 39 mL/min. The respiratory rate needs to be increased by the anesthetist to prevent hypercapnia during a laparoscopic bariatric procedure.
  - Mean arterial pressure is increased during pneumoperitoneum.
  - Obese patients have a greater increase in heart rate during pneumoperitoneum when compared to nonobese.
  - Though the cardiac output is reduced immediately after initiation of the pneumoperitoneum, especially in the obese, it is often transient.
  - Portal venous flow to the liver is reduced, which can lead to transient elevation of liver enzymes. Trauma caused by mechanical retraction of the liver can also have the same effect.
  - Pneumoperitoneum results in decrease in airway compliance and increase in airway pressure. Alveolar arterial gradient of oxygen is not altered.
  - Oliguria occurs during laparoscopy but not during open surgery. Laparoscopic bariatric surgery does not result in changes in blood urea nitrogen (BUN), creatinine, or creatinine clearance.
  - Pneumoperitoneum has been shown to reduce femoral venous flow. The presence of reverse Trendelenberg position has an additive effect on the same. Sequential compression devices are only partly effective in overcoming the reduction in femoral venous flow in morbidly obese patients.

Questions

40. **A surgeon inserting a laparoscopic adjustable gastric band surgery may encounter the aberrant left hepatic artery (LHA). Which of the following statements is <u>TRUE</u> about the aberrant LHA?**
    A. Most commonly arises from the celiac artery and courses through the pars flaccida of lesser omentum.
    B. Division of this artery in the lesser omentum is most often required to place a gastric band.
    C. It arises most commonly from the left gastric artery.
    D. It is highly uncommon with reported rates of <5%.

41. **Arterial supply to the stomach is disrupted when performing a sleeve gastrectomy. It is also important to know their anatomy during other types of bariatric surgery. Identify the <u>TRUE</u> statement about the arterial supply to the stomach.**
    A. Omental necrosis occurs in up to 3% of the cases after sleeve gastrectomy.
    B. The right gastric artery is the second largest artery to the stomach and its division is to be avoided during a sleeve gastrectomy.
    C. The gastroduodenal arises from the right gastroepiploic artery.
    D. The left gastric artery should not be damaged during a sleeve gastrectomy.

42. **A surgeon needs to identify the ligament of Treitz while doing the RYGB. Identify the correct statement about this ligament.**
    A. The only intestinal attachment is the duodenojejunal flexure.
    B. It has no potential hernial spaces related to it.
    C. It is a striated muscle with a tendinous attachment.
    D. It is very closely related to the inferior mesenteric vein.

43. **The stomach mucosa has different distribution of cells that produce different substances. Which of the following statement is <u>FALSE</u> about the same?**
    A. The interstitial cells of Cajal are found in highest number in the fundus.
    B. Ghrelin-producing cells are mainly found in the body of the stomach.
    C. Parietal cells are found in highest concentration in the antrum of stomach.
    D. G cells are most abundant in the antrum of the stomach.

44. **Division of the short gastric vessels during a sleeve gastrectomy can have consequences on the splenic blood supply. Which one of the following statements about such consequences is <u>TRUE</u>?**
    A. Intraoperatively an area of demarcation of the lower splenic pole is seen, which is farthest from the short gastrics.
    B. Progression of the demarcation occurs early, but never occurs postoperatively.
    C. Postoperatively splenic infarction can present with fever and shoulder pain even in the absence of sepsis.
    D. Patient has to be followed up for splenic vein thrombosis for the first 24 hours.

45. **Surgeons have had different opinions on whether the vagus nerve should be preserved during gastric bypass surgery. Identify the <u>TRUE</u> statement about vagal innervation of the stomach.**
    A. The anterior and posterior vagal nerves are formed by the right and left vagal nerves, respectively.
    B. Severing the vagal nerve during LAGB has been shown to cause failure of weight loss.
    C. Severing of the anterior vagus leads to an increased incidence of gallstones.
    D. The vagal nerves are chiefly motor and not sensory.

46. **The blood supply to the distal stomach and duodenum is critical for a successful ileoduodenal anastomosis during BPD. Identify the TRUE statement about vascular supply of the duodenum.**
    A. The supraduodenal artery that supplies the first part of duodenum is frequently absent.
    B. The anemic spot of Mayo corresponds to distribution of superior pancreatico-duodenal artery.
    C. The prepyloric vein of Mayo constantly indicates position of the pylorus.
    D. Right gastroepiploic artery is important for duodeno-ileal anastomosis in BPD and should be preserved to avoid blowout of anastomosis.
    E. The anterior aspect of the duodenal bulb is more vascularized when compared to the posterior aspect.

47. **Vitamin D supplementation and monitoring for its deficiency is essential for post–bariatric surgery patients. Identify the FALSE statement about occurrence of vitamin D and calcium deficiency in a post-bariatric patient.**
    A. Decreased serum phosphorous is found in vitamin D deficiency.
    B. Secondary hyperparathyroidism is easily corrected by vitamin D supplementation.
    C. Looser's zones are areas of lucency seen on radiographs at places where arteries cross over bones.
    D. Osteocalcin as a marker of bone formation is increased in vitamin D deficiency–associated bone disease.

48. **Obesity has an influence on the effect of general anesthesia on the respiratory function, and it is therefore necessary to identify effects of obesity on pulmonary function. Which of the following is TRUE regarding pulmonary function of morbidly obese patients?**
    A. At rest, obese patients have twice the atelectasis of normal patients.
    B. They have a normal residual volume.
    C. They have a normal diffusing capacity of lung for carbon monoxide (DLCO).
    D. Obese patients have increased chest wall compliance.

49. **Vitamin D deficiency is a common problem before and after bariatric surgery. Identify the TRUE statement about vitamin D deficiency and osteoporosis in bariatric surgery patients.**
    A. The primary site of calcium absorption is the duodenum and proximal jejunum.
    B. C-telopeptide is a specific marker for bone formation.
    C. The primary site of absorption of vitamin D is the duodenum and it is not absorbed in the jejunum.
    D. Monitoring 1,25-dihydroxycholecalciferol is recommended for monitoring of vitamin D deficiency.

50. **Bariatric surgery produces altered pulmonary function after establishment of the pneumoperitoneum. Identify the TRUE statement about alteration of pulmonary function during a laparoscopic procedure.**
    A. The alveolar arterial oxygen gradient is decreased.
    B. Pulmonary compliance is decreased.
    C. Airway pressure is decreased due to bronchodilation caused by hypercarbia.
    D. Physiologic dead space is increased relative to tidal volume.

51. **It is important to monitor the urinary output and renal parameters in a bariatric surgery patient. Identify the TRUE statement about changes in renal function seen during a laparoscopic procedure in a patient with baseline normal renal function.**
    A. There is a decrease in urine output.
    B. Creatinine clearance is reduced.
    C. There is an increase in serum creatinine.

D. Serum aldosterone is increased more during laparoscopic gastric bypass when compared to the open technique.

52. **Increased abdominal pressures during a laparoscopic procedure can affect the hemodynamic status of a patient undergoing bariatric surgery. Identify the <u>TRUE</u> statement about the hemodynamic and respiratory status of a patient undergoing laparoscopic bariatric surgery.**
    A. Obese patients have a more pronounced increase in heart rate level when compared to nonobese patients.
    B. Increase in $PaCO_2$ does not occur during laparoscopy in morbidly obese patients.
    C. Both preload and afterload decrease during laparoscopy.
    D. Morbidly obese patients absorb significantly greater CO_2 when compared to nonobese patients.

53. **GERD is an important comorbidity of obese patients. Identify the <u>FALSE</u> statement about pathogenesis of GERD in obesity.**
    A. There is increased incidence of transient lower esophageal sphincter relaxation (TLESR) in obese patients.
    B. Obese patients do not have an increased incidence of hiatal hernia.
    C. Any meal that distends the gastric fundus promotes LES relaxation.
    D. Increased BMI is correlated with increased gastroesophageal pressure gradient.

54. **It is important to understand the various weight definitions used for obese patients. Identify the <u>FALSE</u> statement about various definitions used in obesity.**
    A. Metropolitan life tables are used to calculate ideal body weight based on height and body build.
    B. In nonobese patients, lean body weight = ideal body weight – fat mass.
    C. Percentage of lean body weight is lower in females when compared to males.
    D. A sedentary Caucasian male whose weight is in the normal range has 4% to 6% of his body weight as fat mass.

55. **Implantable gastric pacing devices alter the normal electrical activity of the stomach. Identify the <u>FALSE</u> statement about electrical activity of the stomach.**
    A. Gastric myoelectrical activity consists of two phases – slow waves and spike potentials.
    B. The gastric slow waves are present only after intake of food.
    C. The gastric slow waves do not cause stomach contraction.
    D. The stomach has a pacemaker located on the greater curvature.
    E. The spike potentials are responsible for strong lumen-occluding gastric contractions.

56. **A 35-year-old diabetic woman, with a BMI of 50, underwent laparoscopic gastric bypass surgery and complains of sudden shortness of breath and chest pain. A diagnosis of pulmonary embolism has been confirmed. Which of the following is <u>NOT</u> part of the patient's obesity-related prothrombotic state?**
    A. Platelet dysfunction
    B. Decreased plasminogen activator inhibitor levels
    C. Increased factor VII
    D. Increased tissue factor
    E. Increased fibrinogen

57. **A married couple comes to the clinic for advice regarding their obesity. The husband has a BMI of 32 kg/m^2 with a waist-hip ratio of 1.5. The wife has a BMI of 34 kg/m^2 with a waist-hip ratio of 0.8. Both are concerned regarding the adverse effects of their obesity on their health. The husband is told that he has a greater amount of visceral obesity that leads to a greater risk of diabetes, insulin**

resistance, and hypertension as compared with his wife. Which of the following statements is <u>FALSE</u>?

A. The intra-abdominal adipocytes are more metabolically active than those from other sites.
B. Release of FFAs into the portal circulation has adverse metabolic actions on the liver.
C. Omentectomy is an established treatment for abdominal obesity.
D. Omental fat shows increased inflammation in obesity.

58. **Insulin levels have been found to decrease after bariatric surgery. Identify the <u>FALSE</u> statement about the role of insulin in energy homeostasis and its change after bariatric surgery.**
A. Insulin is a long-term indicator of energy stores.
B. Insulin inhibits feeding at the level of CNS.
C. Gastric banding has not been shown to produce any change in fasting insulin levels.
D. Sleeve gastrectomy increases first phase of meal-induced insulin secretion.

59. **Obese patients have a resistance to the action of insulin due to which hyperinsulinemia is present in the early stages of type 2 diabetes. Identify the <u>FALSE</u> statement of mechanism of insulin resistance in T2DM.**
A. Accumulation of metabolites involved in fatty acid esterification causing an inhibition of insulin signaling.
B. Increased TNF-α levels.
C. Downregulation of glucose transporter (GLUT)-1 receptors.
D. Production of reactive oxygen species (ROS) contributes to insulin resistance.

60. **A volunteer is enrolled in a study to measure the effect of RYGB on insulin sensitivity and secretion. A euglycemic hyperinsulinemic test is performed both before and 1 month after the procedure. Which is a <u>FALSE</u> statement about this test?**
A. It is the gold standard for measurement of insulin resistance.
B. If the patient requires higher rate of glucose infusion to maintain euglycemia during the test, then the patient has a higher insulin resistance.
C. Modification of the technique can be used to measure regional insulin-mediated glucose uptake.
D. It is assumed that the endogenous glucose production is completely inhibited during the technique.

61. **Hypertension is one of the components of the metabolic syndrome. Identify which of the following mechanisms is <u>NOT</u> one of those proposed by which insulin resistance causes hypertension.**
A. Insulin is antinatriuretic.
B. Insulin stimulates production of nitric oxide while it inhibits synthesis of endothelin.
C. Sympathetic overactivity accompanying insulin resistance increases blood pressure.
D. Increased production of ROS due to increased FFAs seen in insulin-resistant states.

62. **Several clinical studies in bariatric surgery have measured insulin resistance change after bariatric surgery. Which one of the following is not a method of assessing insulin resistance?**
A. HOMA-IR
B. Insulin tolerance test (ITT)
C. Euglycemic clamp
D. Intravenous arginine stimulation test (IVAST)

63. The physiologic actions of insulin are essential in the control of the many aspects of glucose and lipid metabolism. Which of the following statements about the action of insulin is <u>FALSE</u>?
   A. Insulin increases the transcription of the GLUT-4 gene.
   B. Insulin inhibits hormone-sensitive lipase.
   C. Insulin stimulates lipoprotein lipase.
   D. High CSF insulin levels have been correlated with insulin resistance in obese patients.

64. Increased triglycerides and decreased HDL cholesterol are seen in obesity and insulin resistance resulting in deleterious effects like atherosclerosis. Identify which of the following is <u>NOT</u> involved in the pathogenesis of the above process.
   A. Increased activity of cholesterol ester transfer protein (CETP)
   B. Decreased activity of lipoprotein lipase
   C. Increase activity of hormone-sensitive lipase
   D. Increased splanchnic lipolysis

65. Peroxisome proliferator–activated receptor gamma (PPARγ) has been implicated in the causation of insulin resistance. Identify the <u>FALSE</u> statement about PPARγ.
   A. PPARγ is a cell membrane receptor.
   B. Fatty acids serve as ligands for PPARγ.
   C. Thiazolidinediones are PPARγ agonists.
   D. PPARγ affects transcriptional activity.

66. Insulin secretion in response to a meal was tested in two individuals; Subjects A and B. The results are plotted in the graph shown below. Which of the following statements regarding the results is <u>FALSE</u>?

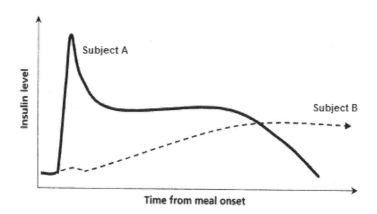

Insulin-secretion profiles at meal time

A. Subject A: First phase peaks at about 10 minutes after a meal.
B. Subject A: Second phase peaks about 20 to 40 minutes after a meal.
C. Subject B: Lacks the first phase.
D. Subject B: Insulin secretion involves only preformed insulin.

ANSWER KEYS

1. A	18. A	35. D	52. A
2. D	19. C	36. D	53. B
3. D	20. C	37. C	54. D
4. A	21. C	38. C	55. B
5. B	22. D	39. B	56. B
6. A	23. C	40. C	57. C
7. C	24. C	41. D	58. C
8. B	25. C	42. D	59. C
9. D	26. C	43. C	60. B
10. A	27. A	44. C	61. B
11. C	28. A	45. C	62. D
12. B	29. B	46. A	63. D
13. B	30. A	47. B	64. D
14. C	31. C	48. A	65. A
15. C	32. E	49. A	66. D
16. C	33. D	50. B	
17. D	34. B	51. A	

ANSWER KEY WITH EXPLANATION
Gastrointestinal Hormones and Adipokines

1. **Answer: A.**

   Melanocortin receptor (MC4R) stimulation causes decreased feeding. α-MSH causes stimulation, and AgRP and NPY cause inhibition of MC4R. Melanocortin receptor mutations are relatively common in obese patients (3–4% of patients) and is the most common cause of genetic obesity.

   References:
   - Farooqi S, O'Rahilly S. Genetics of obesity in humans. Endocrine Rev 2006; 27 (7):710–718.
   - Wardlaw SL. Clinical review 127: Obesity as a neuroendocrine disease: lessons to be learned from proopiomelanocortin and melanocortin receptor mutations in mice and men. J Clin Endocrinol Metab 2001; 86:1442–1446.

2. **Answer: D.**

   D correctly indicates the position of the arcuate nucleus of the hypothalamus. A, B, and C indicate lateral nucleus, paraventricular nucleus, and ventromedial nucleus, respectively, of the hypothalamus.

3. **Answer: D.**

   LEPR (leptin receptors) are present on POMC-, AgRP-, and NPY-producing neurons.

   POMC is proteolytically cleaved to give α-MSH, which is an agonist of melanocortin receptors (M3R and M4R). Ligand interaction results in decreased feeding (anorexigenic).

   AgRP is a potent antagonist of the melanocortin receptors, resulting in increased feeding (orexigenic). NPY, another orexigenic neurotransmitter, is coexpressed with AgRP in the arcuate nucleus.

   AgRP also inhibits the POMC neurons through the neurotransmitter gamma–aminobutyric acid (GABA).

   References:
   - Jobst EE, Enriori PJ, Sinnayah P, et al. Hypothalamic regulatory pathways and potential obesity treatment targets. Endocrine 2006; 29(1):33–48.
   - Beckers S, Zegers D, Van Gaal LF, et al. The role of the leptin-melanocortin signalling pathway in the control of food intake. Crit Rev Eukaryot Gene Expr 2009; 19(4):267–87.

- Fisher SL, Yagaloff KA, Burn P. Melanocortin-4 receptor: a novel signalling pathway involved in body weight regulation. Int J Obes Relat Metab Disord 1999; 23(suppl 1):54–58.

4. **Answer: A.**

Patients with null mutations of POMC have obesity (due to increased appetite). It is well known that activation of POMC neurons causes decreased food intake and negative energy balance. In the same disease there is decreased ACTH secretion causing hypotension and electrolyte abnormalities and decreased α-MSH production resulting in red hair.

Reference:
- Ranadive SA, Vaisse C. Lessons from extreme human obesity: monogenic disorders. Endocrinol Metab Clin North Am 2008; 37(3):733–751.

5. **Answer: B.**

Functional MRI images have revealed increased activity in the nucleus accumbens in leptin-deficient patients even after feeding. Leptin is known to influence dopaminergic pathways that are a part of the reward system providing input to the nucleus accumbens.

References:
- Friedman JM. Leptin at 14 y of age: an ongoing story. Am J Clin Nutr 2009; 89 (3):973S–979S [Epub February 3, 2009].
- Farooqi IS, Bullmore E, Keogh J, et al. Leptin regulates striatal regions and human eating behavior. Science 2007; 317:1355.

6. **Answer: A.**

Ghrelin is transported into the brain by a saturable mechanism by endocytosis in microvessel endothelial cells of the brain. It acts in the CNS by activating the NPY pathway. Ghrelin acts on GRH1a.

It increases gastric emptying and has been found to be promising in clinical trials utilizing ghrelin infusion for gastroparesis.

References:
- Pan W, Tu H, Kastin AJ. Differential BBB interactions of three ingestive peptides: obestatin, ghrelin, and adiponectin. Peptides 2006; 27:911–916.
- Neary MT, Batterham RL. Gut hormones: implications for the treatment of obesity. Pharmacol Ther 2009; 124:44–56.
- Murray CD, Martin NM, Patterson M, et al. Ghrelin enhances gastric emptying in diabetic gastroparesis: a double blind, placebo controlled, crossover study. Gut 2005; 54(12):1693–1698.

7. **Answer: C.**

There is no consensus on the change of ghrelin levels (both in the short as well as the long term) in all types of currently performed bariatric surgeries except sleeve gastrectomy where ghrelin levels have been consistently shown to have decreased after surgery.

Reference:
- Harvey EJ, Arroyo K, Korner J, et al. Hormone changes affecting energy homeostasis after metabolic surgery. Mt Sinai J Med 2010; 77(5):446–465.

8. **Answer: B.**

Both acyl and desacyl ghrelin increase survival and proliferation of the β cells. They also inhibit apoptosis of the same cells. Desacylated ghrelin, the predominant form of circulating ghrelin does not bind to GHr1a unlike the acylated form, thus accounting for the vast majority of differences in the actions of the acylated and the desacylated hormones. The most commonly used assays of ghrelin measure both acylated and unacylated forms of ghrelin. The influence of ghrelin on glucose and insulin levels is controversial.

Reference:

- Granata R, Baragli A, Settanni F, et al. Unraveling the role of the ghrelin gene peptides in the endocrine pancreas. J Mol Endocrinol 2010; 45(3):107–118.

9. **Answer: D.**

The levels of ghrelin are elevated immediately before meals then fall afterward and return to baseline after 2 hours. This is consistent with the role of ghrelin in meal initiation, feeling of hunger/satiety associated with the meals. The levels of ghrelin are decreased in obese patients.

The other choices do not accurately reflect changes in ghrelin levels in the various circumstances mentioned.

Both oral and intravenous glucose can cause release of ghrelin. The suppression of ghrelin by food is partly mediated by the vagus nerve. Gastric distension alone in the absence of nutrients cannot cause release of ghrelin.

References:

- Schmidt PT, Degerblad M, Lindström E, et al. Circulating ghrelin levels after food intake during different phases of the migrating motor complex in man. Eur J Clin Invest 2006; 36(7):503–508.
- Cummings DE, Purnell JQ, Frayo RS, et al. A preprandial rise in plasma ghrelin levels suggests a role in meal initiation in humans. Diabetes 2001; 50(8):1714–1719.

10. **Answer: A.**

GLP-1 is inactivated by DPP-4. This is in contrast to PYY that requires DPP-4 for its activation. GLP-1 is secreted by the ileal L cells in two forms: GLP-1(7-37) and GLP-1 (7-36)amide, the latter being the predominant circulating form. PYY is also secreted by the L cells. GLP-1 has a short half-life of about a few minutes. The insulinotropic activity of GLP-1 is preserved to a large extent in diabetes, that is why GLP-1 analogues are already in clinical use.

References:

- Neary MT, Batterham RL. Gut hormones: implications for the treatment of obesity. Pharmacol Ther 2009; 124(1):44–56 [Epub June 26, 2009].
- Rao RS, Kini S. GIP and bariatric surgery. Obes Surg 2011; 21(2):244–252.
- Salehi M, Aulinger B, Prigeon RL, et al. Effect of endogenous GLP-1 on insulin secretion in type 2 diabetes. Diabetes 2010; 59(6):1330–1337.

11. **Answer: C.**

Incretin effect is defined as the increase in insulin secretion that occurs when the substance is given orally when compared to when it is given intravenously. The calculation of incretin effects from estimates of β-cell secretory responses is based on the assumption that, after glucose ingestion, the endocrine pancreas is stimulated by both the resulting elevation in plasma glucose and the additional stimulation by gastrointestinal (incretin) factors. Isoglycemic intravenous glucose infusions provide a measure of the β-cell secretory responses to the glycemic stimulus without superimposed incretin effects. The difference in β-cell secretory responses ($\int$SR) to both of these stimuli represents the action of incretin factors and is expressed as the percentage of the physiological response to oral glucose, which is taken as the denominator (100%). The formula thus is:

$$\text{Incretin effect} = \frac{\int SR_{\text{oral}} - \int SR_{\text{IV}}}{\int SR_{\text{oral}} \times 100}$$

Reference:

- Nauck MA, Homberger E, Siegel EG, et al. Incretin effects of increasing glucose loads in man calculated from venous insulin and C-peptide responses. J Clin Endocrinol Metab 1986; 63:492–498.

12. **Answer: B.**

GIP and GLP-1 both contribute equally to incretin effect after a meal in healthy subjects.

There is downregulation of GIP receptors in type 2 diabetes and hence presence of "GIP resistance."

GIP increases glucagon secretion, while GLP-1 inhibits the same. This is in contrast to the insulinotropic action of both.

GLP-1 causes delayed gastric emptying, whereas GIP does not affect gastric emptying.

References:

- Nauck MA, Heimesaat MM, Behle K, et al. Effects of glucagon-like peptide 1 on counterregulatory hormone responses, cognitive functions, and insulin secretion during hyperinsulinemic, stepped hypoglycemic clamp experiments in healthy volunteers. J Clin Endocrinol Metab 2002; 87:1239–1246.
- Vilsbøll T, Krarup T, Madsbad S, et al. Both GLP-1 and GIP are insulinotropic at basal and postprandial glucose levels and contribute nearly equally to the incretin effect of a meal in healthy subjects. Regul Pept 2003; 114(2–3):115–121.
- Sancho V, Trigo MV, Martin-Duce A, et al. Effect of GLP-1 on D-glucose transport, lipolysis and lipogenesis in adipocytes of obese subjects. Int J Mol Med 2006; 17:1133–1137.
- Rao RS, Kini S. GIP and bariatric surgery. Obes Surg 2011; 21(2):244–252.
- Meier JJ, Goetze O, Anstipp J, et al. Gastric inhibitory polypeptide does not inhibit gastric emptying in humans. Am J Physiol Endocrinol Metab 2004; 286(4):E621–E625.

13. **Answer: B.**

There is no consensus on the fasting levels of GLP-1 in obesity or in patients who have undergone gastric bypass. Obese patients usually have a decreased post-prandial GLP-1 response when compared with lean subjects. Gastric bypass has been shown to increase postprandial GLP-1 (up to 30-fold increase in incremental AUC).

References:

- Morínigo R, Moizé V, Musri M, et al. Glucagon-like peptide-1, peptide YY, hunger, and satiety after gastric bypass surgery in morbidly obese subjects. J Clin Endocrinol Metab 2006; 91(5):1735–1740.
- Neary MT, Batterham RL. Gut hormones: implications for the treatment of obesity. Pharmacol Ther 2009; 124(1):44–56.
- Korner J, Bessler M, Inabnet W, et al. Exaggerated glucagon-like peptide-1 and blunted glucose-dependent insulinotropic peptide secretion are associated with Roux-en-Y gastric bypass but not adjustable gastric banding. Surg Obes Relat Dis 2007; 3(6):597–601.

14. **Answer: C.**

DePaula et al. have shown an increase in postprandial PYY after ileal transposition associated with a sleeve gastrectomy in humans. PYY increase after BPD has been shown to be greater when compared to RYGB.

The postprandial PYY response after RYGB and sleeve gastrectomy is the same. Sleeve gastrectomy has the additional advantage of decreasing ghrelin levels.

Postprandial PYY response is decreased in obesity. This decreases the satiety effect of the hormone in obese individuals.

References:

- Garcia-Fuentes E, Garrido-Sanchez L, Garcia-Almeida JM, et al. Different effect of laparoscopic Roux-en-Y gastric bypass and open biliopancreatic diversion of Scopinaro on serum PYY and ghrelin levels. Obes Surg 2008; 18(11):1424–1429 [Epub June 10, 2008].
- Peterli R, Wölnerhanssen B, Peters T, et al. Improvement in glucose metabolism after bariatric surgery: comparison of laparoscopic Roux-en-Y gastric bypass and laparoscopic sleeve gastrectomy: a prospective randomized trial. Ann Surg 2009; 250(2):234–241.

- Morínigo R, Vidal J, Lacy AM, et al. Circulating peptide YY, weight loss, and glucose homeostasis after gastric bypass surgery in morbidly obese subjects. Ann Surg 2008; 247(2):270–275.
- DePaula AL, Macedo AL, Schraibman V, et al. Hormonal evaluation following laparoscopic treatment of type 2 diabetes mellitus patients with BMI 20–34. Surg Endosc 2009; 23:1724–1732.

15. **Answer: C.**

PYY is anorexigenic. Hence, it increases levels of POMC and decreases levels of NPY in the brain. The physiological actions of PYY are mediated through the Y2 receptors, a member of NPY family of receptors present in the arcuate nucleus neurons. The Y in PYY stands for tyrosine residue. PYY (1-36) is cleaved by DPP-4 to yield PYY (3-36), which is the biologically active and the predominant form found in the plasma. Fat and protein are the most potent signals for release of PYY. PYY in the circulation can act on the arcuate nucleus, which has a deficient blood–brain barrier, in order to cause satiety effects. PYY also affects other areas in the brain. Though PYY nasal spray showed some initial promise, it has NOT been found to be a promising therapy for obesity.

References:
- Gantz I, Erondu N, Mallick M, et al. Efficacy and safety of intranasal peptide YY3-36 for weight reduction in obese adults. J Clin Endocrinol Metab 2007; 92 (5):1754–1757.
- le Roux CW, Bloom SR. Peptide YY appetite and food intake. Proc Nutr Soc 2005; 64:213–216.

16. **Answer: C.**

Ileal brake is the mechanism by which presence of food in the ileum decreases gastric emptying, increases small intestinal transit time, and reduces food intake. PYY, GLP-1, neurotensin, and oxyntomodulin are the humoral substances involved.

Extrinsic denervation of the jejunoileum abolishes the inhibitory effects of ileal fat on gastric emptying. This demonstrates that neural pathways are involved in the inhibition of small bowel transit and gastric emptying after activation of the ileal brake. Similarly, vagotomy reduced or abolished the inhibitory effects of PYY on pancreatic secretion and food intake and of GLP-1 on gastric acid secretion and food intake.

Reference:
- Maljaars PW, Peters HP, Mela DJ, et al. Ileal brake: a sensible food target for appetite control. A review. Physiol Behav 2008; 95(3):271–281.

17. **Answer: D.**

Low amylin levels are found in both obesity (with impaired glucose tolerance) and diabetes. Meal-stimulated amylin release is more in obesity (with or without impaired glucose tolerance). Though leptin analogues by themselves are not useful in treatment of obesity, the combination of metreleptin and amylin has been found to be more effective in causing weight loss than amylin alone. Amylin decreases glucagon and increases insulin secretion, which is potentially useful in the pharmacotherapy of diabetes.

References:
- Lutz TA.The role of amylin in the control of energy homeostasis. Am J Physiol Regul Integr Comp Physiol 2010; 298(6):R1475–R1484 [Epub March 31, 2010].
- Trevaskis JL, Parkes DG, Roth JD. Insights into amylin-leptin synergy. Trends Endocrinol Metab 2010; 21(8):473–479 [Epub April 21, 2010] (review).
- Reda TK, Geliebter A, Pi-Sunyer FX. Amylin, food intake, and obesity. Obes Res 2002; 10(10):1087–1091.

18. **Answer: A.**

Subcutaneous fat secretes more leptin when compared to visceral fat. Visceral fat also forms 5% to 10% of the total body fat stores. Hence, the chief source of leptin secretion is the subcutaneous fatty tissue. Leptin has been shown to be lower in obese type 2 diabetic patients when compared to obese patients without diabetes. Hyperleptinemia has been correlated with hyperinsulinemia in obese insulin-resistant type 2 diabetic patients. Low leptin levels normally induce positive energy balance. The coexistence of obesity and high leptin levels is due to resistance to action of leptin.

References:

- Fischer S, Hanefeld M, Haffner SM, et al. Insulin-resistant patients with type 2 diabetes mellitus have higher serum leptin levels independently of body fat mass. Acta Diabetol 2002; 39(3):105–110.
- Abdelgadir M, Elbagir M, Eltom M, et al. Reduced leptin concentrations in subjects with type 2 diabetes mellitus in Sudan. Metabolism 2002; 51(3): 304–306.
- Friedman JM. Leptin at 14 y of age: an ongoing story. Am J Clin Nutr 2009; 89 (3):973S–979S.
- Buyukbese MA, Cetinkaya A, Kocabas R, et al. Leptin levels in obese women with and without type 2 diabetes mellitus. Mediators Inflamm 2004; 13(5, 6):321–325.
- Chin-Chance C, Polonsky KS, Schoeller DA. Twenty-four-hour leptin levels respond to cumulative short-term energy imbalance and predict subsequent intake. J Clin Endocrinol Metab 2000; 85:2685–2691.
- Fried SK, Ricci MR, Russell CD, et al. Regulation of leptin production in humans. J Nutr 2000; 130(12):3127S–3131S.

19. **Answer: C.**

Though decreased leptin receptor expression and impaired leptin receptor trafficking can contribute to leptin resistance, their role in actually causing leptin resistance in humans is not well understood. There is evidence that subnormal leptin transport across the blood–brain barrier also contributes to leptin resistance. Adiponectin has not been related.

Reference:

- Morris DL, Rui L. Recent advances in understanding leptin signaling and leptin resistance. Am J Physiol Endocrinol Metab 2009; 297(6):E1247–E1259 [Epub September 1, 2009].

20. **Answer: C.**

Adiponectin has anti-inflammatory, antidiabetic, antihypertensive, and anticancer effects. Low adiponectin levels have been implicated in NASH independent of insulin resistance. Subcutaneous fat produces more adiponectin compared to visceral fat. Obese people have a resistance to actions of adiponectin-like lipolysis.

Adiponectin causes effects like increased glucose uptake, decreased gluconeogenesis (through AMP-activated protein kinase, AMPK), increased fat oxidation (through both AMPK and PPARα), and decreased insulin resistance.

References:

- Ziemke F, Mantzoros CS. Adiponectin in insulin resistance: lessons from translational research. Am J Clin Nutr 2010; 91:258S–261S.
- Dyck DJ. Adipokines as regulators of muscle metabolism and insulin sensitivity. Appl Physiol Nutr Metab 2009; 34(3):396–402.
- Kadowaki T, Yamauchi T, Kubota N, et al. Adiponectin and adiponectin receptors in insulin resistance, diabetes, and the metabolic syndrome. J Clin Invest 2006; 116 (7):1784–1792.
- Lihn AS, Bruun JM, He G, et al. Lower expression of adiponectin mRNA in visceral adipose tissue in lean and obese subjects. Mol Cell Endocrinol 2004; 219 (1–2):9–15.
- Hui JM, Hodge A, Farrell GC, et al. Beyond insulin resistance in NASH: TNF-alpha or adiponectin? Hepatology 2004; 40:46–54.

21. **Answer: C.**

Adiponectin is correlated with insulin, BMI, fat mass, waist-hip ratio, and glucose levels. It is negatively correlated with insulin resistance even after adjustment for BMI, age, and sex. Meal-stimulated adiponectin has been found to be increased in obese patients though basal levels in obese are less than in lean patients. Adiponectin has been found to be increased after all currently performed bariatric procedures including gastric banding.

References:

- Harvey EJ, Arroyo K, Korner J, et al. Hormone changes affecting energy homeostasis after metabolic surgery. Mt Sinai J Med 2010; 77(5):446–465.
- Tschritter O, Fritsche A, Thamer C, et al. Plasma adiponectin concentrations predict insulin sensitivity of both glucose and lipid metabolism. Diabetes 2003; 52 (2):239–243.
- English PJ, Coughlin SR, Hayden K, et al. Plasma adiponectin increases postprandially in obese, but not in lean, subjects. Obes Res 2003; 11(7):839–844.

22. **Answer: D.**

Visceral adipose tissue contributes to hepatic insulin resistance by releasing FFA into the portal circulation. This, in turn, causes an increased production of FFA from the liver, which contributes to peripheral insulin resistance, directly and by increasing myocellular triglyceride.

The conversion of a "lean healthy adipocyte to fat toxic adipocyte" has been implicated in the causation of the metabolic syndrome. Such an adipocyte produces decreased amount of adiponectin and increased amounts of TNF-α, IL-6, and plasminogen activator inhibitor (PAI).

References:

- Brietzke SA. A personalized approach to metabolic aspects of obesity. Mt Sinai J Med 2010; 77(5):499–510.
- Gregor MF, Hotamisligil GS. Thematic review series: Adipocyte Biology. Adipocyte stress: the endoplasmic reticulum and metabolic disease. J Lipid Res 2007; 48:1905–1914.

23. **Answer: C.**

Fats and proteins are potent stimulators for CCK release. Bile acids in the duodenum suppress CCK secretion.

CCK and leptin have a synergistic action. CCK acts on the brain to cause satiety. CCK though reduces the meal size, the meal frequency is increased and no appreciable weight loss is seen in the clinical setting when a long-acting CCK agonist is used.

References:

- Heldsinger A, Grabauskas G, Song I, et al. Synergistic interaction between leptin and cholecystokinin in the rat nodose ganglia is mediated by PI3K and STAT3 signaling pathways: implications for leptin as a regulator of short term satiety. J Biol Chem 2011; 286(13):11707–11715.
- Neary MT, Batterham RL. Gut hormones: implications for the treatment of obesity. Pharmacol Ther 2009; 124(1):44–56.
- Chandra R, Liddle RA. Cholecystokinin. Curr Opin Endocrinol Diabetes Obes 2007; 14(1):63–67.

24. **Answer: C.**

Though an adipokine, resistin is mainly produced in humans by macrophages, monocytes, and bone marrow cells, and thus its main role in humans may be in inflammation rather than in the pathogenesis of obesity and insulin resistance. There is no consensus on the level of visfatin or resistin levels in obese patients or their change after bariatric surgery.

References:

- Ballantyne GH, Gumbs A, Modlin IM. Changes in insulin resistance following bariatric surgery and the adipoinsular axis: role of the adipocytokines, leptin, adiponectin and resistin. Obes Surg 2005; 15(5):692–699.
- Stofkova A. Resistin and visfatin: regulators of insulin sensitivity, inflammation and immunity. Endocr Regul 2010; 44(1):25–36.
- Swarbrick MM, Stanhope KL, Austrheim-Smith IT, et al. Longitudinal changes in pancreatic and adipocyte hormones following Roux-en-Y gastric bypass surgery. Diabetologia 2008; 51(10):1901–1911 [Epub August 15, 2008].
- Botella-Carretero JI, Luque-Ramírez M, Alvarez-Blasco F, et al. The increase in serum visfatin after bariatric surgery in morbidly obese women is modulated by weight loss, waist circumference, and presence or absence of diabetes before surgery. Obes Surg 2008; 18(8):1000–1006 [Epub March 19, 2008].
- Ballantyne GH, Gumbs A, Modlin IM. Changes in insulin resistance following bariatric surgery and the adipoinsular axis: role of the adipocytokines, leptin, adiponectin and resistin. Obes Surg 2005; 15(5):692–699.

Genetics

25. **Answer: C.**

PWS is characterized by short stature, obesity, hyperphagia, hypogonadism, and certain characteristic physical appearances. Obesity starts at 1 to 4 years of age. The Holm's criteria that consist of 8 major, 11 minor, and 8 supportive criteria can be used for the diagnosis of PWS. Clinical criteria may be too stringent and genetic testing is required in most cases when PWS is suspected. This syndrome is due to deletion of paternally derived chromosome 15q (70%), maternal uniparental disomy (25%), and imprinting defect (5%). PWS was the first genetic disorder attributed to genomic imprinting along with Angelman syndrome. DNA methylation test can identify all three defects associated with PWS and hence is 99% sensitive.

References:

- Holm VA, Cassidy SB, Butler MG, et al. Prader–Willi syndrome: consensus diagnostic criteria. Pediatrics. 1993; 91(2):398–402.
- Jin DK. Systematic review of the clinical and genetic aspects of Prader–Willi syndrome. Korean J Pediatr 2011; 54(2):55–63 [Epub February 28, 2011].

26. **Answer: C.**

The cause of the lack of satiety and hyperphagia in PWS is unknown but is likely multifactorial. PWS patients with hyperphagia and excessive obesity have been found to have increased levels of ghrelin, an orexigenic gut hormone, as well as low levels of pancreatic polypeptide, an anorexigenic hormone. Numerous beneficial effects of GH therapy have been documented, including improvement in linear growth, physical appearance, functional muscle mass, and infant neurodevelopment.

Weight control is particularly difficult because of aggressive food-seeking behaviors, lack of satiety, cognitive impairment, and behavioral problems. Although various medications have been tried, and a number of bariatric operations have been performed, the weight loss is limited and does not seem to be long lasting. Calorie restriction remains the cornerstone of weight management in PWS.

References:

- Erdie-Lalena CR, Holm VA, Kelly PC, et al. Ghrelin levels in young children with Prader–Willi syndrome. J Pediatr 2006; 149:199–204.
- Cummings DE, Clement K, Purnell JQ, et al. Elevated plasma ghrelin levels in Prader–Willi syndrome. Nat Med 2002; 8:643–644.
- Zipf WB, O'Dorisio TM, Cataland S, et al. Blunted pancreatic polypeptide responses in children with obesity of Prader–Willi syndrome. J Clin Endocrinol Metab 1981; 52:1264–1266.

- Scheimann AO, Butler MG, Gourash L, et al. Critical analysis of bariatric procedures in Prader–Willi syndrome. J Pediatr Gastroenterol Nutr 2008; 46:80–83.
- Brambilla P, Bosio L, Manzoni P, et al. Peculiar body composition in patients with Prader–Labhart–Willi syndrome. Am J Clin Nutr 1997; 65(5):1369–1374.

27. **Answer: A.**

Geneticist James V. Neel initially proposed the "thrifty gene" hypothesis for diabetes in 1962, and it was later extended to obesity. He reasoned that there must have been selective pressure favoring genes that predispose some individuals to diabetes, and he proposed the existence of thrifty genes. These thrifty genes would promote the efficient utilization of food in times of abundance in order to help hunter-gatherers better survive periods of famine. In the modern Western world of easy access to food (especially high in fat and sugar) and decreased energy output, these genes would then have become detrimental: people with the thrifty gene become obese and develop diabetes because they accumulate energy for a famine that never comes. Although no "thrifty genes" have been identified, leptin has been considered a candidate.

Reference:

- Speakman JR. Thrifty genes for obesity and the metabolic syndrome—time to call off the search? Diab Vasc Dis Res 2006; 3(1):7–11.

28. **Answer: A.**

The pattern of mortality during a famine has been shown to involve the very young and the very old. Obesity rates in these two groups have been historically low. Other arguments against the thrifty gene hypothesis include the following:

The prevalence of obesity in hunter-gatherer populations between famines is low and does not support the hypothesis.

Famines are relatively rare events, occurring about once every century.

Many populations that later developed obesity and diabetes have had no history of famine or starvation.

Reference:

- Speakman JR. Thrifty genes for obesity and the metabolic syndrome—time to call off the search? Diab Vasc Dis Res 2006; 3(1):7–11.

Body Composition

29. **Answer: B.**

DEXA is an acronym for dual-energy X-ray absorptiometry. Photon beams of low and high energy levels are generated by an X-ray tube and measured by a detector. Differential attenuation of the photon beams based on tissue density allows one to quantify body composition in terms of bone, lean tissue, and fat. DEXA is considered the current gold standard for measuring body composition. It is relatively simple when compared with other methods of measuring body composition such as isotope dilution and hydrodensitometry. It has been shown to be accurate, but it may underestimate percent body fat as percent body fat decreases and DEXA has not been well studied in obese patients. Radiation exposure to the patient is very small (approximately 0.3 μSv), less than the unavoidable daily background radiation (approximately 2 μSv).

Reference:

- Mattsson S, Thomas BJ. Development of methods for body composition studies. Phys Med Biol 2006; 51(13):R203–R228.

30. **Answer: A.**

There are many instruments available for measurement of bioimpedance, varying in quality from personal to professional use. Use of BIA is increasing because it is quick, inexpensive, and noninvasive. BIA is based on the measurement of the passage of an electrical current through the body. The body is imagined as a cylinder and impedance is then directly proportional to the length of the cylinder and inversely proportional to the cross-sectional area of the cylinder. Impedance is then used in equations to estimate body fat. There are single, dual, and multifrequency BIA devices. Since the conductor in BIA is human body fluids, measurements may be influenced by electrolyte abnormalities, hydration status of the body, and in disturbances of water balance such as cardiac or renal failure. This is especially true of single-frequency devices and less true for multifrequency devices. Single-frequency devices give output in terms of body cell mass (BCM), extracellular mass (ECM), and fat mass (FM). These measurements are influenced by the hydration status of the body. Multifrequency devices are able to subdivide total body water (TBW) into intracellular (ICW) and extracellular water (ECW), and BCM and ECM can then be estimated taking these fluid shifts into consideration. In general, BIA devices tend to underestimate percent body fat.

Reference:
- Dehghan M, Merchant AT. Is bioelectrical impedance accurate for use in large epidemiological studies? Nutr J 2008; 7:26.

31. **Answer: C.**

Like CT scan, MRI can reliably measure regional fat. Most commonly, a single cross-sectional image is obtained at the interspace between the fourth and fifth lumbar vertebrae. The image is then used to quantitate subcutaneous and visceral fat. Good contrast between adipose and nonadipose tissues is usually accomplished using conventional T1-weighted, spin-echo pulse sequences. T1-weighted images show fat as lighter and water darker. T2-weighted images show water as lighter. MRI is highly accurate but very expensive, and it does take a longer time than CT scan. Most MRI scanners can accommodate patients up to 300 lb and it may be difficult to accommodate super-obese patients.

Proton (1H) and sodium (23Na) MRI protocols have been developed that measure the quality (lipid and sodium concentration) of skeletal muscle tissue.

References:
- Ross R, Goodpaster B, Kelley D, et al. Magnetic resonance imaging in human body composition research. From quantitative to qualitative tissue measurement. Ann N Y Acad Sci 2000; 904:12–17.
- Lee SY, Gallagher D. Assessment methods in human body composition. Curr Opin Clin Nutr Metab Care 2008; 11(5):566–572.

32. **Answer: E.**

Obese individuals are at an increased risk of the metabolic syndrome, a cluster of risk factors for cardiovascular disease and diabetes.

According to American Heart Association (AHA)/updated National Cholesterol Education Program (NCEP) criteria, metabolic syndrome is defined as the presence of at least three or more of the following components:
1. Central obesity (increased waist circumference in men $\geq$102 cm, women $\geq$88 cm)
2. Hypertriglyceridemia ($\geq$150 mg/dL)
3. Low HDL cholesterol level (men <40 mg/dL, women <50 mg/dL)
4. Increased fasting glucose level ($\geq$100 mg/dL) or use of medication for hyperglycemia
5. Hypertension ($\geq$130/85 mm Hg) or use of medication for hypertension

Criteria to diagnose metabolic syndrome have also been provided by WHO, IDF (International Diabetes Federation), and EGIR (European Group for the Study of Insulin Resistance).

References:
- Grundy SM, Brewer HB Jr., Cleeman JI, et al. Definition of metabolic syndrome: report of the National Heart, Lung, and Blood Institute/American Heart Association conference on scientific issues related to definition. Circulation 2004; 109:433–438.

- National Cholesterol Education Program (NCEP) Expert Panel on Detection, Evaluation and Treatment of High Blood Cholesterol in Adults. Third report of expert panel on detection, evaluation and treatment of high blood cholesterol in adults (Adult Treatment Panel III) final report. Circulation 2002; 106:3143–3421.

33. **Answer: D.**

A single slice at the L4-L5 intervertebral level is used to measure the amount of fat, expressed in cubic cm.

Air displacement plethysmography does not require radiation exposure and is also comfortable for the patient. Dilution techniques for measurement of body composition use deuterated or tritated water for measurement of total body water from which other measures of body composition are derived.

The 3D surface imaging system, though useful for assessment of body composition and has a good correlation with air displacement plethysmography, is not used in bariatric surgery.

References:
- Ness-Abramof R, Apovian CM. Waist circumference measurement in clinical practice. Nutr Clin Pract 2008; 23(4):397–404.
- Klein S, Allison DB, Heymsfield SB, et al. Waist circumference and cardiometabolic risk: a consensus statement from Shaping America's Health: Association for Weight Management and Obesity Prevention; NAASO, the Obesity Society; the American Society for Nutrition; and the American Diabetes Association. Obesity (Silver Spring) 2007; 15(5):1061–1067.

34. **Answer: B.**

Many sites of measuring waist circumference have been described: at the level of the superior border of the iliac crest, midpoint between the iliac crest and the lowest rib, at the umbilicus, and at the minimal waist. With any of these, the measurement is taken on the bare abdomen at the end of normal expiration. The reproducibility of the measurement has been shown to be high at all sites. However, the value obtained for waist circumference can vary markedly depending on the site of measurement, particularly in women, and can impact the prevalence of abdominal obesity ranging from 23% to 34% in men and 31% to 55% in women. Most studies use the superior border of the iliac crest or the midpoint between the iliac crest and lowest rib as the site of waist circumference measurement. Waist circumference is a stronger clinical predictor of diabetes and metabolic syndrome than is BMI. BMI > 30 is assumed to correspond to increased waist circumference or central obesity according to WHO and IDF criteria. Waist circumference does measure both SAAT and IAAT (intra-abdominal adipose tissue) together.

References:
- Mason C, Katzmarzyk PT. Variability in waist circumference measurements according to anatomic measurement site. Obesity 2009; 17:1789–1795.
- Klein S, Allison DB, Heymsfield SB, et al. Waist circumference and cardiometabolic risk: a consensus statement from Shaping America's Health. Obesity 2007; 15 (5):1061–1067.

Animal Models of Bariatric Surgery

35. **Answer: D.**

ob/ob mice have an absence of circulating leptin, while *db/db* mice have a mutation of leptin receptor resulting in a truncated leptin receptor. *fa/fa* rats (Zucker fatty rats) have a full length but dysfunctional receptor.

References:
- Margetic S, Gazzola C, Pegg GG, et al. Leptin: a review of its peripheral actions and interactions. Int J Obes Relat Metab Disord 2002; 26:1407–1433.

- Brockmann GA, Bevova MR. Using mouse models to dissect the genetics of obesity. Trends Genet 2002; 18(7):367–376.

36. **Answer: D.**

Because of their large body structure, surgical techniques in pigs can be performed to simulate those done in humans. Although the pig stomach is similar to the human stomach, there are a few differences – the cardia is exaggerated, the fundus is large, the diverticulum ventriculi is a small partially isolated pocket present within the fundus 4 cm distal to the cardia, thickened perigastric membranes, and a small lesser sac is present. Unlike the human small intestine, the pig counterpart has a variable length with an intraperitoneal duodenum, smaller caliber, fragile nature, and mesenteric vascular arcades in the subserosa. The colon is the same caliber as the small bowel, is supported to the dorsal abdominal wall by the mesocolon, has a spiral course, has a left-sided cecum, and lacks a proper transverse mesocolon and appendix.

Reference:
- Rao RS, Rao V, Kini S. Animal models in bariatric surgery—a review of the surgical techniques and postsurgical physiology. Obes Surg 2010; 20(9):1293–1305.

37. **Answer: C.**

The esophagus opens into the lesser curvature of the stomach. The rat stomach has a cardia or forestomach that is continuous with the esophagus and is lined by squamous epithelium. It is thinner and relatively nonmotile. The fundus and pylorus (glandular stomach) have a similar anatomy as humans. The forestomach and the pylorus are separated by a band of tissue called margo plicatus (limiting ridge). The greater and lesser omentum and mesentery have a similar anatomy as humans. The liver has four lobes. Unlike the human intestine, the jejunum has the greatest length but cannot be easily distinguished from the other two segments. The ileum is recognized by the presence of large lymph nodes that appear as small bumps on its surface. Given the small organs of the rat, one needs to use microsurgical instruments and techniques.

Reference:
- Rao RS, Rao V, Kini S. Animal models in bariatric surgery—a review of the surgical techniques and postsurgical physiology. Obes Surg 2010; 20(9):1293–1305.

38. **Answer: C.**

The surgical technique of gastric bypass in pigs is as follows:

A 10- to 30-mL gastric pouch is created using a linear cutting stapler. The pouch can be created using a Baker's tube. A V-shaped pouch can also be created taking advantage of the small lesser sac. Since it is difficult to identify the ligament of Treitz, the duodenum can be followed to the point where it passes behind the colon. The Roux limb can be positioned either antegastric or retrogastric, but it cannot be retrocolic as there is no proper transverse mesocolon. The gastrojejunostomy can be hand-sewn or stapled. Because of the variable length of the intestine, it is better to calculate the length of the Roux and afferent limbs as a fraction of the total intestinal length. The jejunojejunostomy can be done intracorporeally or extracorporeally and can be either hand-sewn or stapled. Gastrostomy (to avoid gastric dilation) and jejunostomy(for postoperative feeding) have been used by some investigators. Also, the staple lines frequently need to be reinforced with sutures due to the thick stomach wall and perigastric membranes. The fragile nature of intestine causes frequent complications due to leakage – this has to be taken into account when using the pig as a survival model. Awareness of the liver and spleen anatomy is also necessary to avoid complications during retraction.

Reference:
- Rao RS, Rao V, Kini S. Animal models in bariatric surgery—a review of the surgical techniques and postsurgical physiology. Obes Surg 2010; 20(9):1293–1305.

39. **Answer: B.**

Type of rat	Metabolic profile
Wistar rats	Nonobese and nondiabetic. Also susceptible to obesity, diabetes, and related metabolic disorders when fed a high-fat diet. Specific components of the Western diet can influence development of obesity in these rats.
Sprague-Dawley	Nonobese and nondiabetic. But when fed a high-fat diet, they develop obesity and impaired glucose tolerance.
Zucker fatty rats (fa/fa)	Obese and nondiabetic. They have a mutation of hypothalamic leptin receptors and also profound hepatic insulin resistance. The hyperinsulinemia reaches peak at the 18th week. Though they have impaired glucose tolerance they do not develop frank diabetes.
Zucker diabetic fatty (ZDF)	Obese and diabetic. They have peripheral insulin resistance due to mutation of GLUT*-4 receptors in skeletal muscle and adipose tissue. They also have impaired glucose-induced insulin release due to mutation of GLUT-2 receptors in β cells and apoptosis of β cells. But the females can increase insulin production to overcome insulin resistance, thus capable of acting as controls.
Goto-Kakizaki	Nonobese diabetic rat model. Have a defect of development of β cells due to absence of growth factors and defective proliferation of β cells due to glucotoxicity. Also have hepatic insulin resistance.
Fisher-344 (F-344)	Nondiabetic and nonobese. But prone to obesity when fed high-calorie diet. Young rats also develop insulin resistance and increased triglycerides when fed high-calorie diet.

Reference:
- Rao RS, Rao V, Kini S. Animal models in bariatric surgery—a review of the surgical techniques and postsurgical physiology. Obes Surg 2010; 20(9):1293–1305.

Applied Anatomy and Physiology

40. **Answer: C.**

Aberrant hepatic arteries are most commonly classified by Michel's classification. Type 5 refers to accessory LHA and type 2 refers to replaced LHA. Type 5 was present in 8% and type 2 in 10% of the cases in Michel's series. Both arise from the left gastric artery and course through pars condensa of lesser omentum. In the series by Hiatt et al., accessory/replaced LHA was present in about 10% of the 1000 cases. During laparoscopy, Douard et al. found ALHA (aberrant left hepatic artery) rate (34%) was higher than in previously reported series.

In a series by Kim et al., 36% of the patients died when LHA was ligated. The ALHA may be the only arterial supply to the left lobe of the liver and its inadvertent ligation, rarely, has led to clinically significant ischemia of the left lobe. Division of this artery is to be avoided during placement of a Lap-Band.

References:
- Hiatt JR, Gabbay J, Busuttil RW. Surgical anatomy of the hepatic arteries in 1000 cases. Ann Surg 1994; 220(1):50–52.
- Kim DK, Kinne DW, Fortner JG. Occlusion of the hepatic artery in man. Surg Gynecol Obstet 1973; 136(6):966–968.
- Nehoda H, Lanthaler M, Labeck B, et al. Aberrant left hepatic artery in laparoscopic gastric banding. Obes Surg 2000; 10(6):564–568.
- Michels NA. Newer anatomy of the liver and its variant blood supply and collateral circulation. Am J Surg 1962; 112:337–347.
- Douard R, Chevallier JM, Delmas V, et al. Laparoscopic detection of aberrant left hepatic artery: a prospective study in 300 consecutive patients. Surg Radiol Anat 2006; 28(1):13–17.

41. **Answer: D.**

The left gastric artery is carefully preserved during a sleeve gastrectomy. The sleeve pouch may not have adequate perfusion after ligation of the left gastric vessels and a total gastrectomy may be required. The stomach can survive with three of the four major arteries ligated. The right gastroepiploic is the second largest artery to the stomach and it arises from the gastroduodenal artery. The right gastric artery usually arises from the hepatic artery but can arise from the gastroduodenal artery. The left gastroepiploic artery arises from the splenic artery. The right gastric artery branches can be divided during a sleeve gastrectomy. There are no published reports of omental necrosis after a sleeve gastrectomy. Hepatic and splenic infarctions have been documented after gastric bypass.

References:

- Yu J, Turner MA, Cho SR, et al. Normal anatomy and complications after gastric bypass surgery: helical CT findings. Radiology 2004; 231(3):753–760.
- Png KS, Rao J, Lim KH, et al. Lap-Band causing left gastric artery erosion presenting with torrential hemorrhage. Obes Surg 2008; 18(8):1050–1052.

42. **Answer: D.**

Ligament of Treitz is made of smooth muscle and is closely related to the inferior mesenteric vein. Paraduodenal hernias can occur in potential spaces related to the ligament of Treitz (hence referred to as Treitz hernias).

The Ligament of Treitz arises from right crus as it passes around the esophagus. It is inserted into the third and fourth parts of the duodenum and less frequently at the duodenojejunal junction.

References:

- Singh NS, Singh MS, Devi ND, et al. Suspensory muscle of duodenum: in human foetuses of Manipuri origin. J Anat Soc India 2003; 52(2):152–154.
- Moore K, Dalley A, Agur A. Clinically Oriented Anatomy. 6th ed. Baltimore: Lippincott Williams and Wilkins, 2010:241.

43. **Answer: C.**

The gastrin-producing G cells are mainly found in the antrum of the stomach. The interstitial cells of Cajal are found in highest number in the fundus. They are regarded as pacemakers of the gastrointestinal tract. Parietal cells are found in the fundus and the body of the stomach, but not in the antrum.

The ghrelin-producing cells are mainly found in the body of the stomach, although they are present in all parts of the gastrointestinal tract. They are only present in the mucosa but not in the myenteric plexus.

Reference:

- Ibba Manneschi L, Pacini S, Corsani L, et al. Interstitital cells of Cajal in the human stomach: distribution and relationship with enteric innervation. Histol Histopathol 2004; 19(4):1153–1164.

44. **Answer: C.**

It has been noted by several investigators that the short gastric arteries can supply a part of the spleen near the upper pole even after splenic artery was ligated. Though not the main supply to the spleen, some patients have an aberration of the blood supply that can compromise the blood supply to the upper pole of the spleen when the short gastrics are divided.

In one series, discoloration of the upper pole of the spleen was seen in 4.1% of the patients and became symptomatic in 0.4% of the patients. The area of demarcation was less than 2 cm in most patients and it is known to progress postoperatively, although this occurs rarely as was seen in the same series in a patient who was evaluated by abdominal CT scan 7 days postoperatively.

Splenic infarction can present with fever and shoulder and back pain, which are also signs of a staple line disruption and sepsis. A surgeon has to inspect the spleen intraoperatively for ischemic changes and consider splenic infarction as one of the differentials in patients presenting with fever and pain postoperatively.

Reference:
- Stamou KM, Menenakos E, Gomatos IP, et al. Clinical implications of sleeve gastrectomy as a source of spleen infarction or ischemia. Obes Surg 2011; 21(10):1490–1493.

45. **Answer: C.**

The vagal nerves divide into several branches around the esophagus. These branches come together again above the esophageal hiatus and form the left (anterior) and right (posterior) vagal trunks. In 50% of patients, there are more than two vagal nerves at the esophageal hiatus.

Near the GE junction, the anterior vagus sends a branch (or branches) to the liver in the gastrohepatic ligament, and continues along the lesser curvature as the anterior nerve of Latarjet. Vagotomy of the anterior vagus may thus cause hypotony of the gallbladder increasing the incidence of gallstones.

Similarly, the posterior vagus sends branches to the celiac plexus and continues along the posterior lesser curvature. The nerves of Latarjet send segmental branches to the body of the stomach before they terminate near the angularis incisura as the "crow's foot," sending branches to the antropyloric region.

Although clinicians are accustomed to thinking about the vagus nerves as important efferent nerves (i.e., carrying stimuli to the viscera), it is important to consider the fact that about 75% of the axons contained in the vagal trunks are afferent (i.e., carrying stimuli from the viscera to the brain). Vagotomy done during a LAGB has been shown to enhance weight loss in some studies, but the data have not been consistent.

References:
- Dempsey DT. Stomach. In: Brunicardi FC, Andersen DK, Billiar TR, et al., eds. Schwartz Principles of Surgery. 9th ed. United States: McGraw-Hill, 2010.
- Martin MB, Earle KR. Laparoscopic adjustable gastric banding with truncal vagotomy: any increased weight loss? Surg Endosc 2011; 25(8):2522–2525.
- Patankar R, Ozmen MM, Bailey IS, et al. Gallbladder motility, gallstones, and the surgeon. Dig Dis Sci 1995; 40(11):2323–2335.

46. **Answer: A.**

The supraduodenal artery is frequently absent.

The anemic spot of Mayo corresponds to the distribution of supraduodenal artery. It may be mistaken for a duodenal ulcer.

The two arterial pedicles (infra- and supraduodenal) reach the bulb on its posterior aspect. Each pedicle is made up of two sorts of blood currents (right and left); the posterior aspect of the bulb seems to be the most vascularized one, explaining, apart from bleeding from gastroduodenal artery erosion, the hemorrhagic character of ulcers of the posterior aspect of the bulb. The predominance of the left-hand currents explains the possible ischemia of the duodenal bulb and/or rupture of the duodenal stump after their interruption.

The left gastric artery is alone sufficient to preserve the arterial supply of the stomach due to its rich submucosal network. When other arteries are sacrificed, no increase in leakage rates was found in BPD-DS patients.

The prepyloric vein of Mayo has not been shown to indicate the position of the pylorus accurately.

References:
- Skandalakis JE, Colborn GL, Weidman TA, et al. Skandalakis Surgical Anatomy. Columbus: McGraw-Hill, 2006.
- Marchesini JB. A safer and simpler technique for the duodenal switch: to the editor. Obes Surg 2007; 17(8):1136.

47. **Answer: B.**

    Increased 25-hydroxy vitamin D levels and decreased calcium and phosphorous levels are found in vitamin D deficiency. A specific radiologic feature of osteomalacia, whether associated with phosphate wasting or vitamin D deficiency, is pseudofractures or Looser's zones. These are radiolucent lines that occur where large arteries are in contact with the underlying skeletal elements; it is thought that the arterial pulsations lead to the radiolucencies. As a result, these pseudofractures are usually a few millimeters wide, several centimeters long, and are seen particularly in the scapula, the pelvis, and the femoral neck. Vitamin D deficiency is associated with increased N-telopeptide (marker of bone resorption), increased osteocalcin (marker of bone formation), or an "uncoupling" effect on bone remodeling. Secondary hyperparathyroidism has been seen frequently (33%) after bariatric surgery. This secondary hyperparathyroidism has been postulated to be due to additional mechanisms (unrelated to vitamin D deficiency) such as a novel mechanism like parathyroid hormone (PTH) resistance or due to parathyroid hyperplasia. Increased PTH after bariatric surgery is not easily corrected by vitamin D supplementation.

    References:
    - Bringhurst FR, Marie BD, Stephen MK, et al. Chapter 346: Bone and mineral metabolism in health and disease. In: Fauci AS, Braunwald E, Kasper DL, et al., eds. Harrison's Principles of Internal Medicine. 17th ed. New York: McGraw-Hill, 2008.
    - Signori C, Zalesin KC, Franklin B, et al. Effect of gastric bypass on vitamin D and secondary hyperparathyroidism. Obes Surg 2010; 20(7):949–952.
    - Strohmayer E, Via MA, Yanagisawa R. Metabolic management following bariatric surgery. Mt Sinai J Med 2010; 77(5):431–445.

48. **Answer: A.**

    The pulmonary function and respiratory mechanics of obese patients are altered by the amount of adipose tissue and its distribution. Chest wall compliance is reduced, and the chest wall musculature is often unable to fully produce anterior excursion. Pulmonary function studies in obese patients typically show a restrictive pattern with decreases in functional residual capacity, expiratory reserve volume, vital capacity, and inspiratory capacity. These changes have also been observed in obese children. In addition, reductions in the forced expiratory reserve volume in 1 second (i.e., FEV1), the forced expiratory flow between 25% and 75% of vital capacity (i.e., FEF25–75), and the DLCO have been noted.

    Reference:
    - Kuruba R, Koche LS, Murr MM. Preoperative assessment and perioperative care of patients undergoing bariatric surgery. Med Clin North Am 2007; 91(3):339–351, ix (review).

49. **Answer: A.**

    The primary site of absorption of calcium is the duodenum and proximal jejunum, while that of vitamin D is the jejunum and the ileum. N- and C-telopeptides are specific markers for bone resorption; osteocalcin is a marker for bone formation. 25-hydroxycalicerferol is monitored to check for vitamin D deficiency.

    References:
    - Allied Health Sciences Section Ad Hoc Nutrition Committee; Aills L, Blankenship J, Buffington C, et al. ASMBS allied health nutritional guidelines for the surgical weight loss patient. Surg Obes Relat Dis 2008; 4(5 suppl):S73–S108.
    - Strohmayer E, Via MA, Yanagisawa R. Metabolic management following bariatric surgery. Mt Sinai J Med 2010; 77(5):431–445.

50. **Answer: B.**

    The alveolar-arterial gradient is unchanged. Airway pressure is increased by 12% to 17%. Pulmonary compliance is decreased by 31% to 42%. The physiological dead space to tidal volume ratio is not affected. Lung compliance is decreased when the pneumoperitoneum is established.

References:

- Perilli V, Sollazzi L, Bozza P, et al. The effects of the reverse Trendelenburg position on respiratory mechanics and blood gases in morbidly obese patients during bariatric surgery. Anesth Analg 2000; 91(6):1520–1525.
- Nguyen NT, Anderson JT, Budd M, et al. Effects of pneumoperitoneum on intraoperative pulmonary mechanics and gas exchange during laparoscopic gastric bypass. Surg Endosc 2004; 18(1):64–71 [Epub November 21, 2003].
- Dumont L, Mattys M, Mardirosoff C, et al. Changes in pulmonary mechanics during laparoscopic gastroplasty in morbidly obese patients. Acta Anaesthesiol Scand 1997; 41(3):408–413.
- El-Dawlatly AA, Al-Dohayan A, Abdel-Meguid ME, et al. The effects of pneumoperitoneum on respiratory mechanics during general anesthesia for bariatric surgery. Obes Surg 2004; 14(2):212–215.

51. **Answer: A.**

In a study of laparoscopic versus open gastric bypass, it was seen that urine output was reduced by 31% to 64% in the laparoscopic group when compared to the open group. There was no change in perioperative levels of BUN and serum creatinine. Serum levels of antidiuretic hormone, aldosterone, and plasma renin activity peaked at 2 hours after surgical incision but there was no significant difference between the open and laparoscopic groups. In a different study by the same authors, it was observed that creatinine clearance in gastric bypass patients was in the normal range during both the first and second postoperative days.

References:

- Nguyen NT, Anderson JT, Ho HS, et al. Evaluation of intra-abdominal pressure after open and laparoscopic gastric bypass. Obes Surg 2001; 11:40–45.
- Nguyen NT, Perez RV, Fleming N, et al. Effect of prolonged pneumoperitoneum on intraoperative urine output during laparoscopic gastric bypass. J Am Coll Surg 2002; 195(4):476–483.
- Magner D, Nguyen NT. Physiology of laparoscopy in morbidly obese. In: Sugerman HJ, Nguyen NT, eds. Management of Morbid Obesity. Philadelphia: Taylor and Francis, 2006.

52. **Answer: A.**

Obese patients have a more pronounced increase in heart rate during laparoscopy, although both heart rate and mean arterial pressure increase in both obese and nonobese patients. $PaCO_2$ increases during laparoscopy by about 9% in morbidly obese. The end-tidal CO_2 increases by 15% during laparoscopy in morbidly obese. Ventilatory adjustments are needed to prevent hypercapnia and acidosis. While preload is decreased, afterload increases during laparoscopy. Mean arterial blood pressure rises with insufflation. Cardiac output has not been found to be decreased in some studies. Cardiac output increases during the procedure due to compensatory mechanisms. The absorption of CO_2 in morbidly obese patients and nonobese patients appears to be similar.

References:

- Magner D, Nguyen NT. Chapter 8: Physiology of laparoscopy in morbidly obese. In: Sugerman HJ, Nguyen N, eds. Management of Morbid Obesity. Philadelphia: Taylor and Francis, 2005.
- Nguyen N, Wolfe B. Physiological effects of pneumoperitoneum on the morbidly obese. Ann Surg 2005; 241:219–226.

53. **Answer: B.**

Obesity is associated with increased TLESR, postprandial gastroesophageal reflux (GER), and esophageal acid exposure. The frequency of TLESR is correlated with increased BMI and waist circumference. TLESR frequency is increased by distension of the gastric fundus, so any meal, regardless of its composition, will have the potential to promote reflux.

There is an association between hiatal hernias and obesity. During inspiration, increased intragastric pressure and the gastroesophageal pressure gradient are correlated with increased BMI.

References:

- Anand G, Katz PO. Gastroesophageal reflux disease and obesity. Gastroenterol Clin North Am 2010; 39(1):39–46.
- Pandolfino JE, El-Serag HB, Zhang Q, et al. Obesity: a challenge to esophago-gastric junction integrity. Gastroenterology 2006; 130(3):639–649.
- Kamat P, Wen S, Morris J, et al. Exploring the association between elevated body mass index and Barrett's esophagus: a systematic review and meta-analysis. Ann Thorac Surg 2009; 87(2):655–662.
- Renehan AG, Tyson M, Egger M, et al. Body-mass index and incidence of cancer: a systematic review and meta-analysis of prospective observational studies. Lancet 2008; 371(9612):569–578.

54. **Answer: D.**

Ideal body weight (IBW) is a measure derived by life insurance companies to describe the weight statistically associated with maximum life expectancy. Metropolitan life tables are used to calculate IBW based on height and body build.

Lean body mass (LBM) is total body weight minus the weight of body fat. LBM includes muscles, bones, tendons, ligaments, and body water. In normal patients, LBW consists of about 80% water for males and 75% water for females. In morbid obesity, LBW is estimated by increasing IBW by 20% to 30%.

A sedentary Caucasian male whose weight is in the normal range has 10% to 15% of his body weight as fat mass. It increases with age and is lower in athletes. Lean body weight is relatively more and fat mass relatively less in males when compared to females.

55. **Answer: B.**

The stomach has intrinsic myoelectrical activity and a native "pacemaker" located in the proximal stomach wall along the greater curvature. This electrical conduction regulates gastric motility. Normal gastric myoelectrical activity consists of two components – slow waves (also called basal electrical rhythm) and spike potentials. The slow wave occurs at regular intervals whether or not the stomach contracts. It originates in the proximal stomach and propagates distally toward the pylorus. The normal frequency of the gastric slow wave is about three cycles per minute (CPM) in humans. The gastric slow wave determines the maximum frequency, propagation velocity, and propagation direction of gastric contractions. When a spike potential (similar to an action potential) is superimposed on the gastric slow wave, a strong lumen-occluding contraction occurs. The gastric slow waves themselves are not sufficient to cause contractions of the stomach. Rather, it is only when the release of stimulatory neurotransmitters from enteric nerve endings is superimposed on these waves of depolarization that an action potential may occur, leading in turn to contraction of the smooth muscle. Various patterns of motility can thus be accomplished depending on whether the stomach is filled with a meal or is in the fasted state.

References:

- Barrett KE. Chapter 8: Gastric motility. In: Barrett KE, ed. Gastrointestinal Physiology. Available at: http://eresources.library.mssm.edu:2059/content.aspx?aID=2307328.
- Shikora SA. Implantable gastric stimulation for weight loss. J Gastrointest Surg 2004; 8(4):408–412.

56. **Answer: B.**

In the Framingham Offspring study it was found that BMI was directly associated with fibrinogen, factor VII, PAI-1, and tissue plasminogen activator (tPA) antigen in both men and women and with von Willebrand factor (VWF) and viscosity in women. In patients with obesity, platelets show an increased activation and a reduced sensitivity to the physiological and pharmacological antiaggregating agents. Tissue factor has been found to be increased in obese patients and in patients with metabolic syndrome.

References:

* Rosito GA. Association between obesity and a prothrombotic state: the Framingham Offspring Study. Thromb Haemost 2004; 91(4):683–689.
* Anfossi G. Platelet dysfunction in central obesity. Nutr Metab Cardiovasc Dis 2009; 19(6):440–449.
* Nieuwdorp M, Stroes ES, Meijers JC, et al. Hypercoagulability in the metabolic syndrome. Curr Opin Pharmacol 2005; 5(2):155–159.
* Ayer JG, Song C, Steinbeck K, et al. Increased tissue factor activity in monocytes from obese young adults. Clin Exp Pharmacol Physiol 2010; 37(11):1049–1054.

57. **Answer: C.**

Waist-hip ratio >0.9 in women and >1.0 in men is abnormal. Insulin resistance, diabetes, hypertension, hyperlipidemia, and hyperandrogenism in women are linked more strongly to intra-abdominal and/or upper body fat than to overall adiposity. Intra-abdominal adipocytes are more metabolically active than those from other depots. Release of FFAs into the portal circulation leads to insulin resistance. Omentectomy is still an experimental therapy as equivocal results have been obtained from the studies done so far. Omental fat biopsies have been shown to have increased inflammation in obese patients.

References:

* Klein S. The case of visceral fat: argument for the defense. J Clin Invest 2004; 113(11):1530–1532.
* Collins D, Hogan AM. The omentum: anatomical, metabolic, and surgical aspects. J Gastrointest Surg 2009; 13:1138–1146.
* Bujalska IJ, Kumar S, Stewart PM. Does central obesity reflect "Cushing's disease of the omentum"? Lancet 1997; 349(9060):1210–1213.
* Fain JN, Cheema P, Tichansky DS, et al. The inflammatory response seen when human omental adipose tissue explants are incubated in primary culture is not dependent upon albumin and is primarily in the nonfat cells. J Inflamm (Lond) 2010; 7:4.

58. **Answer: C.**

Insulin is a long-term indicator for energy stores. Fasting insulin levels are greater in overweight people. Insulin inhibits the NPY/AgRP neurons and thus can decrease feeding. All bariatric surgical procedures decrease fasting insulin levels. In addition sleeve gastrectomy increases first-phase insulin secretion. Though fasting insulin is reduced after LAGB, an increase in incretin effect is not observed.

References:

* Basso N, Capoccia D, Rizzello M, et al. First-phase insulin secretion, insulin sensitivity, ghrelin, GLP-1, and PYY changes 72 h after sleeve gastrectomy in obese diabetic patients: the gastric hypothesis. Surg Endosc 2011; 25(11):3540–3550.
* Harvey EJ, Arroyo K, Korner J, et al. Hormone changes affecting energy homeostasis after metabolic surgery. Mt Sinai J Med 2010; 77(5):446–465.

59. **Answer: C.**

Accumulation of metabolites of fatty acid esterification like diacyglycerol and ceramide impair insulin signaling. In insulin resistance there is decreased translocation to GLUT-4 to the plasma membrane causing decreased glucose uptake.

Mechanisms of insulin resistance include decreased cell membrane expression of GLUT-4 receptors in the skeletal muscle. GLUT-1 is responsible for non-insulin-dependent glucose uptake, while GLUT-4 requires insulin-insulin receptor binding and tyrosine kinase signal pathway activation for normal expression and activity on the cell membrane. GLUT-2 enables passive glucose movement across cell membranes between liver and blood, and for renal glucose reabsorption.

TNF-α induces production of ROS by activation of NADPH oxidase. ROS activates a pathway that interferes with signaling from the insulin receptor.

References:

- Gallagher EJ, Leroith D, Karnieli E. Insulin resistance in obesity as the underlying cause for the metabolic syndrome. Mt Sinai J Med 2010; 77(5):511–523.
- Flier JS. Insulin receptors and insulin resistance. Annu Rev Med 1983; 34:145–160.
- Lele RD. Pro-insulin, C peptide, glucagon, adiponectin, TNF alpha, AMPK: neglected players in type 2 diabetes mellitus. J Assoc Physicians India 2010; 58:30, 35–40.
- Gallagher EJ, Leroith D, Karnieli E. Insulin resistance in obesity as the underlying cause for the metabolic syndrome. Mt Sinai J Med 2010; 77(5):511–523.
- Schinner S, Scherbaum WA, Bornstein SR, et al. Molecular mechanisms of insulin resistance. Diabet Med 2005; 22:674–682.
- Bournat JC, Brown CW. Mitochondrial dysfunction in obesity. Curr Opin Endocrinol Diabetes Obes 2010; 17(5):446–523.
- Rytka JM, Wueest S, Schoenle EJ, et al. The portal theory supported by venous drainage-selective fat transplantation. Diabetes 2011; 60:56–63.
- Barbuio R, Milanski M, Bertolo MB, et al. Infliximab reverses steatosis and improves insulin signal transduction in liver of rats fed a high-fat diet. J Endocrinol 2007; 194:539–550.
- Dresner A, Laurent D, Marcucci M, et al. Effects of free fatty acids on glucose transport and IRS-1-associated phosphatidylinositol 3-kinase activity. J Clin Invest 1999; 103:253–259.
- Aguirre V, Uchida T, Yenush L, et al. The c-Jun NH(2)-terminal kinase promotes insulin resistance during association with insulin receptor substrate-1 and phosphorylation of Ser(307). J Biol Chem 2000; 275:9047–9054.

60. **Answer: B.**

Euglycemic hyperinsulinemic clamp is considered the gold standard for assessing insulin resistance. An insulin plasma level is first maintained at a desired level, and then the rate of glucose infused simultaneously to maintain euglycemia is used to calculate the insulin resistance. It is assumed that, due to the insulin and glucose infusion, the endogenous glucose production is completely inhibited during the technique. The calculation of insulin sensitivity is based on the fact that the rate of glucose infusion to maintain euglycemia is inversely proportional to the insulin resistance, that is, the more the insulin resistance, the less glucose is needed to reach euglycemia. PET in conjunction with an euglycemic hyperinsulinemic clamp has been used to measure regional insulin-mediated glucose uptake.

Reference:

- Monzillo LU, Hamdy O. Evaluation of insulin sensitivity in clinical practice and in research settings. Nutr Rev 2003; 61(12):397–412.

61. **Answer: B.**

Studies have shown that insulin resistance (IR) or hyperinsulinemia is present in the majority of hypertensive patients, suggesting a link between obesity, glucose intolerance, and hypertension. Insulin is a stimulator of the vasodilator nitric oxide (NO) through insulin-mediated PI3K signaling and phosphorylation of eNOS. Under normal circumstances, vasodilatation occurs in the skeletal-muscle vasculature in response to insulin release after eating and promotes glucose disposal. In opposition to NO, endothelin-1 (ET-1) is a potent vasoconstrictor, which is stimulated by insulin activity through the MAPK pathway. NO is an inhibitor of ET-1. However, it has been proposed that in insulin-resistant states, insulin signaling through the PI3K pathway is impaired, leading to decreased NO. In addition, increased cytokines, such as IL-6, along with low adiponectin levels and leptin resistance, cause decreased NO and increased action of ET-1, with the subsequent development of hypertension. FFA can also induce hypertension by increased production of ROS, which increases oxidative stress and decreases NO. Hyperinsulinemia may also lead to increased peripheral vascular resistance due to sympathetic overactivity, volume expansion from its antinatriuretic effects, and increased angiotensinogen II.

Reference:
- Gallagher EJ, Leroith D, Karnieli E Insulin resistance in obesity as the underlying cause for the metabolic syndrome. Mt Sinai J Med 2010; 77(5):511–523.

62. **Answer: D.**

IVAST is used to measure β-cell function.

The hyperinsulinemic euglycemic clamp is the gold standard for measurement of insulin resistance.

The ITT consists of a bolus of 0.1 U/insulin and collections of plasma glucose frequently from 0 to 15 minutes. Plasma glucose $t_{1/2}$ is calculated from the slope of least square analysis of plasma glucose concentrations from 3 to 15 minutes after insulin injection. The rate constant for ITT is given by $0.693/t_{1/2}$ which is a measure of insulin resistance. This test is uncommonly used to measure insulin resistance.

Currently, the most commonly used method in clinical practice and in clinical studies of bariatric surgery is the homeostasis model assessment (HOMA), because of its simplicity. HOMA requires only the measurements of the fasting plasma insulin and fasting plasma glucose. The model is derived from a computer program that assesses the relationship between fasting plasma insulin and plasma glucose levels, in a large population of normally glucose-tolerant individuals. From the data, a simple formula for the calculation of HOMA index for insulin resistance (HOMA-IR) can be used:

HOMA-IR = [fasting plasma insulin (μU/L)/fasting plasma glucose (mmol/L)]/22.5
or
HOMA-IR = [fasting plasma insulin (μU/L)/fasting plasma glucose (mg/L)]/405

References:
- Reaven GM. Insulin secretory function in type 2 diabetes: Does it matter how you measure it? J Diabetes 2009; 1(3):142–150.
- Duseja A, Thumburu KK, Das K, et al. Insulin tolerance test is comparable to homeostasis model assessment for insulin resistance in patients with nonalcoholic fatty liver disease. Indian J Gastroenterol 2007; 26:170–173.

63. **Answer: D.**

Glucose is taken up by the insulin-sensitive GLUT-4, and exercise increases GLUT-4 receptors. The number of these receptors inversely correlates with insulin resistance. Insulin inhibits hormone-sensitive lipase and thus decreases lipolysis in the adipose tissue and prevents the release of FFAs. At the same time, insulin stimulates lipoprotein lipase, thus increases the uptake of FFAs from VLDL. It also decreases HDL by stimulating its breakdown by hepatic lipase and VLDL is exchanged for HDL. Low CSF insulin levels have been shown to correlate with insulin resistance in obese patients.

References:
- Gallagher EJ, Leroith D, Karnieli E. Insulin resistance in obesity as the underlying cause for the metabolic syndrome. Mt Sinai J Med 2010; 77(5):511–523.
- Kern W, Benedict C, Schultes B, et al. Low cerebrospinal fluid insulin levels in obese humans. Diabetologia 2006; 49(11):2790–2792.
- Masharani U, German MS. Chapter 18: Pancreatic hormones and diabetes mellitus. In: Gardner DG, Shoback D, eds. Greenspan's Basic and Clinical Endocrinology. 8th ed. Available at: http://eresources.library.mssm.edu:2059/content.aspx?aID=2633151.

64. **Answer: D.**

The onset of insulin resistance (IR) has a profound effect on lipid profiles. IR results in the increased production of FFAs from adipocytes through loss of its inhibition of hormone-sensitive lipase. Additionally, endothelial lipoprotein lipase function is impaired, both events leading to the increase in circulating FFAs. The increased influx of FFAs to the liver and insulin stimulation of hepatic lipogenesis lead to increased hepatic TG (triglyceride) production in the form of VLDL and steatosis as the TG are stored in the liver. Adipocyte production of cholesterol ester transferase protein allows for the transfer of cholesteryl esters from HDL to VLDL. There is increased clearance of HDL by the kidneys and the liver takes up HDL and produces VLDL, therefore leading to the low HDL and elevated TG levels seen with the metabolic syndrome.

Reference:
- Gallagher EJ, Leroith D, Karnieli E. Insulin resistance in obesity as the underlying cause for the metabolic syndrome. Mt Sinai J Med 2010; 77(5):511–523.

65. **Answer: A.**

PPARγ is present in the cytoplasm and nucleus, but its activity as a nuclear receptor requires association with retinoid X receptor (RXR). Both endogenous substances like fatty acids and eicosanoids and exogenous substances like thiazolidinediones act as ligands for PPARγ. Thiazolidinediones are PPARγ agonists.

Reference:
- Kawai M, Sousa KM, MacDougald OA, et al. The many facets of PPARgamma: novel insights for the skeleton. Am J Physiol Endocrinol Metab 2010; 299(1):E3–E9.

66. **Answer: D.**

Insulin resistance (IR) is a key element in the development of hyperglycemia and T2DM. In normal individuals, ingestion of nutrients results in the secretion of insulin from the pancreatic β cells. Specific triggers for insulin release include glucose, amino acids, FFAs, and gastrointestinal hormones, such as GLP-1. There is a rapid first-phase insulin response that occurs immediately after eating (release of preformed insulin), peaks at 10 minutes, and disappears after approximately 20 minutes. Its effect is to inhibit hepatic glucose production and promote glucose uptake. This is followed by a second-phase insulin response (which involves secretion of newly synthesized insulin), which begins at 15 to 20 minutes and peaks during the next 20 to 40 minutes. In IR and T2DM, the initial β cell abnormality is a loss of the first-phase insulin response, followed by an exaggerated second-phase response. This ultimately leads to hyperinsulinemia.

References:
- Gallagher EJ, Leroith D, Karnieli E Insulin resistance in obesity as the underlying cause for the metabolic syndrome. Mt Sinai J Med 2010; 77(5):511–523.
- Davis SN. Chapter 60: Insulin, oral hypoglycemic agents, and the pharmacology of the endocrine pancreas. In: Brunton LL, Lazo JS, Parker KL, eds. Goodman & Gilman's The Pharmacological Basis of Therapeutics. 11th edn. Available at: http://eresources.library.mssm.edu:2059/content.aspx?aID=958974.

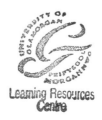